Occup

Health Services
A Guide to Program Planning and Management

Edited by William L. Newkirk, M.D.

Occupational Health Research

and Lynn D. Jones

Division of Ambulatory Care
and Health Promotion
of the American Hospital Association

AHA®
American Hospital Publishing, Inc.,
a wholly owned subsidiary
of the American Hospital Association

The views expressed in this book are those of the authors and editors.

Library of Congress Cataloging-in-Publication Data

Occupational health services : a guide to program planning and management / edited by William L. Newkirk and Lynn D. Jones.
ISBN 1-55648-034-2
1. Occupational health services--Planning. 2. Occupational health services--Administration. I. Newkirk, William L. II. Jones, Lynn Dickey.
[DNLM: 1. Health Planning. 2. Occupational Health Services--organization & administration. WA 412 015]
RC968.023 1989
DNLM/DLC 89-17496
for Library of Congress CIP

Catalog no. 016142

Printed in the U.S.A.

AHA is a service mark of the American Hospital Association used under license by American Hospital Publishing, Inc.

Text set in English Times
2.5M–7/89–0240
3M–3/90–0264

Linda Conheady, Manuscript Editor
Lawrence Denne, Editorial Assistant
Marcia Bottoms, Managing Editor
Peggy DuMais, Production Coordinator
Marcia Vecchione, Designer
Brian Schenk, Books Division Director

Contents

Contributors

John E. Carnes, J.D., is commission counsel for the Maine Human Rights Commission, Augusta, Maine, and is actively engaged in litigation of handicap discrimination cases. His past experience includes writing the *Employment Regulations* of the Maine Human Rights Commission and drafting numerous pieces of legislation dealing with handicap discrimination in employment.

Lisa B. Chace, M.S.N., is administrative director, Center for Occupational Health, Exeter Hospital, Exeter, New Hampshire. In addition, she is adjunct professor in the Department of Nursing at the University of New Hampshire. She consults with hospitals nationwide on the development of hospital-based occupational health services. She has had six years of experience in developing, managing, and marketing hospital-based occupational health services. Before coming to Exeter Hospital, she was instrumental in establishing an occupational health program including on-site nursing at a Boston area hospital. Since 1985, she has concentrated on developing a multidisciplinary team of occupational health professionals who provide the most comprehensive occupational medicine program in New Hampshire.

Marsha Barnhart Eng, M.S., is marketing coordinator, Sentara Health System, Norfolk, Virginia, a diversified ambulatory health services corporation with 10 subsidiaries. Her past experience includes serving as occupational and business health program coordinator for Sentara Health System. Her responsibilities included creating, developing, and delivering comprehensive occupational health programs for area businesses.

Sandra Figler, D.P.H., M.B.A., is vice-president, strategic planning and marketing, Rochester General Hospital, Rochester, New York. Her present affiliations include the Society for Hospital Planning and Marketing and the Academy of Health Services Marketing. Her previous experience includes serving as president of Health Marketing Dynamics in Louisville, Kentucky, a national health care marketing and business development firm with a focus on specialty services and diversification strategies.

Roy K. Gerber, M.B.A., is director, Bethesda Healthcare Inc., the delivery mechanism of Bethesda Hospital's occupational health product line in Cincinnati, Ohio. Mr. Gerber started the occupational health product line in 1983 and currently has overall responsibility for marketing, operations, and development. Mr. Gerber is also president of Optimum Health Systems, Inc., a hospital consulting firm that specializes in occupational health nursing, employee assistance programs, and sales and marketing.

C. Kirby Griffin, M.D., is medical director, Center for Occupational Health, St. Vincent Hospital and Medical Center, Portland, Oregon. He is affiliated with the American College of Occupational Medicine and is on the board of directors for the Northwest Occupational Medicine Association.

Philip S. Hanna, M.P.H., is chief executive officer, MedWork, an emergency and occupational health care facility in Dayton, Ohio, where he is active in program development consulting. He is also chief financial officer and senior manager for a group of 10 emergency medicine specialists. His previous experience at Miami Valley Hospital includes planning and implementing one of the first air ambulance services in Ohio, coordinating a facility expansion and renovation effort, and guiding the hospital in obtaining formal certification as a trauma center and neonatal intensive care unit program. He was project director of Western Ohio Emergency Medical Services, with all program development responsibilities, and also has experience in planning at a health systems agency.

Dean Imbrogno, M.D., is president, MedWork, an emergency and occupational health care facility in Dayton, Ohio. He is a board-certified emergency physician, currently practicing full-time occupational medicine. He is an assistant clinical professor in emergency medicine at Wright State University and is past chairman of the American College of Emergency Physicians occupational medicine committee.

Gary G. Irish, M.P.H., M.B.A., is president, GlenOaks Medical Center, Glendale Heights, Illinois. Mr. Irish's previous affiliations include vice-president, Adventist Health System/North, Hinsdale, Illinois; executive director, Loma Linda OB/GYN Medical Group, Loma Linda, California; director of planning and resource management, Loma Linda University Medical Center, Loma Linda, California; and health planner, Inland Counties Health Systems Agency, Riverside, California.

Lynn D. Jones, M.P.S., is manager, Worksite Health Services, American Hospital Association, Division of Ambulatory Care and Health Promotion, Chicago, Illinois. She is responsible for assisting hospitals in developing and marketing worksite health programs for business and industry. In previous positions with the AHA, she developed, directed, and managed health promotion programs for employees of the AHA and Blue Cross Association.

Frank H. Leone, M.P.H., M.B.A., is founder and president of Ryan Associates, Sudbury, Massachusetts, which provides occupational health consulting services to institutional providers. His past experience includes serving as executive director of a regional trauma center and New England's largest emergency air transport program (University of Massachusetts Medical Center, Worcester, Massachusetts). Mr. Leone was deputy director of the occupational health service at the University of Massachusetts Medical Center for five years.

John Maxfield, M.D., is medical director, Occupational Health, and staff emergency physician at Alexandria Hospital, Alexandria, Virginia. Dr. Maxfield spent six years at Newport Hospital in Newport, Rhode Island, where he was chief of emergency medicine and founder and medical director of the occupational health service. He is also the author of a national survey on occupational medicine and the emergency department. He has contributed to a widely used occupational health computer software product (OHR).

Thomas F. McCoy, D.O., is director of research and development in medical ergonomics, LINK Performance and Recovery Systems, Inc., Portland, Maine. His current projects include writing a text primer on medical ergonomics and developing a vibration threshold device for early detection of C.T.S. in industry. He was the recipient of a grant from the Maine Department of Labor to aid corporations in developing cumulative trauma management programs. He is associate professor of bioengineering at the University of New Hampshire and an assistant professor of anatomy and clinical instructor at New England College of Osteopathic Medicine. At the University of New England, he is developing a postgraduate medical ergonomics certificate program for physicians and allied health professionals.

Terry A. Morton, M.A., is director of marketing, Sentara Enterprises, Norfolk, Virginia, a subsidiary of the Sentara Health System. Sentara is a not-for-profit system with 3 hospitals and 12 urgent care centers that deliver comprehensive health-related services to business and industry. Mr. Morton's responsibilities include marketing, sales, customer service, and program development. His previous experience includes serving as product director for occupational health programs at Sentara.

William L. Newkirk, M.D., is director of research, Occupational Health Research, Skowhegan, Maine, and director of occupational medicine,

Redington-Fairview General Hospital, Skowhegan, Maine. Dr. Newkirk has served on the National Committee on Occupational Medicine of the American College of Emergency Physicians and on the Workplace Safety Commission of the Maine legislature. He is coauthor of *Managing Emergency Medical Services: Principles and Practices* (Reston, VA: Reston Publishing Co. (Prentice-Hall), 1984).

David A. Nicewonger, M.B.A., is workers' compensation specialist, St. Vincent Hospital Center for Occupational Health, Portland, Oregon. He has spoken and taught courses at 1988 and 1989 Occupational Health Research conferences on the development, implementation, and effectiveness of injury management programs.

Peter Orris, M.D., M.P.H., is medical director of Managed Care, The Industrial Health Program, Mount Sinai Hospital, Chicago, Illinois, and attending physician, Cook County Hospital Division of Occupational Medicine, Chicago, Illinois. He is also an associate professor of clinical community health and preventive medicine at Northwestern University Medical School, Chicago, Illinois. His previous experience includes serving as Region V medical officer, National Institute for Occupational Safety and Health, which has offices in Chicago and responsibility for seven midwestern states.

Timothy R. Patten, M.B.A., is vice-president for business development, GlenOaks Medical Center, Glendale Heights, Illinois, and president of Occupational Medicine Network, Inc. (OMNI). His experience includes serving as assistant vice-president of business development, Glendale Heights Community Hospital, Glendale Heights, Illinois. Mr. Patten was responsible for the development of OMNI at Glendale Heights Community Hospital and assisted with the legal structure, negotiated the joint venture agreement, handled program development, and facilitated start-up of the clinic operations.

Barbara Robino, R.N., is vice-president and administrator, Occupational Health Services, Rose HealthCare Centers, an affiliate of Rose Medical Center, Denver, Colorado. She developed and currently manages the WorkComp Plus program, a medical management program for the treatment of work-related injuries and illnesses. She has been instrumental in establishing numerous occupational health programs for employers in Colorado. She is a well-known consultant to hospitals and private industry. Her previous experience includes serving as administrator of the workers' compensation self-insured plan for Associated Grocers of Colorado.

Mark A. Rothstein, J.D., is professor of law and director of the Health Law Institute, University of Houston Law Center, Houston, Texas. In addition, he is adjunct professor of public health, University of Texas School of Public Health. His publications include *Medical Screening and Employee Health*

Costs (1989); *Medical Screening of Workers* (1984); and *Occupational Safety and Health Law* (2nd edition, 1983).

Rob Ryder is director of Interstate Health Services, Inc., a subsidiary of the Penrose/St. Francis Healthcare System, Colorado Springs, Colorado. He is the developer of Profile Systems for Occupational Health, Inc., a division of Interstate Health that provides wellness, employee assistance program, and occupational medicine services to over 250 businesses in Colorado. Profile Systems has won both the Colorado Governor's Award as the outstanding health promotion program in the state of Colorado for employers of 1,000 or more employees and the Healthcare Forum/3M Corporation national award for innovation in health care. Mr. Ryder serves as vice-president on the national board of directors of the Society of Prospective Medicine. He has presented and consulted nationally.

R. Kevin Smith, D.O., is medical director, Occupational Medicine Network, Inc., Glendale Heights, Illinois, a comprehensive, hospital-based occupational medicine program. He is also a consultant for occupational medicine for Drever Medical Clinic, Aurora, Illinois, a multispecialty clinic. His previous experience includes several positions as emergency physician and occupational medicine physician. He was assistant professor of clinical emergency medicine at the University of Illinois. He is a former board examiner for the American Board of Emergency Medicine and served on the board of directors of the American College of Emergency Physicians.

Richard J. Torraco, B.S.N., M.S., is clinical manager of the occupational health nursing program at the Center for Occupational Health, a multiservice occupational health program based at Exeter Hospital, Exeter, New Hampshire. He is responsible for the operations and program development of the occupational health nursing program, which provides a contract service to small and mid-sized employers in southern New Hampshire. In addition to program management, he conducts workplace health and safety evaluations for client companies on a consulting basis. He is an adjunct professor in the Department of Nursing at the University of New Hampshire and Lesley College in Cambridge, Massachusetts.

Richard D. Tucker, J.D., M.H.A., is an attorney with Leen and Emery, Bangor, Maine. His primary concentration is workers' compensation insurance litigation. His previous experience includes positions as resident counsel/ workers' compensation claims manager at Dexter Shoe Company, Dexter, Maine, a major U.S. shoe manufacturer, and associate attorney at Lord, Bissell, and Brook, Chicago, Illinois, where he handled medical malpractice cases and product liability litigation for hospitals and other clients.

Patricia van Horne, R.N., is administrative director of the Industrial Medicine Program at Redington-Fairview General Hospital, Skowhegan, Maine.

She has developed a worksite visit program using nurses as physician extenders in the workplace.

James L. Weeks, Sc.D., is deputy administrator, Department of Occupational Health and Safety, United Mine Workers of America, Washington, DC. He is also a certified industrial hygienist. At the UMWA, he is responsible for conducting research, developing policy, assisting union members, and representing the union in occupational health and safety matters. Prior to working for the UMWA, he directed an occupational health program for Local 201 of the International Union of Electrical Workers in Massachusetts.

Richard C. Williams, M.B.A., M.S., is president, HealthSell, Inc., Cincinnati, Ohio, a health care sales and marketing firm. Mr. Williams is the author of *Managing the Hospital Sales Team* (Chicago: American Hospital Publishing, Inc., 1988) and has been involved in occupational health programs for more than a dozen years as a hospital administrator, manager, and marketing and sales person. He has developed, managed, and evaluated dozens of programs throughout the country.

List of Figures

List of Tables

Acknowledgments

In this book, we have attempted to cover many issues in the rapidly changing field of occupational health. We hope that it provides you with some of the answers you need to establish or expand an occupational health program for your hospital or freestanding clinic.

Many people helped with the development of this book. We are deeply grateful to all of them for their assistance. We would specifically like to thank the following people:

The chapter authors. We are grateful to all of the authors who contributed to this book and shared their experience and expertise—both those whose chapters were included in the final publication and those whose chapters were not.

Educational program participants. To all the physicians, nurses, therapists, marketers, and administrators who have attended educational programs on occupational health that we have organized or taught over the last decade. Your ideas have shaped both the field of occupational medicine and this book.

Hospital occupational health program staff members. To all the people who have endured questionnaires, visits, and phone calls and who have answered endless questions about what works and what doesn't. We couldn't have reached our conclusions without your input, experience, and perspectives.

The Redington-Fairview General Hospital and the hospitals supporting Occupational Health Research. This book is one example of how your long-term financial commitment to developing new approaches to occupational health is improving the care hospitals provide to employers and employees.

The American Hospital Association, whose financial and staff support made this book possible, and in particular, to Dorothy Wilson, whose tireless revisions brought this manuscript together.

We are happy to have been able to play a role in bringing this book to life. During the process, our families have had to endure late meals from distracted spouses and parents. Without their support, this book would not exist.

Chapter 1

Introduction

William L. Newkirk, M.D.
Dean Imbrogno, M.D.
Gary G. Irish, M.P.H., M.B.A.

The Environment Leading to Hospitals' Interest in Occupational Health

Hospitals' interest in occupational health has increased during the past decade—a period of significant changes in the health care market. During the 1980s, occupational health programs have become a frequent diversification strategy for hospitals. Three major trends have helped to create the increased interest in occupational health: the shrinking hospital inpatient market, competition between hospitals and physicians resulting from hospital diversification into ambulatory care and the increase in the supply of physicians, and the shift in power from providers to payers.

The Shrinking Hospital Inpatient Market

Since it hit its peak level in 1981, the hospital inpatient market has significantly declined.[1] In 1987, the number of inpatient days was 223.4 million, a decline of 18.7 percent, or 50 million patient days, since 1981. Although the well-publicized movement to prospective pricing for Medicare patients has had an impact on this trend, admissions of persons under age 65 have also declined 15.7 percent since 1981.[1]

The decline in the inpatient market has profoundly affected hospitals. Hospitals have responded to this change in a variety of ways. Two significant responses have been the following:

- *Increased competition for inpatient referrals.* The competition for inpatient referrals has increased the importance of hospital marketing. A key element of hospital marketing has been to expand major referral sources. Corporations are one of these target sources.

- *Greater diversification into ambulatory care services.* Greater diversification into ambulatory care services has opened new opportunities for profit. According to a 1988 survey, outpatient diagnostic centers, inpatient rehabilitation centers, and outpatient surgery centers have been the three most profitable diversification strategies for hospitals (figure 1-1).[2] Industrial medicine programs have been the fourth most successful strategy, with a success rate of 85 percent. Although these diversification strategies have often improved hospitals' bottom lines, they have also brought hospitals into more direct competition with their medical staffs.

The Competition for Patients between Physicians and Hospitals

Hospitals' increasing diversification into ambulatory care and the resulting competition with medical staffs has occurred during a period when the physician supply has continued to grow (table 1-1). Current estimates indicate that by 1990, there will be 250 physicians for every 100,000 persons, almost twice the number there were in the 1960s.[3]

The increase in the physician supply is altering the traditional physician-hospital relationship. During the period prior to 1981 when the number of hospital inpatient days was continually increasing, physicians and hospitals coexisted in a mutually beneficial economic relationship. The hospitals' source of inpatient admissions was physicians, and the number of physicians and inpatient admissions was growing. As private business entrepreneurs, physicians operated independently in a seller's market. Establishing a new practice was relatively easy because of the substantial excess demand for physicians' services. In addition, few constraints regarding the actual practice of medicine existed. Neither hospitals nor physicians had to actively seek new patients. For a long time, in fact, marketing was considered unethical.

All of that has changed. Hospitals are losing inpatient days and must thus actively seek patients and compete with other hospitals and physicians. Physicians face not only increased competition but also significant constraints in their practices from governmental agencies and managed care systems. As hospitals begin to market managed care programs, they place further constraints on physicians' practices. A 1988 survey indicated that competition for outpatients and physician recruitment were the two major causes of conflict between hospitals and physicians (figure 1-2).[4]

The Power Shift from Providers to Payers

While hospitals, with their declining utilization rates, and physicians, with their burgeoning numbers, have been struggling to determine how to divide up the health care market, the parties that pay for health care services have

Figure 1-1. Diversification Strategies Ranked by Success in Generating a Profit or Breaking Even

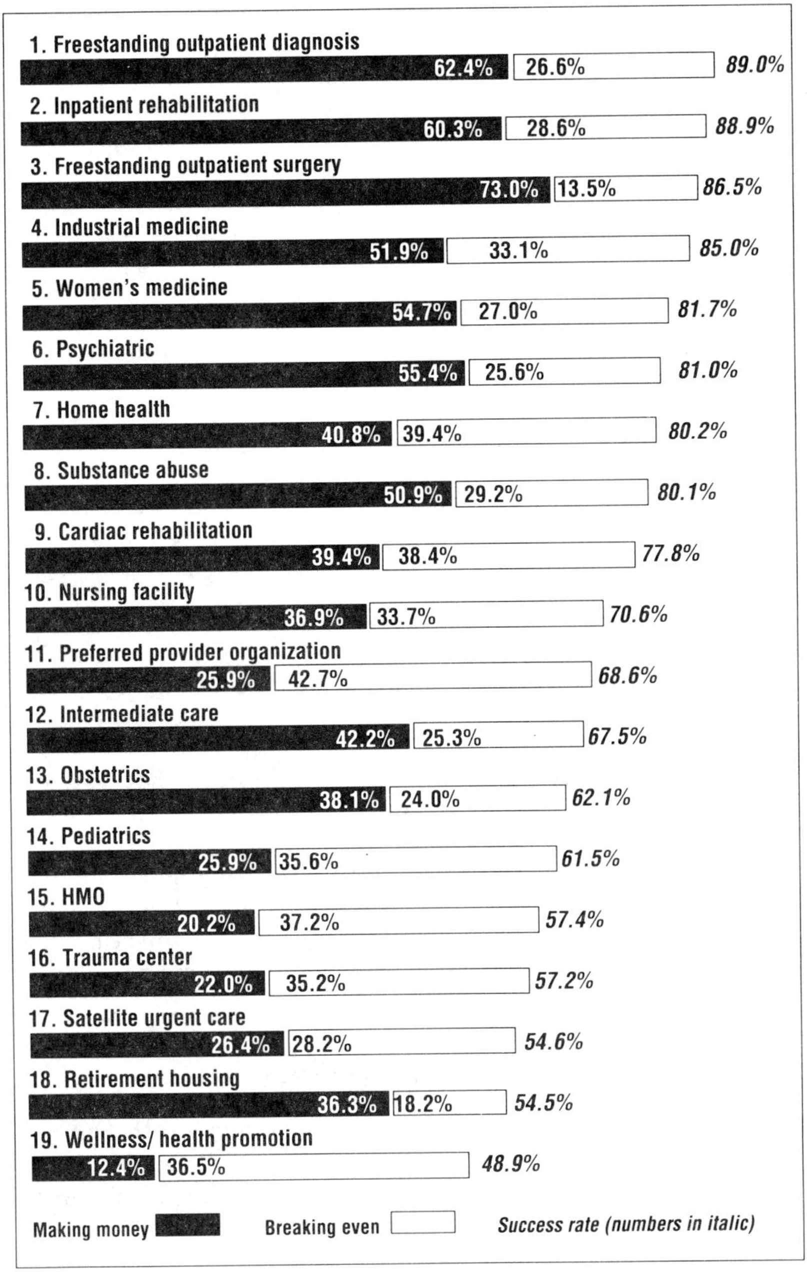

Strategy	Making money	Breaking even	*Success rate*
1. Freestanding outpatient diagnosis	62.4%	26.6%	*89.0%*
2. Inpatient rehabilitation	60.3%	28.6%	*88.9%*
3. Freestanding outpatient surgery	73.0%	13.5%	*86.5%*
4. Industrial medicine	51.9%	33.1%	*85.0%*
5. Women's medicine	54.7%	27.0%	*81.7%*
6. Psychiatric	55.4%	25.6%	*81.0%*
7. Home health	40.8%	39.4%	*80.2%*
8. Substance abuse	50.9%	29.2%	*80.1%*
9. Cardiac rehabilitation	39.4%	38.4%	*77.8%*
10. Nursing facility	36.9%	33.7%	*70.6%*
11. Preferred provider organization	25.9%	42.7%	*68.6%*
12. Intermediate care	42.2%	25.3%	*67.5%*
13. Obstetrics	38.1%	24.0%	*62.1%*
14. Pediatrics	25.9%	35.6%	*61.5%*
15. HMO	20.2%	37.2%	*57.4%*
16. Trauma center	22.0%	35.2%	*57.2%*
17. Satellite urgent care	26.4%	28.2%	*54.6%*
18. Retirement housing	36.3%	18.2%	*54.5%*
19. Wellness/ health promotion	12.4%	36.5%	*48.9%*

Making money Breaking even *Success rate (numbers in italic)*

Numbers to the right of the bars indicate success rates.

Source: Hamilton/KSA, 1988. Reprinted by permission from Sabatino, F. G. The diversification success story continues: survey. *Hospitals* 63(1):27, Jan. 5, 1989.

Table 1-1. Growth in Physician Specialties

Specialty	1986	2010 (projected)
General internal medicine	71,879	102,100
General/family practice	68,437	77,800
Pediatrics	38,631	59,100
Psychiatry	37,440	42,800
General surgery	32,859	34,700
Obstetrics/gynecology	31,882	42,100
Radiology	24,073	32,900
Anesthesiology	23,795	35,700
Pathology	16,387	17,600
Emergency medicine	12,343	22,500

Source: AMA Center for Health Policy Research, 1988. Reprinted by permission from *AHA News*, Aug. 22, 1988, p. 7.

been assuming greater control. Two payer groups have been dominant forces:

- *Governmental agencies* have been controlling care for the elderly and indigent populations through prospective pricing, preadmission certification, and quality-of-care reviews.
- *Corporate America* has been directing care for the employed population. Faced with health benefit costs that are rising at a rate greater than inflation, employers have sought to directly control health care costs, referral patterns, and the provision of health care.

Hospital Occupational Health Programs

Many hospitals have responded to the forces of declining inpatient utilization rates, increases in the physician supply, and expanding payer control by developing occupational health programs directed to meet industrial needs. The rationale is that strong relationships between hospitals and industry strengthen the hospital's position regarding both work-related and non–work-related admissions. Unfortunately, hospitals entering the occupational health services marketplace often have little knowledge of the requirements of an occupational health program.

Figure 1-2. Major Causes of Conflict between Physicians and Hospitals

By Region

Upper Midwest		**Midwest**		**Northeast**	
Physician recruitment	57.7%	Competition for outpatients	61.3%	Competition for outpatients	63.4%
Competition for outpatients	54.3%	Physician recruitment	58.0%	Physician recruitment	55.6%
PRO activities	45.8%	Managed care	51.7%	PRO activities	50.1%
Managed care	37.5%	PRO activities	51.3%	Managed care	43.1%
Designation of priority programs	36.6%	Designation of priority programs	47.4%	Designation of priority programs	42.7%
Board representation	28.7%	Buying physician practices	37.6%	Board representation	37.8%
Buying physician practices	28.5%	Board representation	20.5%	Buying physician practices	27.0%

West		**Southwest**		**Southeast**	
Competition for outpatients	64.1%	Physician recruitment	68.2%	Competition for outpatients	65.5%
Physician recruitment	58.5%	Competition for outpatients	53.0%	Physician recruitment	59.3%
Managed care	56.8%	PRO activities	46.0%	PRO activities	43.5%
Designation of priority programs	46.5%	Designation of priority programs	45.0%	Managed care	41.9%
PRO activities	36.2%	Managed care	44.0%	Designation of priority programs	41.1%
Board representation	29.7%	Board representation	38.0%	Board representation	32.4%
Buying physician practices	22.8%	Buying physician practices	20.4%	Buying physician practices	22.2%

By Hospital Size

200–299 beds		**300–400 beds**		**400 or more beds**	
Physician recruitment	64.4%	Competition for outpatients	65.8%	Competition for outpatients	68.8%
Competition for outpatients	53.4%	Physician recruitment	56.4%	Designation of priority programs	59.0%
PRO activities	50.2%	Managed care	49.5%	Managed care	57.1%
Managed care	38.0%	Designation of priority programs	43.3%	Physician recruitment	53.2%
Designation of priority programs	34.4%	PRO activities	42.3%	PRO activities	40.8%
Board representation	33.1%	Buying physician practices	32.1%	Buying physician practices	32.4%
Buying physician practices	19.6%	Board representation	28.0%	Board representation	23.2%

Note: Upper Midwest includes Iowa, Kansas, Minnesota, Missouri, Nebraska, North Dakota, and South Dakota; Midwest includes Illinois, Indiana, Kentucky, Michigan, Ohio, and Wisconsin; Northeast includes Connecticut, Maine, Massachusetts, New Hampshire, New Jersey, New York, Pennsylvania, Rhode Island, and Vermont; West includes Alaska, Arizona, California, Colorado, Hawaii, Idaho, Montana, Nevada, New Mexico, Oregon, Utah, Washington, and Wyoming; Southwest includes Arkansas, Louisiana, Oklahoma, and Texas; Southeast includes Alabama, Delaware, Florida, Georgia, Maryland, Mississippi, North Carolina, South Carolina, Tennessee, Virginia, Washington, DC, and West Virginia.

Source: Hamilton/KSA, 1988. Data are based on 623 responses. Adapted from Grayson, M. A. Breaking the medical gridlock. *Hospitals* 63(4):32, Feb. 20, 1989.

Components of an Occupational Health Program

In 1916, the American Association of Industrial Physicians and Surgeons, later renamed the American Occupational Medical Association (AOMA), was formed to organize physicians and develop guidelines for industrial medical care. In 1978, AOMA defined the standards of an occupational health program (reprinted as an addendum to this chapter). The organization is now known as the American College of Occupational Medicine (ACOM).

As the ACOM standards indicate, an occupational health program may embrace a broad range of activities. Activities may include those in the following areas:

- *Industrial hygiene.* Industrial hygiene is concerned with chemical or physical agents that affect employees. The industrial hygienist's job is to recognize, evaluate, and control these hazards. A typical job for an industrial hygienist is to evaluate an industrial process, recognize the potential for specific toxic exposures, and measure and monitor these exposures by using engineering controls, personal protective devices, or administrative controls to reduce exposure to safe levels or eliminate it.
- *Safety engineering.* Safety engineering is similar to industrial hygiene except that safety engineering attempts to reduce the likelihood of acute traumatic injury, whereas industrial hygiene attempts to control toxic exposures.
- *Environmental health.* Environmental health is concerned not only with those factors covered by industrial hygiene but also with waste disposal, water quality management, and environmental stressors and toxins.
- *Ergonomics.* Ergonomics is the study of humans at work. It has two distinct components. The first is health physics, which deals with designing facilities to be compatible with human dimensions, capabilities, and limitations. For instance, a health physicist would modify a job that predisposes workers to injuring their backs because lifting is being done in an awkward position. A second component of ergonomics is human factor engineering, which helps workers integrate information to do their jobs better. The human factor engineer focuses on such details as the proper placement of clocks, control panels, levers, and gauges to prevent mistakes in jobs requiring quick reactions in critical situations.
- *Occupational medicine.* Occupational medicine is a complex field that includes areas such as toxicology, epidemiology, biostatistics, orthopedics, and pulmonary medicine. The most important aspect of occupational medicine, and one that distinguishes it from all other medical specialties, is that the practice of occupational medicine requires that the occupational physician have an intimate knowledge

of the workplace. Occupational medicine is a medical specialty organized in 1955 under the American Board of Preventive Medicine. In 1988, there were 1,257 board-certified occupational medicine physicians, far fewer than the current demand. Physicians seeking to specialize in occupational medicine have two avenues open to them: residency training and practice eligibility. In 1988, the United States had 24 residency training programs that graduated about 100 residents annually. Practice eligibility is available to those physicians who have not completed a formal residency but have worked full-time for several years in occupational medicine. Information on the routes to specialty certification is available from the American Board of Preventive Medicine, located at Wright State University in Dayton, Ohio.

Few if any hospital programs provide all of the essential components of an occupational health program outlined by AOMA in 1978 because few hospitals have the expertise to provide the broad range of services required. Instead, hospital occupational health programs evolve in response to market needs and reflect financial reality. At their worst, hospital occupational health programs merely repackage existing weak hospital services and market them under the banner of "occupational health." These programs are rarely successful. Successful occupational health programs are those that are based on a careful assessment of the occupational health needs of the market and provide services customized to meet those needs.

The Occupational Health Market

Understanding how successful hospital occupational health programs are designed requires an understanding of the characteristics that define the occupational health market. These characteristics include the following:

- *The occupational health market is huge and is getting larger.* Medical benefits resulting from workers' compensation have increased from $3.9 billion in 1980 to $8.3 billion in 1986, an increase of 113 percent (figure 1-3). These medical benefits represent about 10 percent of the entire medical indemnity market.
- *Payments in the occupational injury market are legally mandated, and in many states, reimbursement is 100 percent of the medical costs.* Workers' compensation law mandates that almost all employers pay for the medical services related to their workers' injuries. Frequently, the reimbursement rate is set at 100 percent of costs. This high level of reimbursement sharply contrasts with the level of reimbursement in most segments of the hospital market.
- *Seventy percent of workers' compensation payments go to wage replacement—providing wages to injured workers unable to return*

Figure 1-3. Workers' Compensation Medical Benefits, 1980–1986

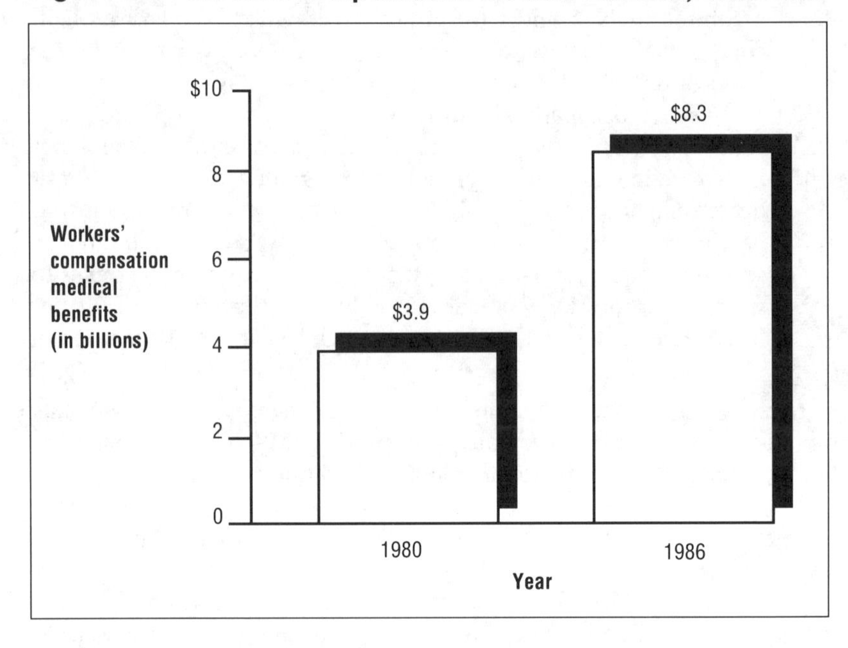

Source: Social Security Administration.

to full-time work. In 1986, companies spent $8.3 billion on medical benefits associated with workers' injuries (figure 1-4). Companies also paid $17.7 billion to workers for missing time from work as a result of their injuries.

- *The injury rate is falling, but the time missed per injury has increased 86 percent since 1972.* In 1972, there were 10.9 injuries per 100 workers. In 1985, there were 7.9 injuries. In 1972, the average injured worker missed 4.4 days as a result of his or her injury. In 1985, the average injured worker missed 8.2 days.[5]
- *Only about 23 percent of injured workers receive payment for lost time.* In 1986, only 22.6 percent of workers' compensation claims were paid for lost time. Those 22.6 percent of cases were responsible for more than 70 percent of workers' compensation costs.[6]
- *The highest rates of injury occur in blue-collar industries.* Workers in blue-collar industries have substantially higher rates of injury than those in manufacturing industries (figure 1-5). Workers in meat-packing plants, for example, have rates of injury 15 times higher than those of insurance or real estate workers.
- *Employers with 100 to 249 employees have the highest rates of injury.* The lowest injury rates are for the smallest and largest employers

Figure 1-4. Workers' Compensation Payments, 1980–1986

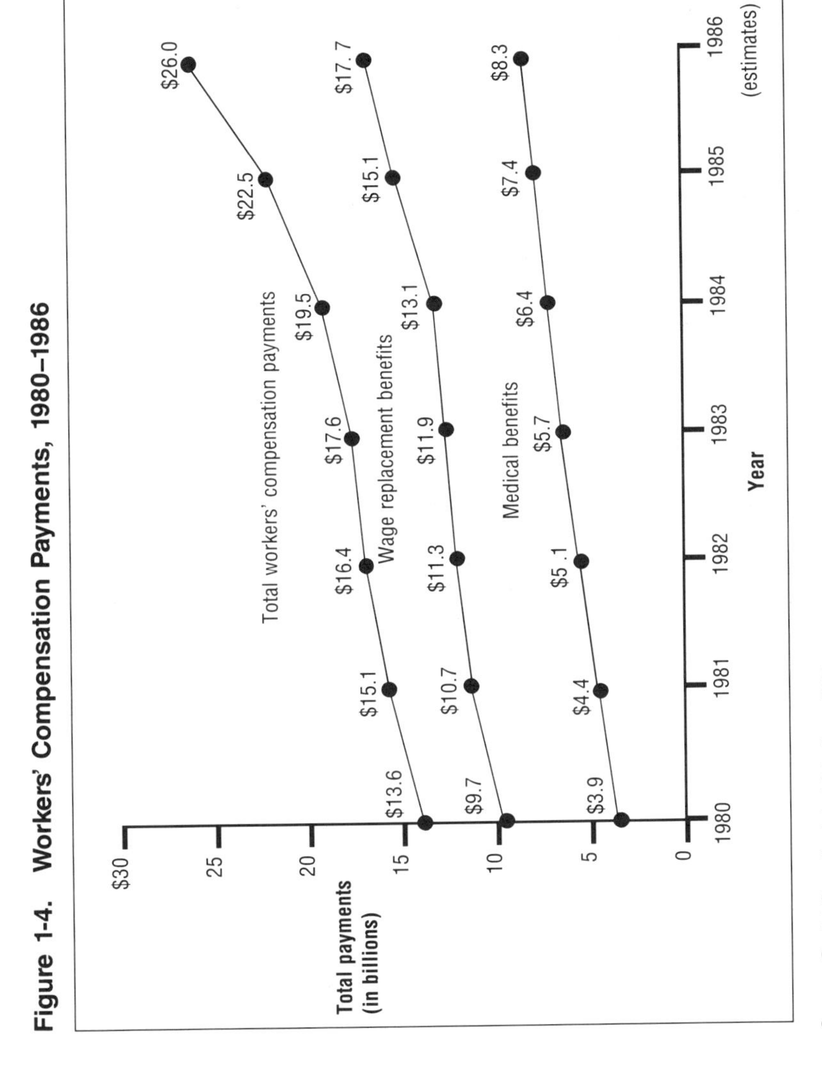

Source: Social Security Administration, 1987.

Figure 1-5. Industry Sectors with the Highest Injury and Illness Rates in 1985

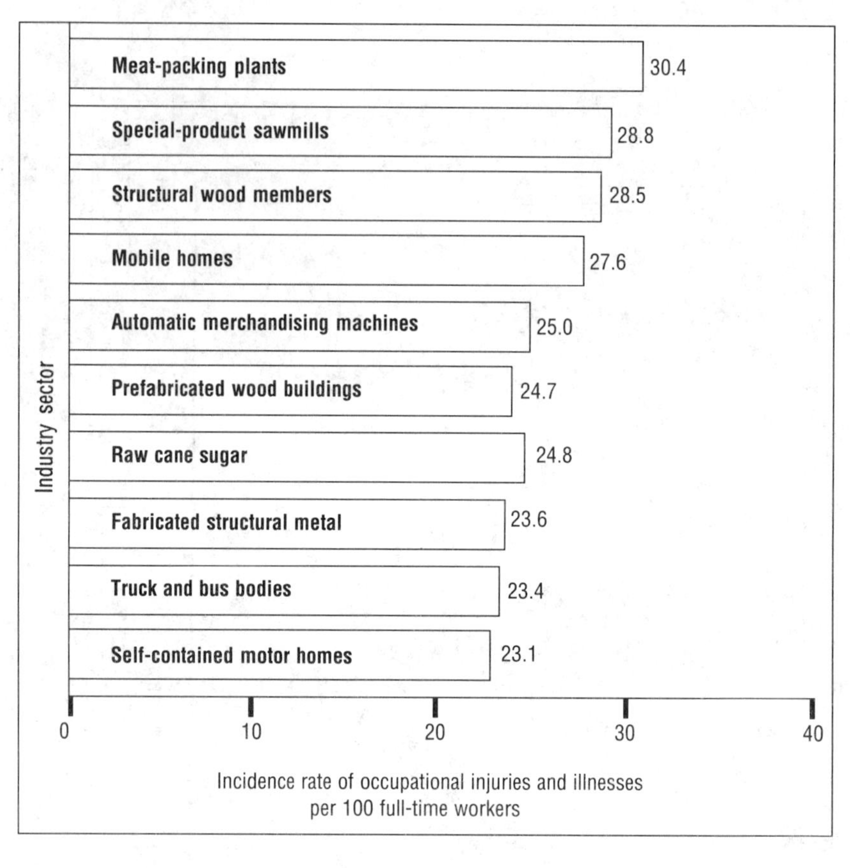

Source: United States Department of Labor, 1985.

(figure 1-6). Large employers may have their own medical departments and as a result are often not a prime target for hospital health programs.

The Current Status of Occupational Health Programs

A 1987 American Hospital Association survey mailed to 6,575 registered U.S. hospitals found that almost one-half (47 percent), or 1,510 of the 3,237 hospitals responding to the survey, had an occupational health program (table 1-2). An additional 13 percent, or 418 hospitals, indicated that they planned to develop a program. Half of the hospitals that had programs had 200 or more beds. Hospitals in the New England, Middle Atlantic, and Pacific regions most frequently reported having occupational health programs.

Figure 1-6. Injury/Illness Rates by Size of Work Force in 1985

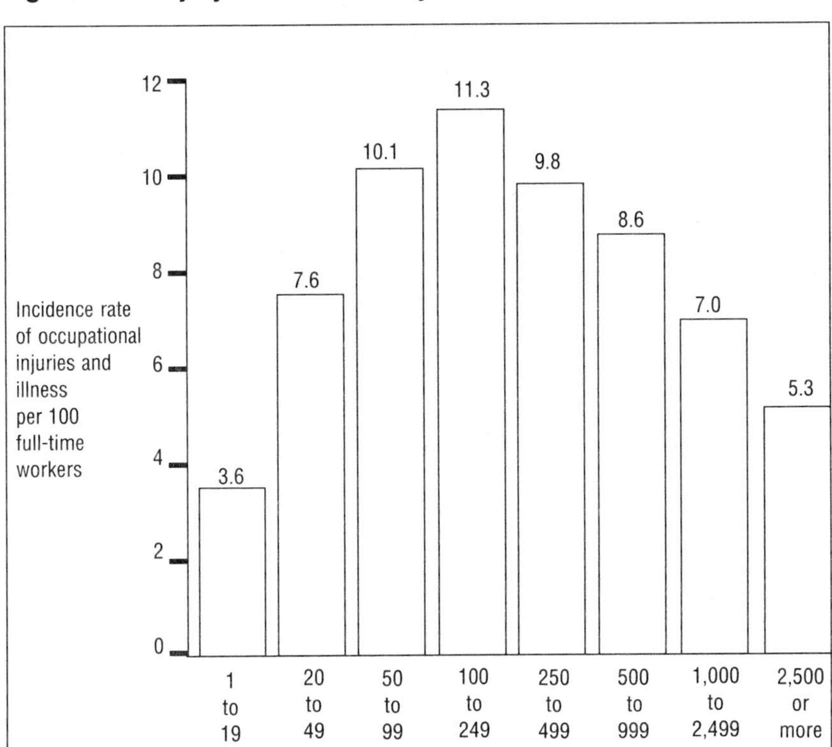

Source: United States Department of Labor, 1985.

Forty-eight percent of hospitals with occupational health programs, or 719 hospitals, provided services to businesses either exclusively or in addition to services provided to hospital employees. Forty-four percent, or 666 hospitals, provided occupational health services only to hospital employees (table 1-3). Hospitals most likely to limit services to businesses had more than 100 beds, were located in the East North Central states, or were in communities with populations of 100,000 to 250,000. Although the largest actual number of hospitals providing industrial or occupational health services only to businesses were community not-for-profit institutions, the investor-owned for-profit hospitals were slightly more likely, percentagewise, to provide occupational services to this market.

Most occupational health services (81 percent) were administered by a hospital department (table 1-4). Only 5 percent were operated by a for-profit subsidiary, and only 1 percent were administered by a hospital foundation.

The distribution of hospitals that reported revenue from industrial or occupational health services is shown in table 1-5. Forty-three percent of

Table 1-2. Status of Industrial or Occupational Health Programs by Hospital Characteristics

	Total		Have Program		Plan Program		No Plans for Program		No Longer Provide		Missing	
Total	3,257	100%	1,510	47%	418	13%	929	29%	15	0%	365	11%
Number of Beds												
6– 24	91	100%	25	27%	7	8%	49	54%	0	0%	10	11%
25– 49	428	100%	126	29%	45	11%	195	46%	0	0%	62	14%
50– 99	706	100%	237	34%	99	14%	279	40%	2	0%	89	13%
100–199	827	100%	397	48%	115	14%	215	26%	3	0%	97	12%
200–299	475	100%	261	55%	74	16%	90	19%	4	1%	45	10%
300–399	294	100%	204	69%	26	9%	39	13%	5	2%	20	7%
400–499	171	100%	104	61%	23	13%	24	14%	1	1%	19	11%
500 or more	245	100%	156	64%	29	12%	38	16%	0	0%	22	9%
Census Region												
New England	172	100%	103	60%	22	13%	29	17%	3	2%	15	9%
Middle Atlantic	369	100%	210	57%	36	10%	83	22%	4	1%	36	10%
South Atlantic	491	100%	233	47%	59	12%	137	28%	0	0%	62	13%
East North Central	582	100%	276	47%	103	18%	144	25%	1	0%	58	10%
East South Central	208	100%	82	39%	25	12%	75	36%	1	0%	25	12%
West North Central	439	100%	164	37%	53	12%	160	36%	1	0%	61	14%
West South Central	355	100%	131	37%	45	13%	138	39%	0	0%	41	12%
Mountain	223	100%	101	45%	26	12%	61	27%	1	0%	34	15%

Pacific	389	100%	206	53%	47	12%	102	26%	4	1%	30	8%
U.S. associated areas	9	100%	4	44%	2	22%	0	0%	0	0%	3	33%
SMSA Size												
Nonmetropolitan	1,356	100%	442	33%	186	14%	551	41%	2	0%	175	13%
Under 100,000	53	100%	28	53%	10	19%	10	19%	0	0%	5	9%
100,000–250,000	328	100%	179	55%	40	12%	79	24%	0	0%	30	9%
250,000–500,000	297	100%	173	58%	39	13%	52	18%	4	1%	29	10%
500,000–1 million	361	100%	193	53%	45	12%	78	22%	3	1%	42	12%
1 million–2.5 million	485	100%	284	59%	65	13%	80	16%	3	1%	53	11%
Over 2.5 million	357	100%	211	59%	33	9%	79	22%	3	1%	31	9%
Control Code												
Government, nonfederal	784	100%	277	35%	102	13%	309	39%	1	0%	95	12%
Nongovernment, not-for-profit	1,976	100%	962	49%	276	14%	512	26%	13	1%	213	11%
Investor-owned, for-profit	322	100%	143	44%	39	12%	96	30%	1	0%	43	13%
Government, federal	155	100%	128	83%	1	1%	12	8%	0	0%	14	9%

Note: Percentages are based upon the row total.

Source: *Final Report: Census of Hospital-Based Health Promotion and Patient Education Programs, 1987.* Copyright 1988 by the AHA Division of Ambulatory Care and Health Promotion.

Table 1-3. Target Audiences of Industrial or Occupational Health Programs by Hospital Characteristics

	Respondents Having Industrial/ Occupational Health Programs		Service Provided to: Businesses Only		Employees Only		Both		Missing	
Total	1,510	100%	298	20%	666	44%	421	28%	125	8%
Number of Beds										
6– 24	25	100%	3	12%	12	48%	3	12%	7	28%
25– 49	126	100%	16	13%	69	55%	22	18%	19	15%
50– 99	237	100%	39	17%	119	50%	57	24%	22	9%
100–199	397	100%	76	19%	165	42%	121	31%	35	9%
200–299	261	100%	63	24%	98	38%	80	31%	20	8%
300–399	204	100%	45	22%	84	41%	69	34%	6	3%
400–499	104	100%	23	22%	43	41%	36	35%	2	2%
500 or more	156	100%	33	21%	76	49%	33	22%	14	9%
Census Region										
New England	103	100%	19	18%	25	24%	51	50%	8	8%
Middle Atlantic	210	100%	45	21%	101	48%	49	23%	15	7%
South Atlantic	233	100%	38	16%	131	56%	46	19%	18	8%
East North Central	276	100%	68	25%	89	32%	98	36%	21	8%
East South Central	82	100%	16	20%	38	46%	20	24%	8	10%
West North Central	164	100%	27	17%	74	45%	47	29%	16	10%

West South Central	131	100%	28	21%	69	53%	18	14%	16	12%
Mountain	101	100%	14	14%	49	49%	28	28%	10	10%
Pacific	206	100%	41	20%	88	43%	64	31%	13	6%
U.S. associated areas	4	100%	2	50%	2	0%	0	0%	0	0%
SMSA Size										
Nonmetropolitan	442	100%	74	17%	222	50%	92	21%	54	12%
Under 100,000	28	100%	4	14%	10	36%	12	43%	2	7%
100,000–250,000	179	100%	46	26%	66	37%	58	32%	9	5%
250,000–500,000	173	100%	31	18%	68	40%	63	36%	10	6%
500,000–1 million	193	100%	40	21%	83	43%	57	30%	13	7%
1 million–2.5 million	284	100%	50	18%	132	47%	77	27%	25	9%
Over 2.5 million	211	100%	53	25%	84	40%	62	29%	12	6%
Control Type										
Government, nonfederal	277	100%	38	14%	158	57%	57	21%	24	9%
Nongovernment, not-for-profit	962	100%	219	23%	352	37%	317	33%	74	8%
Investor-owned, for-profit	143	100%	35	25%	66	46%	31	22%	11	8%
Government, federal	128	100%	6	5%	90	70%	16	13%	16	13%

Note: Percentages are based upon the row total.

Source: *Final Report: Census of Hospital-Based Health Promotion and Patient Education Programs, 1987.* Copyright 1988 by the AHA Division of Ambulatory Care and Health Promotion.

Table 1-4. Organizational Structures of Industrial or Occupational Health Programs by Hospital Characteristics

	Total		Hospital Department		For-Profit Subsidiary		Hospital Foundation		Other		Missing	
Total	1,510	100%	1,222	81%	78	5%	11	1%	86	6%	113	7%
Number of Beds												
6– 24	25	100%	17	68%	0	0%	0	0%	5	20%	3	12%
25– 49	126	100%	105	83%	1	1%	0	0%	7	6%	13	10%
50– 99	237	100%	196	83%	9	4%	2	1%	10	4%	20	8%
100–199	397	100%	316	80%	17	4%	4	1%	22	6%	38	10%
200–299	261	100%	213	82%	16	6%	1	0%	17	7%	14	5%
300–399	204	100%	174	85%	17	8%	1	0%	4	2%	8	4%
400–499	104	100%	78	75%	8	8%	2	2%	11	11%	5	5%
500 or more	156	100%	123	79%	10	6%	1	1%	10	6%	12	8%
Census Region												
New England	103	100%	79	77%	12	12%	2	2%	3	3%	7	7%
Middle Atlantic	210	100%	181	86%	9	4%	2	1%	5	2%	13	6%
South Atlantic	233	100%	196	84%	9	4%	0	0%	9	4%	19	8%
East North Central	276	100%	220	80%	19	7%	2	1%	14	5%	21	8%
East South Central	82	100%	72	88%	1	1%	1	1%	4	5%	4	5%
West North Central	164	100%	135	82%	4	2%	1	1%	14	9%	10	6%
West South Central	131	100%	109	83%	4	3%	0	0%	8	6%	10	8%
Mountain	101	100%	77	76%	6	6%	0	0%	7	7%	11	11%

Pacific	206	100%	150	73%	14	7%	3	1%	21	10%	18	9%
U.S. associated areas	4	100%	3	75%	0	0%	0	0%	0	25%	0	0%
SMSA Size												
Nonmetropolitan	442	100%	362	82%	12	3%	3	1%	24	5%	41	9%
Under 100,000	28	100%	24	86%	2	7%	0	0%	1	4%	1	4%
100,000–250,000	179	100%	149	83%	13	7%	2	1%	4	2%	11	6%
250,000–500,000	173	100%	137	79%	11	6%	0	0%	12	7%	13	8%
500,000–1 million	193	100%	155	80%	11	6%	2	1%	14	7%	11	6%
1 million–2.5 million	284	100%	223	79%	15	5%	1	0%	23	8%	22	8%
Over 2.5 million	211	100%	172	82%	14	7%	3	1%	8	4%	14	7%
Control Code												
Government, nonfederal	277	100%	227	82%	6	2%	2	1%	21	8%	21	8%
Nongovernment, not-for-profit	962	100%	774	80%	64	7%	8	1%	49	5%	67	7%
Investor-owned, for-profit	143	100%	116	81%	8	6%	1	1%	5	3%	13	9%
Government, federal	128	100%	105	82%	0	0%	0	0%	11	9%	12	9%

Note: Percentages are based upon the row total. Total includes only those respondents that provide industrial or occupational health.

Source: *Final Report: Census of Hospital-Based Health Promotion and Patient Education Programs, 1987.* Copyright 1988 by the AHA Division of Ambulatory Care and Health Promotion.

Table 1-5. Revenue Status of Industrial or Occupational Health Programs by Hospital Characteristics

	Total		Yes		No		Missing	
Total	1,510	100%	651	43%	749	50%	110	7%
Number of Beds								
6– 24	25	100%	3	12%	14	56%	8	32%
25– 49	126	100%	25	20%	84	67%	17	13%
50– 99	237	100%	85	36%	143	60%	9	4%
100–199	397	100%	168	42%	188	47%	41	10%
200–299	261	100%	141	54%	107	41%	13	5%
300–399	204	100%	105	51%	90	44%	9	4%
400–499	104	100%	56	54%	45	43%	3	3%
500 or more	156	100%	68	44%	78	50%	10	6%
Census Region								
New England	103	100%	63	61%	30	29%	10	10%
Middle Atlantic	210	100%	89	42%	104	50%	17	8%
South Atlantic	233	100%	79	34%	140	60%	14	6%
East North Central	276	100%	161	58%	104	38%	11	4%
East South Central	82	100%	26	32%	51	62%	5	6%
West North Central	164	100%	71	43%	80	49%	13	8%
West South Central	131	100%	40	31%	80	61%	11	8%
Mountain	101	100%	35	35%	58	57%	8	8%
Pacific	206	100%	87	42%	98	48%	21	10%
U.S. associated areas	4	100%	0	0%	4	100%	0	0%
SMSA Size								
Nonmetropolitan	442	100%	138	31%	262	59%	42	10%
Under 100,000	28	100%	17	61%	9	32%	2	7%
100,000–250,000	179	100%	94	53%	71	40%	14	8%
250,000–500,000	173	100%	92	53%	76	44%	5	3%
500,000–1 million	193	100%	91	47%	89	46%	13	7%
1 million–2.5 million	284	100%	114	40%	150	53%	20	7%
Over 2.5 million	211	100%	105	50%	92	44%	14	7%
Control Code								
Government, nonfederal	277	100%	87	31%	170	61%	20	7%
Nongovernment, not-for-profit	962	100%	504	52%	389	40%	69	7%
Investor-owned, for-profit	143	100%	55	38%	80	56%	8	6%
Government, federal	128	100%	5	4%	110	86%	13	10%

Note: Percentages are based upon the row total. Total includes only those respondents that provide industrial or occupational health.

Source: *Final Report: Census of Hospital-Based Health Promotion and Patient Education Programs, 1987.* Copyright 1988 by the AHA Division of Ambulatory Care and Health Promotion.

hospitals, or 651 hospitals, reported that their services generated revenue. Large institutions (200 or more beds), community not-for-profit organizations, or those in metropolitan areas with populations of less than 500,000 or more than 2.5 million were most likely to report revenue. The New England and East North Central census regions reported the highest percentages of revenue-producing services. Respondents least likely to report that occupational health generates revenue were small institutions or those in nonmetropolitan areas.

Principles of Successful Occupational Health Program Design

A successful hospital occupational health program is designed around three principles:

- *It concentrates on acute injury treatment and follow-up.* Almost without exception, profitable occupational health programs feature injury treatment as their core service. Injury treatment is a legally mandated corporate expense, it meets the most pressing current need of industry, and it is a service whose volume often exceeds the resources of the local medical community.
- *In addition to injury treatment, its product line provides services that meet corporate needs and have a synergistic relationship with one another.* The occupational health product line frequently contains six components: acute injury treatment, employee screening, health promotion, worksite nursing, employee assistance, and rehabilitation.
- *It provides services that may reduce the amount of time an injured worker is disabled, thereby significantly reducing workers' compensation expenses.* As noted earlier in this chapter, lost time per injury has increased 86 percent since 1972, and payments for lost time amount to about $17.7 billion per year.

Although these three principles characterize successful programs, developing a successful program involves much more than understanding and applying these principles. This book is designed to cover the topics necessary to understand occupational health program development.

Overview of This Book

Part one of this book describes the elements of a hospital occupational health services product line. In chapter 2, the concept of a product line and the importance of synergy among services in the product line are introduced. Understanding these concepts provides a foundation for learning about the individual elements of the product line.

The first element in the occupational health services product line, acute injury treatment and case management, is the subject of chapters 3 and 4.

In chapter 3, the importance of having injury treatment be the centerpiece of the occupational health services product line is stressed. The chapter covers the basic elements of successful treatment programs for injured workers and reviews the workers' compensation system. Chapter 4 describes how to set up a tracking system for injured workers and how tracking can be used as a marketing tool.

Chapters 5, 6, 7, and 8 cover the second element of the occupational health services product line, employee screening. Employee examinations performed in occupational situations are different from the routine physical examinations performed by hospitals. In chapter 5, the Occupational Safety and Health Administration (OSHA) is described, and its history and standards-setting process are explained. The chapter reviews the ways hospital occupational health programs relate to OSHA standards in the areas of record keeping, personal protective devices, and medical surveillance. Chapter 6 reviews the legal issues relating to preemployment screening. The chapter emphasizes the importance of understanding job risks while making preemployment assessments and limiting preemployment inquiries to job-related functions. Chapter 7 presents the complex issues involved in establishing a drug-testing program for employees. Chapter 8 reviews the controversies surrounding employee testing for acquired immunodeficiency syndrome (AIDS).

The third element of the occupational health services product line is worksite programs. Chapter 9 discusses the advantages and importance of worksite programs from the perspective of industry and questions how occupational health programs can effectively function without an intimate knowledge of the workplace. This chapter also reviews the role of the occupational health nurse and the nurse's role in the workplace.

The fourth element of the product line, health promotion, is discussed in chapter 10. From a profit perspective, health promotion has proved to be one of the weaker hospital diversification strategies as a stand-alone product, but it can strengthen the product line, provide an entree into some companies, and offer promise for future reduction in illness and injury rates.

The fifth element of the product line, employee assistance programs (EAPs), is addressed in chapter 11. With the recent trend toward drug testing, EAPs are becoming increasingly important as part of a company's comprehensive approach to substance abuse.

The sixth and final element of the product line is rehabilitation. From an industry perspective, rehabilitation programs are important because they address the problems of the small portion of the injured worker population that accounts for a disproportionate amount of the workers' compensation expense. Chapter 12 reviews the elements that characterize successful rehabilitation programs.

In the chapters in part two, operational issues that affect hospital occupational health programs are described. The first operational issue is marketing and sales. Chapter 13 provides a framework for developing a marketing plan for an occupational health program. Chapter 14 reviews sales strategies that are effective in presenting the occupational health services product line to industry.

The second group of operational issues includes program staffing, organization, and location. Chapter 15 covers the nuts and bolts of establishing an occupational health program. Chapter 16 reviews the framework for determining whether a freestanding clinic makes sense.

The third operational issue is developing positive medical staff relationships. Chapter 17 reviews the four development phases through which all new projects pass. It provides guidelines for steps that can reduce medical staff resistance to a new occupational health program. One method of reducing resistance is a hospital–physician joint venture. Chapter 18 discusses how a hospital can determine whether a joint venture makes sense.

New technology, the fourth operational issue, plays an important role in hospital occupational health programs. Chapter 19 discusses the pros and cons of applying computers to resolve problems in occupational health programs. Chapter 20 analyzes the current issue of expensive high-technology equipment.

The last operational issue involves the provision of hospital occupational health services in an ethical manner. Chapter 21 focuses on the often-conflicting demands occupational health places on occupational health physicians. Chapter 22 reviews the ethical and quality issues that face hospital occupational health programs from the labor perspective.

The final section of the book provides, in chapter 23, a case study of how the product line and operational forces can be merged into a successful, comprehensive occupational health program. Chapter 24 concludes the book with a discussion of unresolved issues and trends for the future.

For many hospitals, an occupational health program is an integral part of their plan for long-term viability. This book summarizes the strategies that have proved successful in this regard.

References

1. Gallivan, M. Margins drop, utilization improves in 1987. *Hospitals* 62(9):40, May 5, 1988.
2. Sabatino, F. G. The diversification success story continues: survey. *Hospitals* 63(1):26, Jan. 5, 1989.
3. Martinsons, J. N. U.S. MD glut limits demand for FMG physicians. *Hospitals* 62(3):67, Feb. 5, 1988.
4. Grayson, M. A. Breaking the medical gridlock. *Hospitals* 63(4):32–37, Feb. 20, 1989.
5. Calculation based upon 1985 United States Department of Labor data reprinted in *Marketing to Employers,* Vol. 2, *Occupational Health Programs.* Washington, DC: Health Care Advisory Board, July 1988, p. 7.
6. Health Care Advisory Board. *Marketing to Employers.* Vol. 2, *Occupational Health Programs.* Washington, DC: HCAB, July 1988, p. 57.

*Addendum: Scope of Occupational Health Programs and Occupational Medical Practice**

This statement was prepared by the Occupational Medical Practice Committee of the American Occupational Medical Association: Bruce W. Karrh, M.D., Chairman; Bruce H. Bennett, M.D.; Caesar Briefer, M.D.; Robert M. DeuPree, M.D.; William G. Mays, M.D.; James W. Mitchell, M.D.; Robert H. Moore, M.D.; Billie H. Shevick, M.D.; W. Lloyd Wright, M.D. The statement was approved by the AOMA Board of Directors at its meeting April 20–21, 1979, in Anaheim, Calif.

Introduction

Occupational medicine as a specialty and the practice of occupational medicine have undergone many changes in recent years. These have been caused largely by changing expectations of society in general, and employed persons in particular, as exemplified by legislation directed toward providing a safe and healthful workplace, such as the Occupational Safety and Health Act and the Toxic Substances Control Act. There has also developed great concern over the chronic health effects of long-term exposures to low levels of chemical and physical agents. The result has been to increase the demands on the time of occupational physicians while requiring that they be more knowledgeable and experienced in both clinical and occupational medicine, toxicology, epidemiology, industrial hygiene, and administration.

While there has been a change in the demands on physicians practicing occupational medicine, the scope of occupational medical practice has also enlarged, resulting in an increase in the components and services of an occupational health program.

An occupational medical program must, as a minimum:

- Obey all relevant laws and regulations
- Take all feasible steps to keep industrial operations and/or products from having an adverse effect on the health of employees, customers or the public
- Accept responsibility and assist in the provision of necessary care in cases where health is harmed due to industrial operations and/or products

The specific contents of an occupational health program will be largely determined by the functions of the work organization and the specific workplace activities and potential hazards present.

---

*This article is reprinted from the *Journal of Occupational Medicine* [21(7):487–89, July 1979], with permission of the American College of Occupational Medicine (formerly the American Occupational Medical Association).

Comprehensive occupational health programs require the skills of persons trained or experienced in a variety of disciplines, including clinical and occupational medicine, industrial hygiene, toxicology, epidemiology and biometry, occupational health nursing, safety engineering, and human factors engineering. Such a program requires an organizational structure that insures communication and coordination of activities between these various, seemingly diverse, but interdependent, skills. The exact organizational relationship necessary to fulfill the various responsibilities varies between companies and can only be generalized in this document.

The organization must report at a management level high enough to assure that top company management is fully informed of all significant occupational health activities, problems and concerns so that appropriate action can be taken where necessary to assure a safe and healthful workplace.

An occupational health program should not be used as a means to further the specific interests of management or unions but to provide methods and procedures to assist in providing a safe and healthful workplace for all concerned.

Records which are developed for retaining the data from an occupational health program—medical data on employees, exposure data on employees or groups of employees, work assignment data, toxicology and industrial hygiene data, and epidemiological data—must be kept in such a way as to insure the degree of confidentiality the data require. Procedures for preserving this confidentiality, yet allowing access to those with a bona fide need to know, must be developed.

Employees who are the subject of medical or exposure records should be informed of the existence and contents of these records. Likewise, employees should be informed of the appropriate toxicologic and epidemiologic data which are pertinent to their potential workplace exposures.

This document will list those components and services which are considered a necessary or essential part of all occupational health programs and those which are desirable if time and availability of medical and paramedical personnel permit. These latter are elective components of an occupational health program.

Occupational Health Program

A. Essential Components

1. *Health evaluation of employees.* Employees should be fully informed of the results of each evaluation, whether or not abnormalities are detected. When abnormalities, or questionable abnormalities, are detected, the employee should be informed and referred to the personal physician or appropriate referral physician for further diagnostic evaluation or treatment. Evaluations should be carried out on the following occasions:
   (a) *Pre-assignment*—Health status, including assessment of emotional status, should be assessed prior to making recommendations to

management regarding the assignment of an employee to a job to assure that the person can perform the job safely and efficiently without endangering the person's safety or health and that of others. This recommendation shall be based on any or all of the following:
  (1) Medical history
  (2) Occupational history
  (3) Assessment of the organ systems likely to be affected by the assignment
  (4) Evaluation of the description and demands of the job to which assignment is being considered

(b) *Periodic*—The health status of the employee should be periodically reviewed where there is a likelihood that workplace exposures or activities could have an adverse health effect. This review may be limited to those organs or systems most likely to be affected.

(c) *Post-illness or injury*—The health status of an employee should be reevaluated following absence from work due to illness or injury to assure that the individual has sufficiently recovered from the illness or injury to perform the job without undue risk of adverse health or safety effects to the individual or others, and that the employee is not taking any medication which increases the risk of illness or injury due to the workplace.

(d) *Termination and retirement*—The health status of an employee should be evaluated at the time of termination or retirement. The employee should be informed concerning his or her health status and advised of any adverse health effects due to the job.

2. *Diagnosis and treatment of occupational injuries or illnesses, including rehabilitation.* Occupational injuries and illnesses should be diagnosed as promptly as practical and treated as appropriate within the capabilities of the workplace medical facility. The occupational health personnel for a workplace are uniquely qualified to diagnose occupational illnesses and injuries because of their knowledge of the workplace. The occupational physician should also be knowledgeable regarding rehabilitation programs and facilities in the area. Frequently the workplace can be used for rehabilitating employees, especially where selective work can be provided.
3. *Emergency treatment of nonoccupational injury or illness.* The occupational health program should provide treatment for emergency conditions, including emotional crises, which occur among employees while at work. This treatment may only be palliative and to prevent loss of life and limb or, where personnel and facilities are available, may be more definitive.
4. *Education of employees in potential occupational hazards which may be specific to the job, instruction on methods of prevention and on*

recognition of possible adverse health effects. Every employee should know the potential hazards involved in each job to which he or she is likely to be assigned. This instruction must include methods of recognizing and preventing possible adverse health and safety effects from the workplace. The employee must be instructed to report any adverse health effect to his or her supervisor and to the occupational medical personnel.

5. *Evaluation of programs for the use of indicated personal protective devices—ear plugs, safety spectacles, respirators, etc.* The occupational health personnel should develop techniques and expertise to assist management in properly fitting personal protective devices, determining that the devices provide adequate protection to employees, and educating the employees in proper utilization and care of the equipment.
6. *Assist management in providing a safe and healthful work environment.* Occupational health personnel should periodically inspect and evaluate the workplace, looking for potential health and safety hazards. Management should be informed when such hazards are found and, where expertise exists, make recommendations for abatement of the hazard.
7. *Toxicological studies on chemical substances which have not had adequate toxicological testing.* Occupational health personnel should advise management on the adequacy and significance of toxicological test data pertinent to the workplace. Where adequate data do not exist, occupational health personnel should recommend appropriate resources for testing.
8. *Biostatistics and epidemiology when adequate data are available and a need exists to evaluate the experience of persons at risk.* The occupational health program should assure that data on employee work experiences and exposures and medical occurrences are accumulated and retained. When appropriate, these data should be used to conduct epidemiological studies to assess the effects the workplace may have had or is having on the employees.
9. *Maintenance of occupational medical records.* The occupational health program must maintain occupational medical records on each employee, documenting the reasons for and the results of all physical examinations and visits to the medical facility. Ideally, these records should contain data sufficient to reproduce a chronology of the employee's medical occurrences, illnesses, and injuries. These data must be maintained confidentially. Procedures for preserving this confidentiality, yet allowing access to those with a bona fide need to know, must be developed.
10. *Immunization against possible occupational infection.* Where employees work jobs with potential exposures for which there is an effective immunization, this protection should be provided to the employee.

11. *Participate with management in planning, providing, and assessing the quality of employee benefits.* The occupational health personnel are best qualified to assist management in evaluating employee health benefits and the costs of such benefits.
12. *Assist in interpretation and/or development of governmental health and safety regulations.* Occupational health personnel are uniquely qualified to assist in interpreting and developing these regulations and to assure they effectively provide the necessary protection to the employee in a manner that is cost effective and best utilizes professional occupational safety and health personnel.
13. *Periodic evaluation of the occupational health program.* This is necessary to assure the program meets its objective effectively. The mechanism for this assessment will vary, but may exist in the program itself.

B. Elective Components of Occupational Health Programs

1. *Palliative treatment of disorders to allow completion of workshift or for condition for which an employee may not ordinarily consult a physician.* Personal medical care may be provided to employees where suitable medical care is not available in the community. This may include early diagnosis, definitive treatment and follow-up, but only under certain appropriate and limited conditions.
2. *Repetitive treatment of nonoccupational conditions prescribed and monitored by personal physician (physiotherapy, routine injections, etc.) or if the employee's personal physician approves this approach.* This provides a service to the employee, the personal physician and the employer by minimizing the time the employee must be off the job, the expense to the employee and the personal physician's time.
3. *Assistance in rehabilitation of alcohol or drug dependent employees or those with emotional disorders.* The workplace provides a unique opportunity to provide this type of assistance to employees and their families.
4. *Health education and counseling (for example, mental health, hypertension control, diabetes control, obesity, physical fitness, smoking cessation programs, etc.).* The workplace provides a unique opportunity for effective health education and health maintenance programs. These may include health counseling for employees and their family members. Occupational health personnel should assist employees by offering advice and counsel regarding the personal health care the employee or family member receives from the local medical community.
5. *Assist management in control of illness-related absence from job.* Occupational health personnel are uniquely qualified to assist management in assessing the reasons for an employee's poor performance or absence from work due to illness or injury and in determining when they are well enough to return to work safely.

6. *Disaster preparedness planning for the workplace and, when appropriate, the community.* Occupational health personnel should assist management in preparing a plan for disaster preparedness. Since community facilities and health and safety personnel are such an essential part of dealing with an emergency at the workplace, such planning should be done in conjunction with that of the local community.
7. *Immunization against nonoccupational infectious diseases.* Frequently the workplace is equipped to provide appropriate immunizations for international travelers and for other nonoccupational conditions.

Summary

The goal of an occupational health program is to insure a safe and healthful workplace. The role of the occupational health professional is to assist in providing this safe and healthful workplace. Although this document is to provide a compilation of the necessary and important parts of an occupational health program, it does not detail how these programs should be structured or how each will function. More assistance on the details can be obtained from suitable reference materials, such as those on the attached brief list, or by consultation with persons trained or experienced in this field.

Bibliography to Addendum

Howe, HF: Organization and operation of an occupational health program, three parts. *J. Occup. Med,* 17(6,7,8), 1975.

American Medical Association: *Scope, Objectives and Functions of Occupational Health Programs.* AMA Department of Environmental, Public and Occupational Health, 535 North Dearborn Street, Chicago, IL 60610, Dec. 1971.

Occupational Medicine, Principles and Practical Applications, C. Zenz (Ed.). Chicago: Year Book Medical Publishers, Inc., 1975.

The Industrial Environment—Its Evaluation and Control. U.S. Department of Health, Education, and Welfare, Public Health Service, Centers for Disease Control, National Institute for Occupational Safety and Health, 1973.

Encyclopaedia of Occupational Health and Safety, Volumes I and II. International Labour Office. Geneva: McGraw-Hill Book Co., 1974.

Part 1

Occupational Health Services Product Lines

Chapter 2

The Product Line Concept

Rob Ryder

In an occupational health services market that is becoming increasingly competitive and volatile, the most effective and efficient way to operate and coordinate all occupational health services may be through a product line structure. A *product line* is a group of services or programs that have similar markets and service objectives and are centrally administered independent of other hospital departments.

The Occupational Health Services Product Line Model

Major programs in an occupational health services product line most commonly include occupational medicine and rehabilitation, employee assistance programs (EAPs), and wellness services. In addition, some providers have successfully expanded their services to include experiential education, organizational development programs, and child care services. All of these services target the corporate community as their primary market and are designed to improve employee health or quality of life or both.

Each major program in the product line has its own manager and maintains its own operations. However, the objective of the product line is to create a synergy between the programs that is of benefit to all. A product line manager who is equally invested in all of the programs provides central leadership, and all program managers report to that person.[1] This model prevents the redundancy of functions such as marketing, budgeting, and resource utilization and avoids some of the turf battles inherent between programs that compete for common markets. The success of all programs is ultimately determined by the performance of the product line as a whole. Therefore, all program managers should be interested in assisting one another instead of competing with one another.

Figure 2-1 provides a sample organizational chart for an occupational health services product line and a listing of product and service placement within major programs. Product placement within programs is usually an evolutionary process that is driven by product content and availability of resources within each program. Conflicts that arise around product placement are decided by the product line manager. However, as with the larger product line, the services that make up a program should be synergistic in nature and logically associated by content.

Profitability and the Product Mix

The primary financial goal of the occupational health services product line is to ensure that the product line as a whole is profitable. However, every program or every product within each program will not necessarily be profitable.

The core of the successful occupational health services product line will be the occupational medicine program; within this program, the injury and illness treatment product is the determinant for long-term financial success. The injury and illness treatment product may not be the most profitable product, but it is the most stable and carries with it the greatest volume. Because the treatment of occupational illnesses and injuries is mandated by law, the injury and illness treatment product will always be the highest and best understood occupational health priority for most corporations. Rarely, however, will treatment be the most profitable product in the product line because of price regulations, contractual considerations, and labor intensiveness associated with treatment. Despite this fact, the profitability of the occupational health services program as a whole will depend on the program's ability to deliver an occupational medicine injury and illness treatment component.

Four primary criteria should be considered when deciding whether and where to place a given product in the occupational health services product line. Products should be able to do the following:

- *Make a financial contribution.* Products meeting this criterion are likely to consistently produce a profit that is significant enough to (1) contribute to a positive bottom line and (2) support value-added products, such as wellness programs, that are not profitable. Many high-margin products (for example, executive physicals) do not meet this criterion because they do not consistently provide enough volume to significantly affect the overall bottom line.
- *Generate referrals.* Products meeting this criterion are likely to produce a significant number of referrals for the hospital and its medical staff. This criterion plays a prominent role in determining the product mix for a hospital-based occupational health services product line;

Figure 2-1. Product Line Organizational Chart

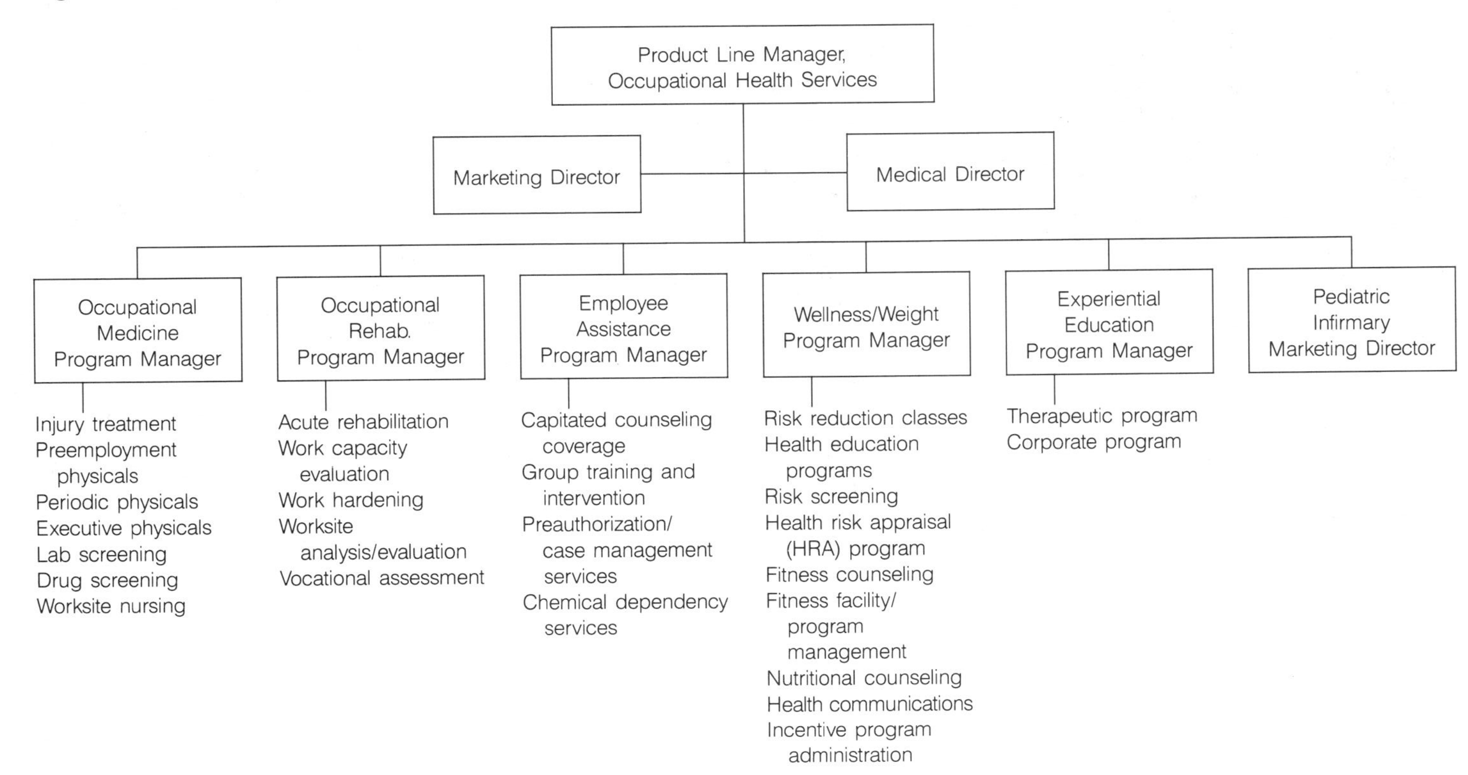

therefore, a system for tracking referrals and referral-generated revenue must be set up. A product line based on the referral criterion and without a referral tracking system is extremely vulnerable during times of economic trouble in the health care industry as a whole.

- *Add value to other occupational health services products.* Products meeting this criterion may not be profitable themselves but may help other products to be more profitable or salable. The mere availability of a product meeting this criterion often creates a marketing differential that facilitates the sale of a more profitable core service, such as an EAP or an occupational medicine program. For example, an EAP that can offer nutritional counseling by a registered dietitian in addition to the usual EAP mental health counseling services may have a significant market advantage over other traditional EAP competitors. The loss sustained by the wellness program employing the dietitian (who is also used for weight-loss classes, executive physicals, and so forth) may be more than offset by the profits from additional business won by the EAP because it can offer nutritional counseling on its menu of available services. Quantifying the contribution made by value-added products is difficult. However, to the occupational health services product line they can spell the difference between success and failure, particularly in a competitive market, and should never be discounted or disregarded.
- *Offset fixed expenses.* Most core products in an occupational health services product line (for example, injury treatment and follow-up, EAP counseling, acute rehabilitation) require, at a minimum, a fixed amount of labor and capital resources regardless of business volume. If core product resources can be used to deliver other products, then fixed expenses are offset and the product line is more profitable. Products meeting this criterion should at least break even and should not interfere with the delivery of the core services they seek to support.

Figure 2-2 summarizes how the program–product mix of one occupational health services product line meets the criteria listed above. This particular product line produces an annual return on revenue of approximately 10 percent. For this service, the financial contribution criterion rates highest in the core products. Other products are characterized by high ratings in the market-value and expenses-offset categories.

No magic formula for a successful product mix exists. A successful mix of products is driven primarily by the market being served. However, without strong core products within the major programs, the construction of a successful occupational service product line is virtually impossible.[2]

Packaging and Cross-Selling within the Product Line

Because the overall performance of the product line is paramount, one service can be used to sell another. For example, within a product line, a sick-child

Figure 2-2. Program–Product Mix of an Occupational Health Service

3 = If properly managed, program/service is likely to meet the criteria
2 = If properly managed, program/service might meet the criteria
1 = Even if properly managed, program/service is unlikely to meet the criteria
Core = Core service that generates fixed expense

	Makes a Financial Contribution	Generates Referrals	Adds Market Value	Offsets Fixed Expenses
Occupational Medicine Program (overall)	3	3	3	
Injury treatment	2	3	3	Core
Preemployment physicals	2	2	3	3
Periodic physicals	2	2	3	3
Executive physicals	2	2	3	3
Lab screening	2	2	3	1
Drug screening	2	3	3	1
Worksite nursing	2	3	3	1
Occupational Rehabilitation Program (overall)	3	2	3	
Acute rehabilitation	3	2	3	Core
Work capacity evaluation	2	2	3	3
Work hardening	2	1	3	3
Worksite analysis/evaluation	2	2	3	3
Vocational assessment	3	1	3	1
Employee Assistance Program (overall)	3	3	3	
Capitated counseling coverage	3	3	3	Core
Group training and intervention	2	3	3	3
Preauthorization/case management services	2	2	3	3
Chemical dependency services	3	3	3	3
Health Promotion/Wellness Program (overall)	1	2	3	3
Risk reduction classes (for example, smoking, weight, stress)	2	1	3	3
Health education programs	1	1	3	3
Risk screening (for example, blood pressure, cholesterol)	2	3	3	3
Health risk appraisal (HRA) program	2	2	3	3
Fitness counseling	1	2	3	3
Fitness facility/program management	3	1	3	2
Nutritional counseling	2	3	3	3
Health communications (for example, newsletter)	1	1	3	1
Incentive program administration	2	1	3	2
Pediatric Infirmary Program	1	2	3	1
Experiential Education	3	1	3	1

care program (pediatric infirmary) may be provided at no registration cost to employees of companies who contract for EAP services. This service usually costs $2 per employee per year. Similarly, companies that are enrolled in the occupational medicine program may receive a 10 percent discount on the per capita rate for EAP services. In this way, the services help support and sell one another by creating market differentials that are difficult for competitors to match. The marrying of EAPs and occupational medicine is particularly attractive because, as detailed in chapter 11, the EAP provides a tool that actually helps reduce costs incurred through the occupational medicine program.

However, within a product line, programs should not be bundled so tightly that corporate clients feel they are being made to accept and pay for a service they do not want. If a company only wants occupational medicine and not an EAP, that is fine. During the course of the relationship that develops when providing occupational medicine services, the occupational medicine staff will have many opportunities to point out to a company the need for and value of an EAP. Once the credibility of the first program is established, selling another service becomes easier.

An occupational medicine program is probably an easier entree into a company than an EAP because the former is better understood. However, this is not always the case. The pediatric infirmary program at Penrose–St. Francis Health System (Colorado Springs, Colorado) has produced as many leads for both the EAP and the occupational medicine program as any other service within the occupational health product line has.

Keys to Marketing and Development Success

The marketing and business development of an occupational health services product line need not be complicated, expensive, or labor intensive. Three keys will help ensure that this is the case:

- *Use a person (or persons) who intimately knows all product line services to accomplish all initial marketing and to coordinate all follow-up marketing.* Having such efforts coordinated increases opportunities for cross-selling within the product line. Marketing occupational health services involves more corporate relations than sales. The fewer contact people a corporate client has to work with within the product line, the quicker a relationship or partnership develops between the client and all components of the product line. The person who coordinates the marketing must be empowered and knowledgeable enough to make product packaging and pricing decisions for all components of the product line in order to best meet the overall needs of the corporate client as well as to best serve the product line as a whole. The ability to act quickly is imperative in a competitive market. Once relationships are established and client needs are determined, much of the follow-up marketing can be accomplished by program managers or staff. Follow-up should always be coordinated centrally to ensure that all products are working in sync.

- *Listen carefully to and act on what customers think they need, not what staff members think they need.* The best marketing resources of the occupational health services product line should go into activities, such as focus groups and educational programs, that allow clients and prospective clients opportunities to voice their needs and dissatisfactions. These types of activities allow for multiple contacts with minimal resources (unlike cold calling), provide follow-up opportunities with participants (everybody wants to know what the reaction has been to their suggestions), and provide a solid basis for corporate relationship building and program ownership. In addition, focus groups and educational programs are indicative of a style of doing business that is appreciated by many businesses today. One warning, however: Staff members should never ask for suggestions if they do not plan to act on what they hear.
- *Ensure that all employees from each program in the product line are aware of and are to some degree involved in all other services in the line.* This third key is perhaps the most important. Over time, it is the line employees (for example, doctors, nurses, technicians, counselors, secretaries, exercise instructors, and so forth) who will make the connections between services and have the visions for new products that will keep all services competitive and viable. These people ultimately have more contact with the corporate client than any marketing person could possibly have, and in the context of their work they will be the ones who help the corporate client to see the connections that will ultimately sell other services in the product line. Fostering this kind of product-line-wide awareness and ownership among employees is, however, no easy task. It requires the following:
  - Regular formal and informal communication between program managers
  - Regular gatherings of all product line employees for the sharing of successes and failures
  - A willingness on the part of product line management staff to allow unprecedented employee initiative
  - Communication among line employees and management and entrepreneurial and intrapreneurial risk taking by line employees
  - An organizational philosophy that expounds a constancy of purpose (for example, extraordinary customer service and responsiveness) that is understandable and applicable to all products in the line

  Without these components, the product line is just another bureaucratic structure that is bound to create barriers instead of synergy among programs.

The Central Product Line Management Team

An essential ingredient to the success of the product line concept is the central product line management team. This group works for all programs in the product line and is responsible for maintaining the congruency of the product line and providing direction for the product line as a whole. The product line management team should be small and able to react quickly to the needs of any program within the product line or to the needs of the product line as a single entity.

A basic product line management team consists of a product line manager or administrator and a product line marketing director. In certain circumstances, the team may be expanded to include a finance manager and a medical director. Each of these functions may have a limited number of support staff (for example, clerical, sales/marketing staff); however, this staff should be kept to a minimum. As a general rule, the resources of the product line should go into delivering the products, not into administrative functions. The nature of the central product line management team must be facilitative, not bureaucratic.

Accountability for the overall success of the product line rests with the product line manager, who must be a person of vision, creativity, and leadership and who must not be overly invested in any given product line program. The product line manager should be astute in the area of hospital and corporate politics and have a good business background (for example, budgeting, financial, or marketing skills). In addition, the product line manager should be one who is excited by entrepreneurial opportunities and is a competent communicator with both employees and customers. He or she must be flexible, have a good sense of perspective, and be able to laugh at the follies of bureaucracy. Finally, and probably most important, the product line manager must be confident and yet humble enough to attribute all product line successes to the employees and managers at the points of service delivery.

The following are the key responsibilities of the product line manager and the central product line management staff:

- *Be constantly aware of the business status of all product line programs.* For the product line to be successful, no program can operate in isolation. The product line management team must always know "which services are hot and which are not" in order to properly facilitate synergistic relationships between product line programs.
- *Develop and promulgate product line philosophy.* A product line is in essence its own company, with its own identity and characteristics. These characteristics must be shared by all components of the product line in order to maintain credibility with the market as well as with staff members. Noted business consultant W. Edwards Deming refers to this as "constancy of purpose," or the single focus or goal

upon which all business decisions and behaviors are based (for example, extraordinary customer service and responsiveness).[3]

- *Supervise all product line program managers.* Central supervision and evaluation of program managers ensures constancy of purpose and reduces interprogram squabbles.
- *Devise an overall marketing strategy and oversee and coordinate the marketing for all programs.* A centralized marketing effort ensures that all programs benefit from marketing efforts and exposures and prevents embarrassing redundancies of effort in the marketplace.
- *Constantly explore connections and synergies between product line programs and services and prevent redundancies.* The product line management team should be alert for redundancies within the product line as well as within the hospital system as a whole.
- *Facilitate regular communication among all product line managers.* Managers should meet on at least a biweekly basis to share successes and failures, exchange information about the market, assist one another in problem solving, and explore connections between programs.
- *Facilitate periodic gatherings of all product line employees.* Employees from all programs should feel that they are on the same team. Monthly meetings of all employees provide the opportunity for the sharing of information, successes, and failures; for team building; and for reinforcement of the product line philosophy.
- *Create a work climate that allows and encourages employee initiative and risk taking.* The product line management team must exhibit a can-do attitude in helping employees get what they need (or perceive that they need) in order to carry out the product line philosophy at the point of service delivery. This attitude often requires both creativity and risk taking on the part of the product line management team. Creativity and risk taking are desirable characteristics that will be embraced by line employees when they are visibly modeled by those in leadership positions.
- *Participate in all negotiations, business deals, and service or product development projects that involve more than one program in the product line.* This action ensures that the health of the overall product line is protected and that services or products are not inappropriately excluded or forgotten as opportunities unfold.

Product Line Problems

The product line model is particularly useful for hospitals that need to assemble or coordinate a series of already existing services into an efficient and marketable unit. It provides a structure that can be put together rapidly, does not dictate immediate change in program operations or staffing, and is far less "bloody" (in terms of managers' egos or even jobs) than, for instance, a merging of departments may be. This scenario is, however, not without its problems.

Physical Proximity

When existing programs are put together in a product line, their facilities may not be located near one another. To develop the kind of employee communication and involvement discussed in this chapter is far more difficult when product line programs are located across town from one another. Although having an EAP and an occupational medicine program share a common entrance and a waiting room is not desirable for confidentiality reasons, having them as next-door neighbors would be very desirable. Not only would such an arrangement facilitate better communication between programs, but it would also improve service and convenience for clients who are referred from the occupational medicine program to the EAP. Even though proximity of program facilities is not always possible in the early stages of product line development, it should always be a goal that is actively pursued.

Product Line Size

Another problem that can come with the success of a product line is size. The more programs and employees that are added to a product line, the more problems there will be in keeping everybody focused and working together for the good of the whole program. Symptoms of size problems include budgetary competition and whining (for example, "EAP always has to discount more than occupational medicine, so its bottom line doesn't look as good"), reduced communication among programs, and duplication of effort in both program development and marketing. An example of the last problem would be when unbeknownst to each other, the wellness and occupational rehabilitation programs both develop a program for sufferers of chronic lower-back pain. When these kinds of situations begin to manifest themselves, the product line manager should redouble efforts in the areas of program philosophy and purpose. A key responsibility of the product line manager is to anticipate and address these types of problems.

Financial Incentives and Competition

Although maintaining a cost center for each program in the product line is probably necessary for monitoring and business diagnostic purposes, the determination of incentives and bonuses should be based at least in part on the performance of the product line as a whole. In addition, non–revenue-producing contributions by any program to overall product line success must be recognized and celebrated in ways that are visible to all employees. These strategies eliminate much of the financial competition among programs.

One alternative to maintaining separate cost centers is to effect transfers of funds between cost centers to compensate programs for services that benefit other programs in the product line. At best, this strategy is difficult to implement because it is often difficult to attach a monetary amount to value-added types of services. At worst, this strategy creates a bureaucratic nightmare that spends significant program resources and energy on internal issues and detracts from service delivery to the customer.

Relationship with the Hospital

If not closely monitored, a hospital can destroy its occupational health services product line by using up product line resources for its own employees' health or for hospital program needs. The hospital should, in fact, be one of the product line's largest and most loyal customers, but the key word here is *customer.* The hospital and the occupational health services product line must have a contractual business relationship. The hospital's use of the services of the occupational health services product line is both appropriate and desirable. The product lines of occupational health services can be used to support such hospital programs as weight-loss services for gastric bypass patients, fitness services for cardiac rehabilitation patients, psychiatric and chemical dependency programs, and occupational medicine and rehabilitation services for employee health. However, the hospital should pay for these services as would any other corporate client.

Services that can be economically offered to the corporate market can be used to enhance traditional hospital programs. For example, outdoor experiential education offered to corporate clients might also be combined as a part of the hospital's existing chemical dependency treatment program. The addition of this component, which would not have been feasible without the cumulative volume supplied by the corporate market, can give the hospital's existing program a distinct competitive advantage. However, if the hospital does not reimburse the occupational health services product line for the use of its services or resources, it will become a drain on the product line's bottom line and threaten the ability of the product line to adequately deliver services to other clients.

Future Trends

In some quarters of the hospital industry, a notion persists that occupational health services may be the health care "cash cow" of the future. However, a 1988 survey indicated that only 52 percent of hospital-affiliated occupational medicine programs and 12 percent of hospital-affiliated wellness programs show a profit.[4] These figures are unlikely to change dramatically over the next several years because the field of occupational health services is becoming increasingly regulated and competitive. However, occupational health services can fill an important market niche for most hospitals in most communities. Therefore, ways must be found for occupational health services to support one another in meeting community and corporate needs as well as hospital needs.

In the future, a marriage of the various types of occupational health services may be inevitable. As a result of a growing trend toward managed care systems in the occupational medicine field, models for the provision of occupational medicine may be developed that are similar to HMOs. Under these conditions, the push toward rapid recovery and prevention, which will mandate the inclusion of EAP and health promotion strategies in the routine delivery of occupational services, may become even greater than it is in the late 1980s. The occupational health services product line of the future may in fact be its own company providing comprehensive occupational health services in a systemized way in order to maximize profits under a capitated fee system. In this scenario, EAPs and wellness programs may no longer be called EAPs and wellness programs. However, they will functionally exist as they currently do and expand on their present capabilities.

Just as employees' work lives cannot be separated from their private lives, neither can the interventions that address the various aspects of those lives be separated. Ultimately, like it or not, occupational medicine, EAPs, and health promotion are all part of the same whole. Hospital turf battles, politics, or product-definition agendas keep these services separated in the short term. However, the current evolution of the occupational medicine field indicates that the successful programs of the future will overcome these obstacles and integrate all occupational health services into an economical and efficient product line approach.

References

1. Folger, J. C., and Gee, E. P. *Product Management for Hospitals: Organizing for Profitability.* Chicago: American Hospital Association, 1987.
2. Health Care Advisory Board. *Marketing to Employers.* Vol. 2, *Occupational Health Programs.* Washington, DC: HCAB, July 1988.
3. Walton, M. *The Deming Management Method.* New York City: Dodd, Mead & Co., 1986.
4. Sabatino, F. G. The diversification success story continues: survey. *Hospitals* 63(1):26–32, Jan. 5, 1989.

Chapter 3

Injury Treatment Services

John Maxfield, M.D.

The centerpiece of the occupational health services product line is the injury management program. Among the 113 hospital-based programs surveyed from across the country by the American Hospital Association in 1985, 75 percent reported that they cared for the injuries of their clients.[1] Among 46 respondents to a 1988 survey, 93 percent said that they provided this service.[2] According to a recent Health Care Advisory Board report, "Without exception, all of the profitable occupational health programs. . .are designed around comprehensive injury treatment and case management services," and not only perform as the lead point for other program offerings but generate two-thirds to three-quarters of the direct revenues.[3]

The reasons are simple. Employers are required by law to meet the health needs and preserve the financial security of their employees in two ways:

- Through compliance with Occupational Safety and Health Administration (OSHA) regulations governing health screening and surveillance
- By covering the direct costs and associated lost wages incurred through medical care of injuries and occupational illnesses

Most employers do not have frequent dealings with OSHA, but injuries on the job are a daily occurrence. Thus, an occupational health program that treats injuries is assured, by law, of a steady supply of clients.

All states and the District of Columbia require employers to cover the cost of medical treatment of injuries—usually at 100 percent of charges—for as long as such coverage is needed.[4] In most statutes reviewed,[5-11] this cost was found to be according to prevailing fees (and subject to utilization review in Virginia),[12] although in Rhode Island, for example, Medicare sets the standard.[13] In Missouri, payment beyond 90 days must be by special order of the Workers' Compensation Commission.[14] Thus, in most states, those who care for workers' injuries find themselves in a better position in terms of reimbursement than those who rely on health insurance for reimbursement for treatment of non-work-related problems.

Each injured worker brings not only his or her own health problem but also his or her employer's manpower problem. Practitioners who fail to consider this issue are losing business to those who do. As long as employees are out of work (after a brief waiting period), their employers must pay them, usually at two-thirds of their wages. This payment is tax-free[15-21] and at least in some instances,[22,23] exempt from the claims of creditors. The resulting need to document the need for time off with pay not infrequently pits the employer against the employee, and the practitioner becomes the referee. The stakes are high: on average, wage replacement accounts for 70 percent of the cost of the injury.[24]

Thus, in a number of important ways, the care of the injured worker is different from patient management in other settings:

- An injury at work is as much a social event as a medical one.
- The medical history and to a lesser extent the physical examination are of considerable legal import.
- The diagnosis, except in long-term disability cases, is not usually of central importance.
- The treatment plan is intimately entwined with the issue of employability.
- Information management is key.

The occupational health services program that effectively manages the treatment of injured workers can expect to benefit in a number of ways. Businesses view competence in handling workers' injuries as an indicator of how well the program, and by inference, the hospital, can perform in other areas, both in areas related to other occupational health products and in more general aspects of health care delivery. For example, one medical center performed more than 24,000 preemployment physicals in 1986–87, without being the least expensive provider in the area, because "...our injury treatment program serves as a feeder."[25] Patients who are impressed with the efficiency and professionalism of their care may choose the program's sponsoring facility for their future nonoccupational health care needs. Furthermore, program referrals keep the medical staff supportive of the program and concomitantly less likely to oppose other hospital programs in the future. For example, 3 to 10 percent of injured patients seen in this setting are referred for follow-up, usually to orthopedists.[26]

The focus of this chapter is treatment of the work-related injury. Injury treatment is part of the larger concept, injury management. The other component of injury treatment is tracking, which is the topic of chapter 4. The following sections summarize the basic legal principles that define covered workers and the assessment of liability, key strategies in the management of injured workers' cases, and operational features of an injury treatment program.

Legal Determination of Covered Workers

In years past, tort law defined issues surrounding liability for worker injury. The result served no one but the legal profession and tended to bring workers and their dependents to ruin. The current system is a compromise greatly to the advantage of the employee. The theory is summed up nicely in the Code of Virginia, although the wording is remarkably similar from state to state:

> The question of negligence of the employer is eliminated. . .the assumption of risk. . .and contributory negligence are abolished, and the rules of evidence are laxly enforced—so laxly that an award may be made on hearsay evidence alone, if credible, and not contradicted.[27]

Whether an injury is compensable often depends on facts ascertained in the medical history. These facts can be useful in two ways: either by diverting the aspiring claimant from pursuing an inappropriate claim or, more commonly, by documenting the facts as presented at the time so that compensability can be more accurately determined in the future. Three issues need to be kept in mind:

- By whom is the worker employed, if employed at all?
- Is the claim an injury?
- Is compensation for the injury disallowed?

Employment Status

In attempting to answer the question, "By whom is the worker employed, if employed at all?" several points from the Code of Virginia are illustrative.

> [An employee is] every person. . .in the service of another under any contract of hire. . .except one whose employment is not in the usual course of the. . .business. . .of the employer.[28]
>
> Nothing in this Act contained shall be construed to make . . . the employee of an independent contractor the employees of the person or corporation employing or contracting with such independent contractor.[29]
>
> A casual employee, such as a domestic, is not usually an employee; the employer would have to have developed a payroll of more than $15,000 per year, the employee would have to be one of three or more

regular such employees, or the employer and employee would have to have had an agreement to be bound by the Act.[30]

> Whenever an employee. . . shall at the time of the injury be in the joint service of two or more employers subject to this Act, such employers shall contribute to the payment of such compensation in proportion to their wage liability.[31]

In general, such issues are addressed similarly in other states, particularly with regard to domestics and seasonal labor. Having some familiarity with the law in this regard can direct paperwork more appropriately, possibly eliminate some paperwork altogether, and in general save time for the program's secretary, the employer, the employee, and the insurer.

Definition of Injury

The practitioner seldom has to directly answer the question, "Is the claim an injury?" However, documenting the employee's version of events close to the time of injury can be of inestimable value should the matter be challenged later. The key elements in defining an *injury* as it is understood in workers' compensation law are that the incident:

- Occurred by accident
- Arose out of employment (refers to cause of injury)
- Occurred in the course of employment (refers to time, place, and circumstances under which the accident occurred)

With regard to the cause of injury, "risks to which all persons similarly situated are equally exposed and not traceable in some special degree to the particular employment" are excluded.[32] For example, in *Memorial Hospital v. Hairston,* the court concluded:

> Where claimant was walking on a flat surface in a well-lighted area, the circumstances did not show that the fall resulted from any condition peculiar to the work environment, or any physical condition afflicting claimant; rather, she inexplicably wound up on the floor, injured but conscious. The court concludes that the circumstances of the present case are not such that the only rational inference to be drawn is that the fall arose out of claimant's employment.[33]

Similarly, injuries resulting when a patient is assaulted by a coworker for reasons unrelated to the victim as an employee are definitely not compensable.[34]

With regard to the determination of whether the injury occurred in the course of employment, employees generally are not compensated if injured going to or from work unless:

- The means of transport or time consumed is paid for by the employer

- The way used is the sole and exclusive means of ingress or egress or the route is constructed by the employer
- The employee is doing something for the employer while en route[35]

Disallowed Injuries

Several reasons for disallowing payment exist, and the various states are fairly uniform in this.[36-42] Three of these reasons can be documented in the medical history and physical examination:

- Intentional self-inflicted injury
- Injury growing out of attempt to injure another
- Injury due to intoxication

The extra time involved in documenting these points in the medical history is minimal. However, the dividends for employers, employees, and insurers are considerable.

Key Strategies in the Management of Injured Workers' Cases

The key to cost-effective management of work-related injuries is not in cutting corners on medical expenses but in concentrating on reducing lost-work time. To appreciate the various strategies available, it is helpful to have an understanding of the insurance system. Employers usually have one of several choices, depending on what is available in their states:

- Private insurance
- State-run insurance fund
- Group self-insurance
- Self-insurance[43-49]

Many states also have a second injury fund, which covers certain types of injuries superimposed on previous injuries. The money in this fund generally comes from a tax on premiums collected by the insurers.

Whether employers have a stake in how much lost-work time they experience is largely related to how directly their premiums are experienced rated. Employers who insure themselves obviously feel savings in lost-work time most directly. Those using other methods will appreciate savings to varying degrees.

Over time, most employers benefit significantly from strategies that cut lost-work time. One such strategy is to minimize utilization of insurance. In most instances, compensation commences not on day 1 but on days 3 to 7, depending on the state.[50-56] Expenses for the uncovered period are usually covered by sick leave or vacation time or out of the worker's pocket. They are covered retroactively by insurance only in the event that the disability extends beyond a set number of days. By the simple expedient of limiting time off to a period less than this critical number of days whenever possible, the number of claims can be greatly reduced. For example, a patient who is told she can return to work on Saturday, which happens to be the last day of the period before compensation commences, but who is off until Monday because she works a five-day week, could not institute a claim. Attention to this sort of detail saved one hospital client of an occupational health program $25,000 in premiums over a two-year period.

A key strategy is that of *light duty.* Even placing the injured worker in a totally unproductive job can result in enormous savings. Consider the following scenario: A worker feels a twinge of back pain on Friday and then calls on Monday to say he cannot get out of bed. His employer does not believe him and tells him to stay away until his doctor gives him a clean bill of health. His doctor prescribes 10 days of bed rest and then sends him to an orthopedist, who is unable to see him for three weeks. Meanwhile, his employer has forgotten him. The worker, who never liked his employer anyway, stays at home suffering the consequences of continuing immobility and seeks redress in the form of compensation benefits or a permanent partial award.

If this situation had been handled properly, this worker would have reported to the workplace in any capacity if at all possible, received almost daily attention in any event, and returned to full duty as soon as practicable. Implementation of such an approach at a shoe manufacturing company outside of Boston resulted in the following benefits:

- The number of claims dropped by 53.4 percent.
- The number of days lost per injury dropped by 53.5 percent.
- The compensation cost per claim was reduced by 75.7 percent.
- The medical costs were reduced by 68.4 percent.
- The average total cost per claim was reduced by 74.8 percent.[57,58]

Workers' compensation costs in 1977–79 for this company had exceeded $200,000. The program was instituted in 1980. In 1981–82, workers' compensation costs were less than $20,000.

Of course, the best strategy is to have the injured employee return to work, provided that the return is medically appropriate. To employ this strategy effectively requires adherence to the fundamental tenet of occupational medicine: Know the job the worker is performing. If direct knowledge is not at hand, a telephone call to the employer or foreman is often rewarding. Some occupational health programs formally analyze the various jobs at their regular clients' worksites according to performance parameters and environmental demands. Employees with disabilities are rated similarly, thereby permitting the matching of disabilities and jobs. The technique, still in its infancy, is at this time more applicable to chronic than to acute disabilities, but it holds promise.[59]

The reporting requirements of workers' compensation law can create seemingly endless amounts of paperwork.[60-66,67] Employees must report to employers; employers to the insurers and the Workers' Compensation Commission, physicians to the employee, employer, and insurer, if requested, and so forth. An occupational health program can endear itself to all parties and make the entire system run more efficiently by collating and furnishing the required information as a matter of routine. A computerized data base with flexible reporting capabilities is admirably suited to this task, as will be discussed in chapter 4.

The types of reports generated should be tailored to requirements, according to statute, or per individual request. With a computerized data base, such information can be abstracted with little effort beyond that needed to design the report in the first place. This willingness to customize is important, as is timeliness of the delivery of the information (within 24 hours). Some practitioners routinely send the actual medical record, dictated, to the employer and to the insurer along with any reports. Having all of this information at hand from the outset can save days of unnecessarily compensated time and, in general, make claims handling a more expedient affair. The willingness to customize and provide timely information pays dividends for the program when grateful insurers steer employers to its door.

Operational Features of an Injury Treatment Program

The success of an injury treatment program will depend in part on certain key operational features: the expediency and continuity of service, convenience, the continuity of management, communication, and the setting. Each of these five aspects of program operation is examined in the following pages.

The Expediency and Continuity of Service

Lack of expediency is the most frequent complaint about emergency department care. Solving this problem is a sine qua non in a competitive market, whatever the setting for the program. Even if the care were free, a worker sitting in a waiting room is an expense. Successful strategies for enhancing service expediency include the following:

- Streamline admissions.
- Keep company and employee data bases.
- Develop a call-ahead policy so that the process precedes the patient.
- Register patients after they are seen. (Although this may be heretical, experience shows that this works, altering patients' perceptions

of their care and decreasing turnaround time, particularly in an emergency department.)
- Cross-train staff in clinical and administrative duties.
- Schedule non–injury-treatment services as much as possible.
- If the program is located in an emergency department, consider developing a "fast-track" system that minimizes the time an injured worker spends in the emergency department. A fast track can provide expedited sign-in procedures and priority treatment and testing.

It is also highly desirable to have a contingency plan for after-hours injuries. In most instances, this plan will necessitate some arrangement with an emergency department. A relationship with the emergency department can create some problems (as indicated later in this chapter under the heading "The Setting"); however, clients cannot be left to sink or swim during late hours, and thus the issue of after-hours care must be addressed.

Convenience

Convenience can be expressed in terms of the accessibility of services to the individual worker as well as in terms of the ease of information exchange between the program and employers. The most successful programs are located within 10 minutes of their clients,[68] and none of this time should be spent looking for a parking space. The importance of customizing paperwork for individual employers has been discussed as one aspect of employer or payer convenience. Billing procedures can also be examined for convenience. For example, of programs queried in a recent survey, 88 percent engaged in consolidating billing for at least some of their clients.[69] Some are even including their consultants' fees in the bill.

The Continuity of Management

Continuity in the medical management of injured workers is essential if a program is attempting to reduce the amount of time they miss from work. In the best program model, a single physician directs all care for an injured worker. When specialty consultation is necessary, the physician selects a consultant who agrees to see the injured worker promptly. The consultant should be highly competent and understand the specific issues involved in the care of injured workers. If possible, the consultant should see the patient in the occupational health clinic so that tracking the injured worker's care is easier.

Three problems arise when programs try to ensure continuity of care:

- *Multiple physicians direct care.* As stated in the preceding paragraph, a single physician should direct care for the injured worker. Certain program designs make this difficult. In an emergency department, for example, the injured worker usually sees the physician on duty.

If the worker returns to the emergency department for follow-up visits, the worker is likely to see a different physician. Under these circumstances, care often becomes fragmented and the direction of care becomes unclear.

- *A nonselective referral list is used.* In some hospitals, referrals to specialty physicians are made by using a call list. A physician on the call list may not be the most competent person to handle the injured worker's problem and, in addition, may not understand the details of an injured worker's care. As a result, the quality and continuity of care are jeopardized. Whenever possible, occupational health programs should carefully limit the panel of physicians to whom they refer patients. In addition, the program should make its expectations for the referral physicians clear—setting them down in writing if possible.
- *Care is delivered at multiple sites.* The more sites at which the care is delivered, the more difficult it is to coordinate the care. The best programs limit the number of sites at which care is delivered by having consultants see workers in the occupational health clinic instead of in the offices of individual physicians.

Communication

Of central importance to the efficient and effective operation of the injury treatment program is contact between the clients and the program via a single outside telephone line to a minimum number of program personnel, preferably one person. The operational motif is *one-stop shopping* for all occupational health needs, with brokering as necessary. Ideally, a telephone call regarding diagnosis and disposition is made to the employer when an employee is discharged, with a formal report, and possibly the medical record as well, following within 24 hours. The suggested content for the report is discussed in chapter 4, as is the importance of continued communication until the patient returns to full employment. Involving employers in the treatment process from beginning to end must be the foundation of any successful occupational health program.

The Setting

The setting chosen for an occupational health facility will be influenced by several factors. A program entirely independent of the hospital is the most flexible and can establish the desired consultant relationships with relative impunity. However, such a program may have difficulty arranging the kind of 24-hour coverage it would like, and it would have the expense of providing ancillary services that a hospital-based program would not. Moreover, an independent program cannot claim the authority by association that a hospital-sponsored service can.

Choices of setting among current hospital-based programs have been varied, and many have several sites.[70] Approximately two-thirds are in the hospital proper; half of these are in the emergency department, and the other half are in an associated fast track. A high percentage of programs are located in separate buildings on the hospital grounds. A smaller number are located in community facilities, mobile units, or industrial sites.

Starting an occupational health program in an emergency department is tempting. A comparatively small initial investment is required, so little is lost if the program fails. Occupational health can bolster a faltering fast track. Small emergency departments can employ personnel more cost-effectively if these employees can also staff an occupational health service. A well-run program encourages those who use the occupational health service (employees and their contacts, employers and their contacts) to return for emergency care as well. In addition, the medical staff may be more accepting of an occupational health program that is part of the emergency department because of the relatively noncompetitive role the emergency department traditionally plays.

Among respondents to the 1988 survey,[71] the breadth of program offerings from emergency department–based programs was as rich and varied as those from programs that were not based in emergency departments, and surprisingly, just as many (79 percent) did at least some of their own follow-up. However, of 20 programs that had at some time used the emergency department as a base of operations, six left, and four of those that left cited problems with the emergency department as figuring in their decision. Of the remaining fourteen, four had complaints but stayed anyway. Complaints were that the emergency department is not efficient, that the environment is too chaotic, that provision of care is too fragmented, that physicians and nurses in the emergency department are not cooperative, and that emergency department staff could not track patients adequately.

Staff attitude problems in an emergency department setting are inevitable. Emergency department nurses may regard such duties as preparing well patients for physical examinations to be an imposition. They are often harried by more urgent cases and therefore may not always be courteous, especially because some may regard injured workers as malingerers.

Implementing a one-stop–shopping telephone number is difficult if there is more than one secretary, which is likely in an emergency department setting. Efficient handling of information requires (1) identifying all occupational health patients, (2) identifying all charts of these patients, (3) accurately identifying the company involved, and (4) promptly routing the charts to an occupational health secretary. Accomplishing all of this reliably in an emergency department is next to impossible.

Continuity of care problems limit the effectiveness of emergency-department–based programs. First, as mentioned before, it is difficult to establish a single emergency department physician to direct the care for an injured worker. Care is generally provided by the physician on duty. Second, emergency departments generally make specialty referrals based on a mandatory, nonselective call list, which can direct injured workers to physicians poorly suited to handling work-related problems. Third, it is difficult to centralize care in the emergency department. Specialty consultation is generally delivered in physicians' offices, which makes tracking injured workers more difficult than when care is provided in a single clinic. These three problems can seriously hamper the ability of an emergency-department–based program to promptly and effectively return injured workers to work.

Finally, contrary to the belief currently in vogue, emergency medicine physicians are not ideally suited to the practice of occupational medicine. The medical aspects of injury treatment make up a small part of occupational medicine and a smaller part of occupational health. An emergency medicine physician could broaden his or her background sufficiently to succeed as a partner in establishing and maintaining an occupational health service, but such actions require significant time and effort.

From testimony nationwide, it is evident that occupational health services can find a niche in emergency departments. However, setting up occupational health services in a separate clinic is almost certainly preferable if the market clearly can and will support such a venture. Despite careful marketing efforts, it is not easy to demonstrate sufficient support for a separate clinic, and the safer tack of operating within an emergency department may be more reasonable at the beginning. Whatever the decision regarding the physical site of the program, most program developers would agree with the following statements as guiding principles for success:

- Physicians should have an interest in occupational health and be willing to invest the time to become knowledgeable in the field. At the very least, physicians should be able to provide reliable backup to specialists in occupational medicine.
- The manager employed should be highly motivated and skilled, a person who will be the driving force for the program and for whom the program is a primary responsibility. This goal may not be able to be realized on day 1, but it should be accomplished as quickly as possible.
- Clerical help should not be fragmented, and if it is not full-time at the outset, some method should be arranged so that one-stop shopping can be offered and reliable communications maintained.
- Care *must* be expedient. For many emergency departments, such care can only be realized through a fast track.
- Methods must be devised to reliably channel patients and paperwork through the system.

References

1. Jones, L. *Profile of Hospital Occupational Services.* Chicago: American Hospital Association, 1986.

2. Maxfield, J. Occupational health and the emergency department, 1988 (submitted for publication).
3. Health Care Advisory Board. *Marketing to Employers.* Vol. 2, *Occupational Health Programs.* Washington, DC: HCAB, July 1988, p. 17.
4. Health Care Advisory Board, pp. 17–33.
5. The Industrial Commission of Virginia. The Virginia Workers' Compensation Act and 1987 Cumulative Supplement, 65.1-1 to 65.1-163, 17.116.04 to 17.116.09, 19.2-305 to 19.2-368.18. Charlottesville, VA: Michie Co., 1982, 1987.
6. *General Laws of Rhode Island*, Vol. 5, 28-29-1 to 28-37-31. Charlottesville, VA: Michie Co., 1986.
7. *Annotated Missouri Statutes,* Vol. 15, 287.010 to 287.800. Kansas City: Vernon Law Book Co., 1965.
8. *Annotated Code of Maryland,* Vol. 8, 101-1 to 101-102.
9. *District of Columbia Code,* Vol. 7, 36-301 to 36-345. Charlottesville, VA: Michie Co., 1985.
10. *Maine Revised Statutes Annotated,* Vol. 16A, 39-1 to 39-196. St. Paul: West Publishing Co., 1978.
11. *Code of Alabama,* Vol. 15, 25-4-1 to 25-5-231. Charlottesville, VA: Michie Co., 1986.
12. The Industrial Commission of Virginia, cited in reference 5.
13. *General Laws of Rhode Island,* cited in reference 6.
14. *Annotated Missouri Statutes,* cited in reference 7.
15. The Industrial Commission of Virginia, cited in reference 5.
16. *General Laws of Rhode Island,* cited in reference 6.
17. *Annotated Missouri Statutes,* cited in reference 7.
18. *Annotated Code of Maryland,* cited in reference 8.
19. *District of Columbia Code,* cited in reference 9.
20. *Maine Revised Statutes Annotated,* cited in reference 10
21. *Code of Alabama,* cited in reference 11.
22. The Industrial Commission of Virginia, cited in reference 5.
23. *General Laws of Rhode Island,* cited in reference 6.
24. Health Care Advisory Board, pp. 17–33.
25. *Ibid.,* p. 22.
26. *Ibid.*
27. The Industrial Commission of Virginia, 65.1-1. Notes from the Code, cited in reference 5.
28. *Ibid.,* 65.1-4.
29. *Ibid.,* 65.1-5.
30. *Ibid.,* 65.1-28.

31. *Ibid.,* 65.1-80.
32. Richmond Mem. Hosp. v. Crane, 222 Va. 283, 278 S.E. 2d 877 (1981), cited in reference 5.
33. Memorial Hosp. v. Hairston, 2 Va. App. 677, 347 S.E. 2d 527 (1986), cited in reference 5, 1987 Supplement.
34. Hopson v. Hungerford Coal Co., 187 Va. 299, 46 S.E. 2d 392 (1948), cited in reference 5.
35. The Industrial Commission of Virginia, 65.1-7. Notes from the Code, cited in reference 5.
36. The Industrial Commission of Virginia, cited in reference 5.
37. *General Laws of Rhode Island,* cited in reference 6.
38. *Annotated Missouri Statutes,* cited in reference 7.
39. *Annotated Code of Maryland,* cited in reference 8.
40. *District of Columbia Code,* cited in reference 9.
41. *Maine Revised Statutes Annotated,* cited in reference 10.
42. *Code of Alabama,* cited in reference 11.
43. The Industrial Commission of Virginia, cited in reference 5.
44. *General Laws of Rhode Island,* cited in reference 6.
45. *Annotated Missouri Statutes,* cited in reference 7.
46. *Annotated Code of Maryland,* cited in reference 8.
47. *District of Columbia Code,* cited in reference 9.
48. *Maine Revised Statutes Annotated,* cited in reference 10.
49. *Code of Alabama,* cited in reference 11.
50. The Industrial Commission of Virginia, cited in reference 5.
51. *General Laws of Rhode Island,* cited in reference 6.
52. *Annotated Missouri Statutes,* cited in reference 7.
53. *Annotated Code of Maryland,* cited in reference 8.
54. *District of Columbia Code,* cited in reference 9.
55. *Maine Revised Statutes Annotated,* cited in reference 10.
56. *Code of Alabama,* cited in reference 11.
57. Fitzler, S., et al. Attitudinal change: the Chelsea back program. *Occupational Health and Safety* 51(2):24–26, 1982.
58. Fitzler, S., et al. Chelsea back program: one year later. *Occupational Health and Safety* 52:52–54, 1983.
59. Newkirk, W. L., Palazole, R., Keller, M., and Washburn, J. *SYSTOC 3.0.* Skowhegan, ME: Occupational Health Research, 1987.
60. The Industrial Commission of Virginia, cited in reference 5.
61. *General Laws of Rhode Island,* cited in reference 6.

62. *Annotated Missouri Statutes,* cited in reference 7.
63. *Annotated Code of Maryland,* cited in reference 8.
64. *District of Columbia Code,* cited in reference 9.
65. *Maine Revised Statutes Annotated,* cited in reference 10.
66. *Code of Alabama,* cited in reference 11.
67. Jenkins v. Lowe's of Norfolk, Inc., 50.1.C 149, cited in reference 5.
68. Health Care Advisory Board, pp. 17–33.
69. Maxfield, cited in reference 2.
70. Maxfield, cited in reference 2.
71. *Ibid.*

Chapter 4

Injured Worker Tracking

David A. Nicewonger, M.B.A.

Injured worker tracking is an active process in which all aspects of an injured worker's treatment are monitored and evaluated from the time of initial treatment to the day the individual is declared medically stable or returned to full work capacity. The tracking component and the treatment component described in chapter 3 form an *injury management* program. The absence of effective tracking causes unnecessary delays in treatment, more lost workdays, and consequently, increased claim costs.

To the frustrated employer who sees the cost of workers' compensation rising, the apparent problem is the cost of medical care. Few employers are aware of the savings that can be realized through the effective management of their injured workers. Those employers who are aware of the advantages of tracking their injured employees become discouraged if injured workers are uncooperative in providing relevant medical information. Even if the information is available to them, most employers are uncertain how to use it to best meet the interests of the company and the injured worker.

By assisting businesses with injury management and tracking, health care providers can remove the barrier between themselves and industry and open the door for other occupational health services. This chapter discusses how to organize a high-quality tracking program that meets the needs of both the injured worker and business and industry while enhancing other occupational health services.

Objectives of a Tracking Program

The first and most important step in developing a tracking program is to establish objectives for the program. Objectives should be aimed at meeting the needs of those individuals who will have an interest in the tracking program. Because the overall purpose of a tracking program is to assist business and industry with injury management, program objectives should address the business community's needs and concerns as well as the interests of the insurance community, physicians, and the injured workers.

The development of program objectives begins with assessing what these four groups want a tracking program to accomplish. Various studies have identified six general objectives applicable to any tracking program:

- Provide excellent and optimal health care to the ill or injured worker
- Improve the efficiency and quality of information for the employee, employer, insurance carrier, and physician
- Coordinate employee treatment and rehabilitation to facilitate optimal recovery and return to work
- Reduce costs for the employer and insurance carrier by decreasing claims and time lost from work and by maintaining productivity levels
- Promote referrals to the medical staff that support the program
- Increase the business community's knowledge, familiarity, and utilization of the medical staff and health care facility for both occupational and nonoccupational health care needs

Providing excellent health care is a basic objective for any health care provider. The reason for including such an obvious concept in the objectives of a tracking program is to emphasize the importance that business and industry place on the quality of medical services provided to their injured workers. A tracking program makes it possible to monitor the effectiveness of the treatment plans used by various physicians and provides employers with information to select physicians who can best meet their specific health care needs.

Improving the quality and efficiency of information to all interested parties is the central focus of any tracking program. Better communication with health care providers is a universal concern of all employers. When an employee is injured, the employer wants and needs feedback regarding the prognosis for the employee's return to work and any medical restrictions the employee will have after returning to the job. If employers do not have this information, they cannot make effective decisions regarding staffing needs during the employee's period of injury. Similarly, the insurance company needs the most current information possible to make the most cost-efficient decisions regarding the management of workers' compensation claims. Finally, whenever several physicians from different specialties are involved in the care of an injured worker, coordinated communication is crucial to the efficient recovery of the patient.

Expensive, but avoidable, delays often occur during the treatment of an injured worker. For example, after completing a therapy program, a patient may be uncertain of what the next step should be. Consequently, the patient may wait several days before following up with a physician. A tracking program sees to it that the patient is contacted immediately after therapy has been completed and guides him or her to the next step in the treatment plan. In the extreme case where an injured worker is content to fall through cracks in the system and collect payment for lost time, a tracking program can signal the treating physician, employer, and insurance carrier of the need to take action to guide the injured worker back into a treatment program. Tracking the injured worker enables all aspects of care to be coordinated and avoids expensive delays and duplication of services.

Cost savings are closely related to the coordination of care and to improved communication. Claims costs are lower if, by decreasing the delays in treatment, the health care provider is able to increase the rate of recovery so that injured workers can return to their jobs with fewer lost workdays. Additionally, the prompt return of workers to their regular duties is more productive for employers than a vacant position or a temporary replacement. Even more savings can be realized through prompt, accurate communication of work restrictions to employers. Through open lines of communication, the employer and treating physician often can arrange modified or light-duty work that the employee can perform. In addition, if the insurance carrier is able to manage claims more effectively as a result of more efficient communication, it can decrease its costs of administering claims.

The final two objectives are closely interrelated. A tracking program can encourage employers to direct more of their injured workers to a medical facility that provides such a service. An increase in the patient base of the occupational health program can also result in more medical staff referrals. In particular, specialists such as orthopedists and neurologists, who have a desire and willingness to treat injured workers, can significantly increase referrals to their practice. In addition, the number of patients seeking medical care for nonoccupational illness and injuries will increase as a result of expanded community exposure. For many injured workers, the treatment received for work-related injuries may be their first contact with the health care facility and its staff. If patients think that they are receiving efficient and high-quality care, they are more likely to seek treatment for nonoccupational injuries and illnesses at that facility.

Designing a Tracking Program

Once the objectives of the tracking program are established and understood by all involved parties, the next task is to design a tracking program that meets these objectives in an efficient, cost-effective manner.

Selecting the Method of Tracking

A tracking system may be manual or computerized. The method chosen has significant implications for the quality of the program as well as for the capabilities and expense of the program.

Manually tracking injured workers requires that a system of log books and patient files be used to monitor treatment progress. The tracker must rely on these systems to flag patients needing attention on any given day and to determine the next treatment step. One problem with this approach is that if a patient's data are misfiled, treatment follow-up delays can result or patient follow-up can be completely forgotten. Another problem is that the system focuses only on the worker's injury, with little or no attention given to the job site or the patient's history of prior injuries. Identifying relationships between the injury and the job or seeing trends in the types of injuries sustained within a specific department of a given company is difficult with a manual tracking system. To do any of these additional assessments requires that data be manually extracted from each file. This work is extremely labor intensive; as the program grows, tracking large numbers of patients from multiple companies becomes unmanageable with a manual system.

To do more than monitoring patient files and telephoning patients to remind them of appointments, the health care provider needs a computerized system. A computerized tracking system can integrate injured workers' demographic data into a computer along with information about their injuries and corresponding treatment. Multiple work-related injuries show up as separate subfiles within the patient's computer file. In addition to patient and injury information, data files can store information regarding employers, insurance carriers, and physicians. Even job-risk information about particular jobs within a specific company can be entered in the file.

Once this information is in the computer files, it can be extracted in a rapid, organized manner. For example, a computer can supply the tracker with a listing of all patients scheduled for follow-up examinations on a given day along with the names of physicians scheduled to see those patients. A computerized system can also generate lists of patients needing specialized attention; for example, it can indicate which patients need to be called to check on their progress after their first week back on the job. By using a computer to provide the tracker with these types of lists, the provider is unlikely to lose data or forget any necessary patient follow-up.

In addition to providing an efficient flagging system for the tracker, a computerized system can simplify communication between the employer, insurance carrier, and treating physicians. Because records of an injured worker's treatment and progress are in the computer along with employer and insurer information, the computer becomes a central information center for all interested parties. The computer can also create relationships between files so that specific tasks can be performed. For example, the provider can study injury trends within a particular company or monitor the effectiveness of the treatment plans of individual physicians to improve referrals to those physicians who have the best success with a particular type of injury. The possibilities of cross-referencing data files and manipulating data are virtually limitless and are invaluable to the quality of a tracking program.

One final point regarding computerized systems is whether to create a system or to purchase a system that has already been developed. The answer to this question varies with each occupational health program. Before making the decision, the provider should consider the nature and complexity of the tasks to be accomplished. The cost of developing software can be prohibitive and frustrating. Also, the provider faces the risk that customized software may still not perform all of the tasks desired. A variety of commercial software programs are available. These programs are quite diverse in complexity, and so finding a package that meets the specific needs of the program is not impossible. The discussion of tracking systems in the remainder of this chapter assumes that the provider is using a computerized system for tracking.

Establishing a Data Base

Once the provider has decided on the tracking method, it can determine the source of the data and the methods for collecting those data. The quality of the tracking and of the information provided to employers is only as accurate as the data base.

Data collection has two separate phases. The first phase consists of obtaining initial information regarding any injury. This information includes patient demographic data as well as employer and insurance information. The method for accomplishing this task varies from one occupational health program to another. Some programs may use an initial interview or admission form that is completed by the patient. In states that require initial injury reports, the data can be extracted from those forms. In either case, initial data collection should be part of the admissions process, and the information obtained should be formatted to facilitate entry into the computer at a later time.

Another crucial aspect of the initial collection of data is the identification of all of the on-the-job injuries that are treated in the facility. Obtaining this information is fairly simple for the independent occupational health clinic that only treats on-the-job injuries. However, urgent care clinics that treat both occupational and nonoccupational injuries must have some organized system of identifying which injuries are work related. The problem becomes more complex in a large hospital, where the patient may enter the system at multiple locations, for example, in the emergency or occupational health departments. In such situations, policies must be adopted and followed to ensure that every on-the-job injury is entered into the tracking program. Any patient not properly entered into the tracking program is, in effect, a failure of the program and has the potential of damaging the reputation and credibility of the program.

The second phase of obtaining data is the collection of follow-up information. The key here is accuracy and timeliness. No employer or insurance carrier is interested in data that are inaccurate or that are not available when they are needed. The health care provider has two major sources for follow-up information: the treating physician and the injured worker. Both sources are important in obtaining a full understanding of the recovery process. On the one hand, the patient is not likely to provide any detailed technical medical information. On the other hand, physicians are more likely to provide information that is strictly related to the patient's medical status; physicians may not even discuss with the patient any interpersonal work problems, such as a conflict with a supervisor who resents creating special conditions for the temporarily impaired worker. Although such personal problems and the feelings of the patient are not important to tracking (and the tracker must be careful to limit involvement in such matters), the knowledge of that information is important to understanding the overall recovery process or the patient's reluctance to follow the established treatment plan.

To effectively obtain follow-up data from the patient and treating physician, the tracker must start communicating with them as early as possible regarding a particular case. Patients should be informed early in their treatment that the tracking program exists, that it is a resource used throughout their recovery process, and that someone within the tracking program may be in contact with them in the future.

The best way to provide this information is through a brief letter given to patients when they are discharged after their initial visit. This letter should describe the tracking program and explain how the patient can contact someone within the tracking system.

The tracker should contact the patient by telephone within 24 to 48 hours of the initial visit. This initial contact establishes communication with the patient and allows patients to ask any questions they may have regarding their claims or the instructions given to them by their physicians. The person making the call should verify that the patient's condition is improving and should either make sure that the appropriate arrangements for follow-up care have been made or offer to assist the patient in obtaining a follow-up appointment. This contact is also a good time to get an assessment of the quality of care patients believed they received during their initial visit.

After the initial phone contact with the patient, additional follow-up contacts can be made on a routine basis to ensure that everything is going well and that the treatment plan is being followed. The computer can be programmed to signal the tracker when it is time to call the patient. Any significant finding from a phone contact with the patient should be entered into the computer just as any information about follow-up treatment by a physician would be entered.

Although the follow-up data obtained from the patient are important, the employer and the insurance carrier are more interested in follow-up data from the physician regarding the medical status of the injured worker. Therefore, a good system of communication must be developed between the treating physician and the tracker. When the treating physician's office is located within the occupational health clinic, the communication between physician and tracker can become a routine part of the clinic operation. However, when the patient is treated by a specialist from outside the occupational health clinic, the provider must establish systems through which data collection can take place.

When physicians who are not affiliated with an occupational health clinic encounter a tracking program, they are often reluctant to accept the tracking program. Most physicians view a tracking program as additional work for their staff with no benefit to their practice. Several approaches can be used to encourage physician cooperation. First, the provider should explain how an effective tracking program can benefit physicians' practices through more referrals and exposure. The next step is to illustrate to the physicians and their staffs how the information network of a tracking program can assist them in dealing with employers and insurance carriers. If the tracking program is providing patient data to those parties, then the physician's office should receive fewer information requests. An additional advantage to physicians in working with the tracking program is that they become part of a communication network among treating physicians. When a patient is referred to a physician who is not in the occupational health clinic, that physician can then look to the tracker to supply background data needed for the initial evaluation of the patient. Computerized tracking can generate a report with those data and have it sent to the consulting or referred physician at the time of referral. This type of report also assists the physician's office staff in identifying which patients are being actively tracked.

After physicians and their staffs see that the tracking program can be helpful to them, their reluctance to cooperate usually dissipates. However, after they agree to work with the tracking program, providers must still develop a system for collecting data in a timely manner. Because all offices are organized and run differently and because no office will cooperate if the tracking system causes problems, the person in charge of the tracking system should meet with the office manager or nurse in each office. Once the importance of and reason for prompt feedback of follow-up data are understood, the physician's office staff can suggest the best system for providing the information without disrupting their office routine. At first, the tracker may have to work with 10 different systems for 13 offices. However, when office staff people are asked how they want to handle the exchange of information, they usually ask for suggestions of how other offices do it. The end result is roughly three or four different systems, ranging from telephone calls to transcription to using a tracking form that can easily be completed at the end of treatment and sent to the tracker (figure 4-1). The key is flexibility on the part of the tracker, who must realize that how the information is obtained is less important than the timeliness of the process.

A good follow-up system requires that the tracker have a good system of flagging the records of those patients who will require some attention on any given day. Two lists that can be computer generated are particularly useful in ensuring that the tracker is able to stay on top of all of the cases.

Figure 4-1. Example of a Tracking Form

Patient's name: ______________________ Physician's name: ______________________

Treatment date: ______________________ Next visit: ______________________

Physician: ______________________

Treatment:

Work Status (indicate one):

________ Released for work on: ________

________ Released for light duty (indicate limitations):

____

Disposition:

________ Off work (indicate anticipated time off work):

____

The first is simply a list of those patients who either have follow-up appointments with physicians that day or who need to be telephoned that day to check on their progress or to direct them to the next step in their treatment. By printing such a list at the start of each day, the tracker can initiate all of the steps necessary to ensure that the follow-up data are collected and entered into the system.

The second list does not need to be created every day but should be generated two to three times per week. This list contains all patient files that are open and active and includes the current status and treatment plan for each patient. This list should be reviewed by the tracker and the medical director of the occupational health program. This system accomplishes two things:

- It ensures that the tracker will not lose track of or forget about a patient because of an oversight or an incorrect entry.
- It provides the medical director of the occupational health program with the opportunity to review the current treatment plan for each patient and to take any needed action if the treatment seems to be ineffective or inappropriate.

Distributing the Information

After the tracking program is designed and after data collection and an active process of tracking injured workers have been started, the tracker should focus on supplying the data to employers and insurance carriers. Employers who have had to struggle with obtaining bits and pieces of information regarding the status and prognosis of an injured employee find this routine feedback to be a tremendous service. The tracker can use several methods to provide this service. Each method is valuable in different situations.

Telephone Follow-Up

The time it takes to pick up the telephone and talk to an employer about an injured worker is invaluable, especially from a public relations point of view. Such contact with health care providers helps dispel the view that providers are distant and unapproachable. Although telephoning the employer each time the patient is seen may not be necessary or even practical, such contact may be appropriate at several stages of the treatment process.

Probably the most crucial time to call the employer is within 24 hours of the initial treatment of an injured worker. This initial contact is important for two reasons:

- *Some employers may not be aware that they have an employee seeking medical treatment for an on-the-job injury.* This situation is particularly true for large companies or for employers that have no clear policy regarding the reporting of work-related injuries. Notifying these employers of the initial injury treatment is important so that they can take the necessary steps to conform with state workers' compensation laws and OSHA regulations.
- *At the time employers become aware of an injury to a worker, they are faced with the uncertainty of when that worker will return to his or her regular duties.* Therefore, decisions must be made about shifting schedules, hiring temporary replacements, or delaying a project. The sooner the employer knows the status of the injured worker and the worker's prognosis for return to work, the quicker the employer can make the most effective decisions with the least impact on production. Therefore, the initial telephone contact within 24 hours of initial treatment becomes an extremely valuable service to businesses.

Another stage of treatment at which a telephone contact with the employer is appropriate is at the time of the patient's release to either regular or modified work duties. The employer can then anticipate the worker's return and make effective decisions regarding production. If the patient is being returned to modified or restricted duty, the employer needs to have a full and clear understanding of the worker's limitations so that the employer can make any necessary adjustments to accommodate the worker.

One other time when a telephone call is valuable is in determining the availability of light-duty jobs at the company or the employer's willingness to make special accommodations in order to get the worker back to some form of work. Without input from the employer, the physician may assume that the patient is unable to return to work and may therefore hold off on releasing the patient to work. For example, if the patient has sprained a knee, the physician will usually take the person off of work if the regular duties of the job require extensive walking. However, a call to the employer may reveal that for the duration of the injury, the employer is willing to shift people and place the injured worker at a desk job. In such a case, one telephone call saves money in lost time and productivity.

One final issue regarding phone calls is who should make them. If the treating physician has the time and is willing to do it, he or she is the best person to make the contact. However, the reality is that few physicians have the time to make calls. If the communication between the physician and the tracker is good, then the tracker is usually the person who makes the telephone contact. The best practice is to have only one or two people telephone employers, especially when contact is first being established, because the consistency of the same person calling provides a certain level of comfort. Such consistency becomes less important once the employer is fully familiar with the occupational health program.

Written Reports

Although the telephone contact is a valuable service to business and industry, it is not practical to call every time the patient is treated. However, especially in long-term cases, employers want and need to know how their injured workers are doing. The answer to providing routine reporting is to create a hard-copy report that can be sent to the employer on a weekly basis. A sample of such a report is shown in figure 4-2. In this example, the employer is provided with information regarding current diagnosis, current status, and number of days the worker has been off the job, as well as other information that may be of value. In receiving such a report on a weekly basis, the employer is updated on the status of any injured workers who are being tracked. Also, the knowledge that someone is watching each patient file and tracking the injured workers is reassuring to an employer who otherwise has no idea of what is going on.

At first, routine written reports may seem more labor intensive than telephone calls after every treatment. However, a computerized tracking program can automatically generate reports such as the one in figure 4-2. Once the report is created, the only labor involved is to run the program each week and put the printed reports in envelopes. Reports can be set up so that they can be folded and placed in a window envelope. The time involved is minimal, and it does not take significantly more labor or time to produce 50 reports than it does to produce 10.

To some people, it seems that tracking and reporting data to business and industry focuses a lot of energy on a service that generates no direct revenues. However, the occupational health program's patient base can be

Figure 4-2. Example of a Written Report on an Injured Employee

Summary of ill and injured workers for the week of 01/23/89 through 01/29/89.

The ABC Widget Company

12345 Main Street

Suite 200

Portland, OR 09725

Employee's Name: Doe, Jonathan C.

Nature of Injury: Right knee, effusion, cellulitis

Status: Release—Desk work only

Treating Physician: D. J. Bonecutter

Next Scheduled Date of Treatment: 02/02/89

Number of Days on "Off Work" Status: 9

Date of Injury: 01/09/89

Released for Work on: 04/19/89

increased when employers start directing their injured workers to the facility so that they can take advantage of the tracking service. In addition, an effective tracking program can open the doors for marketing other occupational health programs. The reason is related to the way that many businesses look at the medical community.

When asked, almost any employer will say that the cost of maintaining a healthy work force and the expenses of workers' compensation have gotten out of hand. Because of the distance the medical community has maintained from the business community and because of all the publicity regarding rising health care costs, business leaders often believe that the health care community is responsible for the rise in workers' compensation costs. This perception by businesses makes marketing health care services to them very difficult. When health care representatives approach an employer to market an occupational health service, they often encounter skepticism toward health care providers. By providing tracking services and demonstrating to employers how such services can help save them money, the providers can make employers more receptive to other occupational health service offerings.

Using Tracking as a Basis for Marketing

If tracking is to be used as a marketing tool, the program must be applied to all patients who come in contact with the occupational health program.

The trackers in some programs argue that tracking all cases is a waste of time and effort. Subsequently, they only track those injured workers from businesses with which the occupational health program has some formal agreement. However, this approach makes it difficult, if not impossible, to expand the number of companies that use the tracking program.

The first task in any marketing plan is to identify those businesses or individuals that would most benefit from a tracking program and would be most likely to use the service. By loading data on all cases into the computer, the provider can organize and extract information on the number and type of injuries for any single employer or group of employers. With these data, the provider can identify those companies that seem to have a higher risk of injury and, in particular, those companies that have a higher incidence of long-term, temporary disabling injuries. These companies are the ones that would most benefit from reductions in lost-work time and tighter case management. Once a company has been targeted for marketing, the tracker should pay special attention to tracking any injured workers from that company and should communicate and report to the employer just as if the employer were already a client.

A marketing person trying to sell the tracking program to a company that has no experience with what tracking can do may have difficulty convincing the employer that a tracking system can actually reduce losses. However, once a case has been tracked and the employer has experienced better communication and decreased losses, getting an employer's commitment or support is much easier. The initial arrangement with a new employer does not have to be a contract. It may simply be an agreement that the employer will direct all of its injured workers to the facility in exchange for tracking all of its injured employees and providing the employer with a report.

After reaching an agreement and tracking a large number of employees for a certain period, the employer and the occupational health program will begin to develop a good working relationship. The employer's distrust of the medical community will disappear, and the employer may become more receptive to other programs, such as preplacement examinations or medical surveillance. By tracking all of a company's employees, the provider can collect enough data to provide a better picture of the occupational health needs of the company. These data can be of value when marketing other programs because they consist of real numbers that specifically reflect an employer's business operation. Having employer-specific data also helps the provider design an individual package of services to address the specific problems within a business, rather than trying to sell a generic package of services that may not meet the employer's needs. Therefore, the key to effectively using a tracking program to market an occupational health program is to develop and carefully manage good data to increase an employer's trust in the program.

When selling a tracking program to an insurance company, the provider must understand that an insurer has two essential objectives: convenience and tighter claims management. Insurance carriers are as frustrated as employers with the difficulty of obtaining accurate, up-to-date information about a patient whose claim they are managing. Insurance companies find it easier to contact one place that can provide them with all of the data regarding an insured employee regardless of who the treating physician may be.

Easier access to patient information allows insurance companies to manage the claim more efficiently by reducing their administrative costs. Additionally, because the insurance carriers are the ones that are making payments for lost-work time, the concepts of tighter injury management and closely monitored treatment plans that result in reduced lost time are appealing.

Some people may wonder why they should market the concept of injury tracking to the insurance community. The answer is tied to the insurance carrier's desire to reduce the cost of as many claims as possible. If insurance companies see that an occupational health tracking program can help them reduce claims costs, they are more likely to encourage the businesses for whom they provide coverage to contact the occupational health facility and participate in the tracking program. Alternatively, insurance companies may give the tracker the names of people from companies that could benefit from the tracking service. In either case, the insurance carrier is essentially referring patients to the occupational health program and increasing the exposure and reputation of the program to the business community.

Summary

The key to utilizing a tracking program as a tool to increase the community visibility of the occupational health program and to enhance its marketing is to design a tracking program that meets the needs of business and industry. By providing a service that gives employers prompt, accurate information and that reduces losses through tighter claims management, a tracking program creates visibility and credibility for the entire occupational health program.

A tracking system is attractive to employers because it does not incur additional expenses and because the benefits are apparent within a short period of time. A tracking program can enhance trust and communication between the health care provider and a company. As a result, the employer may be more receptive to using other services that the occupational health program may provide.

Chapter 5

Employee Screening: OSHA Compliance Services

Peter Orris, M.D., M.P.H.
William L. Newkirk, M.D.

Employee screening is an important part of the occupational health services product line and may embrace a wide variety of activities. Many hospitals offer routine physical examinations as one of their occupational health services. From a health promotion perspective, routine physical examinations can be an effective tool. Hospitals often fail to understand, however, that employee examinations performed in many occupational situations differ significantly from routine physical examinations, and the requirements for conducting the examinations or using the information obtained are regulated by often-confusing legal standards.

This chapter reviews the roles hospital occupational health services programs can play in helping employers comply with Occupational Safety and Health Administration (OSHA) requirements for keeping records, assessing medical suitability of employees for the use of personal protective devices, and conducting medical surveillance. Understanding OSHA's role in the workplace can help occupational health programs design appropriate products and services. Subsequent chapters review preemployment screening and handicap and discrimination regulations (chapter 6), drug testing in the workplace (chapter 7), and the controversies surrounding acquired immunodeficiency syndrome (AIDS) testing (chapter 8). A hospital occupational health program that wishes to provide employee screening must prepare its approach to all of these services that employers may look to the program to provide.

The Purpose of the Occupational Safety and Health Administration

Before 1970, three forces attempted to ensure safe workplaces:

- *State and local governments.* State and local governments attempted to advise and regulate industry with regard to safety hazards and employee risks. There was tremendous variation among states in this effort. Strong regulation occurred in some states (for example, California, Michigan, and Massachusetts); no regulation in others (such as Texas).
- *Insurance companies.* Forces in the private sector, such as insurance companies, sought to improve safety in the workplace through consultation programs and rate incentives.
- *Industry-based groups.* Industry-based groups sought to fill the vacuum and arrive at reasonable guidelines for safe work practices.

These three groups could not do an adequate job. As a result, in 1970 Congress passed the Occupational Safety and Health Act. Under the act, two federal agencies and the states play separate but interlocking roles:

- *Occupational Safety and Health Administration (OSHA).* A part of the Department of Labor, OSHA is responsible for promulgating and enforcing occupational health and safety standards.
- *National Institute of Occupational Safety and Health (NIOSH).* A part of the Department of Health and Human Services, NIOSH is responsible for carrying out research to develop new standards and to train health industry professionals.
- *States.* The states have the right to assume the primary responsibility for enforcing occupational safety and health regulations if they develop a suitable plan for enforcement that is approved by the Secretary of Labor.

To get OSHA started, Congress allowed OSHA two years to adopt industry "consensus" standards. In the interest of speed, OSHA adopted existing standards of such groups as the American National Standards Institute (ANSI), the National Fire Prevention Association (NFPA), and the American Congress of Governmental Industrial Hygienists (ACGIH), making no significant deletions immediately even though problems existed. The standards were complex and often obsolete. For example, one standard prohibited the use of ice in drinking water. This rule dated from a time when ice was cut from possibly contaminated rivers. The industry groups that had developed the standards expected them to be flexible guidelines; however, OSHA's initial actions turned them into inflexible standards. Because of these problems and others, OSHA removed 927 of these standards in 1978.

After this initial grace period, OSHA was required to follow a nine-step process for initiating further standards. This process is outlined in section 6(b) of the Occupational Safety and Health Act. This time-consuming process has slowed the approval of new standards to a snail's pace. The paperwork requirements of this process are enormous. For example, the hearing record for OSHA's carcinogen standard is over 250,000 pages long.

The Occupational Safety and Health Administration is responsible for developing, funding, and in some cases, providing educational programs for workers and management. It provides funding for management and union groups to conduct educational programs through its training directions grants. It also conducts courses at its training center in Des Plaines, Illinois, for plant, corporate, and union health and safety officials. A list of these resources may be obtained through the regional OSHA offices (see appendix A) or from the OSHA Training Institute at 1555 Times Drive, Des Plaines, Illinois 60018.

The standards and news regarding the standards-setting process as well as other relevant information about governmental regulations can be found in the Bureau of National Affairs Safety and Health Reports. The publications, although expensive, can help to answer questions about governmental regulations. For information, contact the Bureau of National Affairs, 1231 25th Street, NW, Washington, DC 20037.

Hospital Occupational Health Programs and OSHA

In their process of complying with OSHA requirements, industries often utilize hospital occupational health programs for assistance with record keeping, assessment of fitness for personal protective devices, and medical surveillance.

Record Keeping

Under the Occupational Safety and Health Act of 1970 (P.L. 91-596), records of the types, extent, and outcomes of many workplace injuries and illnesses must be kept and maintained by companies of 11 or more employees for five years. Although the records to be kept are fairly simple for employers to develop and maintain for themselves, occupational health services programs might consider assisting employers in their record-keeping obligations.

The OSHA log (Form No. 200, the Bureau of Labor Statistics Log and Summary of Occupational Injuries and Illnesses) is the basic form used to summarize data on a company's occupational injuries and illnesses. This form or log containing comparable information in a similar easy-to-read format should be maintained by the company, and although it does not have to be filed with OSHA, it must be available for OSHA inspections.

Employers must record information about every occupational death; every nonfatal occupational illness; and those nonfatal occupational injuries that involve one or more of the following: loss of consciousness, restriction of work or motion, transfer to another job, or medical treatment (other than first aid). Definitions of these terms appear on the reverse side of the form. Each recordable case must be entered on the log within six workdays after the company learns of its occurrence. The summary data reported on the form (with the specific employees' names and other identifying data removed) must be posted in each establishment where notices to employees are customarily posted. The form has spaces to record a brief description of the injury or illness, the number of workdays lost, the number of days of restricted work activity, and the date of death, if applicable.

This summative log is supplemented by a second, more detailed OSHA form (Form No. 101, the Bureau of Labor Statistics Supplementary Record of Occupational Injuries and Illnesses). For each case, Form 101 or a similar written report is used to record data about the accident or exposure to occupational illness (place of accident or exposure, whether it was on the employer's premises, what the employee was doing when injured, and how the accident occurred); about the occupational injury or illness (description of the injury or illness, including part of body affected; name of the object or substance that directly injured the employee; and date of injury or diagnosis or illness); and about other pertinent facts (name and address of physician, name and address of hospital, if applicable, date of report, and name and position of person preparing the report).

Record-keeping requirements in medical surveillance can be more difficult for employers. In cases involving exposure to asbestos, for example, the employer is required to keep the employee's medical surveillance record for the duration of his or her employment plus 30 years!

Personal Protective Devices

When workers are exposed to toxic substances above the allowable amount, the company must respond with engineering controls, work practice controls, or personal protective devices. Engineering controls involve mechanical means designed to reduce the exposure. The toxic substance may be eliminated, contained, diverted, diluted, or collected at the source. Work practice controls involve altering the way the worker performs the job so that exposure can be limited or reduced. Personal protective devices isolate the employee from the emission source. The best example of a personal protective device is a respirator.

Companies may contact occupational health programs to have them assess their workers for the medical suitability of the use of personal protective devices. The OSHA requirement for asbestos surveillance (29 CFR 1910.1001), for example, states:

> No employee shall be assigned to tasks requiring the use of respirators if, based upon his or her most recent examination, an examining physician determines that the employee will be unable to function wearing a respirator, or that the safety or health of the employee or other employees will be impaired by the use of a respirator.

Medical Surveillance

Medical surveillance is the most important area in which employers will use occupational health programs to fulfill OSHA requirements for their companies. Medical surveillance is required for a limited number of dangerous substances, such as asbestos, carcinogens, vinyl chloride, inorganic arsenic, lead, coke-oven emissions, cotton dust, acrylonitrile, ethylene oxide, and formaldehyde. As a rule, OSHA regulations specify certain tests that must be performed as part of the surveillance. A good example of this is the inorganic arsenic standard. This standard requires that workers provide a work history and undergo a chest X ray, nasal and skin examinations, a sputum cytology, and other tests that a physician believes are appropriate. This type of recommendation is fairly representative of OSHA's approach to physician examinations.

Regarding physician examinations, OSHA fails to clarify three areas. First, there are rarely any medical criteria to be used by physicians in performing the examinations, and with few exceptions, there are no required qualifications for physicians performing the examinations. Second, although OSHA explicitly requests that certain procedures or examinations be performed, it does not exclude the employer or physicians from performing other evaluations. As in the case of arsenic, tests can include "other examinations which the physician deems appropriate. . . ." (*Federal Register* 29 C.F.R. 1910.1018.) Third, there is little information on how the information gained by these examinations can and cannot be used in the employer's decision making.

Hospital occupational health programs should perform medical surveillance only if they plan to take the time to learn the details of the required screening. The hospital should ensure that the companies for whom it is screening are also aware of the OSHA requirements. The requirements themselves are listed in Volume 29 of the *Code of Federal Regulations.*

National Institute of Occupational Safety and Health (NIOSH)

Because the OSHA standards-setting process is so slow, many toxic substances do not have appropriate OSHA standards. In those circumstances, it is useful to review NIOSH's recommendations, called "criteria documents." These criteria documents delineate the available scientific knowledge about a hazard, its risks, and its abatement. These and other NIOSH publications are available through the National Technical Information Service or the Government Printing Office. To secure a catalog or inquire about publications, contact NIOSH, DSDTT, Publications Dissemination, 4676 Columbia Parkway, Cincinnati, Ohio 45226-1998.

The National Institute of Occupational Safety and Health maintains a large multidisciplinary professional staff to engage in research and investigations of health and safety hazards. Through industrywide studies, NIOSH selects an industry and a specific exposure that need evaluation. Through its Health Hazard Evaluation Program, it responds to requests for evaluation of specific workplaces and their health problems. It also conducts continuing medical surveillance of occupational disease in the United States. In the laboratory, NIOSH develops methods for the evaluation of industrial toxins by creating standard laboratory procedures for environmental and biological monitoring. Finally, it tests and certifies personal protective equipment destined for use in the workplace.

The agency responds to telephone calls for advice on occupational medical problems and requests for information concerning specific chemicals. It maintains a library with over 200 data bases and can access the world's literature in occupational health. This resource is available to physicians with specific requests at 800/35-NIOSH. If more recent information is needed, the library can refer inquiries to specific researchers who are actively involved in the area of concern.

Additionally, and perhaps more practically, the NIOSH-maintained data base, NIOSHTIC, a cousin to the National Library of Medicine's MEDLINE, is available for access by private citizens. This data base, which is easily searched by novices, contains references and abstracts covering environmental and chemical data as well as disease causation, prevention, and treatment data. It may be accessed by modem through DIALOG, 3460 Hillview Avenue, Palo Alto, California 94304 (800/3-DIALOG), or on laser disc from the Canadian Center for Occupational Health and Safety, 250 Main Street, East Hamilton, Ontario L8N 1H6 Canada (416/572-2981). The data are updated quarterly and cover most questions generated by a hospital-based occupational medical practice.

The National Institute of Occupational Health and Safety funds educational resource centers (ERCs) at major academic institutions (appendix B). These centers provide multidisciplinary professional education in occupational health. Each contains a residency or fellowship training program for physicians, a master's nursing program, training for industrial hygienists and safety engineers, and a wide variety of short-term specific training programs for practicing professionals.

To determine the cause of a workplace health problem when requested by an employer, employees, or an authorized collective bargaining organization, NIOSH performs health hazard evaluations (HHEs). The investigators conducting such studies have the same right of entry into a plant and access to records as OSHA inspectors do. The results of these studies are published, with protected confidentiality of the participating employees, as findings of fact. Recommendations for control of identified hazards are included. However, NIOSH cannot levy fines or compel abatement. If conditions exist that do not meet an OSHA standard, NIOSH informs OSHA of this situation for its review. A copy of the HHE request form is shown in appendix C.

Conclusion

Screening for occupational health purposes differs from screening for routine physical examinations. Occupational health programs need to understand the standards of the Occupational Health and Safety Administration (OSHA) if they wish to perform screening mandated by law. The OSHA standards-setting process is slow and cumbersome, however, and certain toxic chemicals will not be covered by OSHA standards. In those situations, the National Institute of Occupational Safety and Health can be of assistance in providing information on a substance's toxic effects, biological surveillance, and abatement.

Appendix A. Regional Offices of the Occupational Safety and Health Administration

Region I:
16-18 North Street
1 Dock Square Building, 4th Floor
Boston, MA 02109

Region II:
1515 Broadway (1 Astor Plaza)
Room 3445
New York, NY 10036

Region III:
Gateway Building, Suite 2100
3535 Market Street
Philadelphia, PA 19104

Region IV:
1375 Peachtree Street, N.E.
Suite 587
Atlanta, GA 30367

Region V:
230 South Dearborn Street
32nd Floor, Room 3244
Chicago, IL 60604

Region VI:
55 Griffin Street, Room 602
Dallas, TX 75202

Region VII:
911 Walnut Street, Room 406
Kansas City, MO 64106

Region VIII:
Federal Building
1961 Stout Street
Denver, CO 80294

Region IX:
P.O. Box 36017
11349 Federal Building
San Francisco, CA 94102

Region X:
Federal Office Building
909 First Avenue, Room 60003
Seattle, WA 98174

Appendix B. Educational Resource Centers of the National Institute of Occupational Safety and Health

University of Alabama at Birmingham
School of Public Health
University Station Birmingham
Birmingham, AL 35294

Labor Occupational Health Program
University of California
2521 Channing Way
Berkeley, CA 94720

University of Southern California
Institute of Safety & System Management
Room 116
University Park
Los Angeles, CA 90089-0021

University of Illinois
Educational Resource Center
817 South Wolcott
MC 78
Chicago, IL 60612

Harvard School of Public Health
622 Huntington Avenue
Boston, MA 02115

Johns Hopkins School of Hygiene and Public Health
615 North Wolfe Street
Baltimore, MD 21205

Center for Occupational Health and Safety
St. Paul–Ramsey Medical Center
640 Jackson Street
St. Paul, MN 55101

University of North Carolina
Occupational Safety & Health
109 Conner Drive
Chapel Hill, NC 27514

Mt. Sinai School of Medicine
Occupational Safety & Health
Box 1057
One Gustave Levy Place
New York, NY 10029-6574

University of Cincinnati
Occupational Safety & Health
234 Goodman Avenue
Cincinnati, OH 45267

Texas Educational Resource Center
University of Texas
Health Science Center at Houston
School of Public Health
P.O. Box 20186
Houston, TX 77025

Rocky Mountain Center for Occupational & Environmental Health
Building 512
University of Utah
Salt Lake City, UT 84112

Northwest Center for Occupational Health & Safety
Department of Environmental Health
University of Washington, SC-34
Seattle, WA 98195

Appendix C. Form for Requesting a Health Hazard Evaluation

U.S. DEPARTMENT OF HEALTH AND HUMAN SERVICES
NATIONAL INSTITUTE FOR OCCUPATIONAL
SAFETY AND HEALTH
REQUEST FOR HEALTH HAZARD EVALUATION

This form is provided to assist in registering a request for a health hazard evaluation with the U.S. Department of Health and Human Services as provided in Section 20(a)(6) of the Occupational Safety and Health Act of 1970 and 42 CFR Part 85. (See Statement of Authority on Reverse Side.)

Establishment Where Possible Hazard/Problem Exists ______________

Address
Street ______________________ Telephone __________
City ______________ State ________ Zip Code ________

---

1. Specify the particular building or worksite where the possible hazard/problem is located. ______________________

   ____

2. Specify the name, title, and phone number of the employer's agent(s) in charge. ______________________

   ____

3. What Product or Service does the Establishment Produce? ________

   ____

4. Describe briefly the possible hazard/problem which exists by completing the following:
   Identification of Toxic Substance(s) ______________________

   Trade Name(s) (If Applicable) _______ Chemical Name(s) _______

   ____

   ____

   Manufacturer(s) ______________________

OMB No. 0920-0102
Expires 7/31/89

Does the material have a warning label? _____ Yes _____ No. If yes; attach copy of label or a copy of the information contained on the label.

Physical Form of Substance(s): [ ] Dust [ ] Gas
[ ] Liquid [ ] Mist [ ] Other

How are you exposed? [ ] Breathing [ ] Swallowing [ ] Skin Contact

Number of People Exposed __ Length of Exposure (Hours/Day) __

Occupations of Exposed Employees ______________________________

____

5. Using the space below describe further the nature of the conditions or circumstances which prompted this request and other relevant aspects which you may consider important, such as the nature of the illness or symptoms of exposure, the concern for the potentially toxic effects of a new chemical substance introduced into the workplace, etc.

____

____

____

6. (a) To your knowledge has this substance been considered previously by any Government agency? _______ (b) If so, give the name and address of each. ______________________________

____

(c) and, the approximate date it was considered. _______________

7. (a) Is a similar request currently being filed with or under investigation by any other Government (State or Federal) agency? _______ (b) If so, give the name and address of each. ______________________

____

8. Requester—The undersigned Requester believes that a substance (or substances) normally found in the place of employment may have potentially toxic effects in the concentrations used or found.

____

Signature ______________________________ Date __________

Typed or Printed Name ____________________ Phone: Home—_______

Address
Street ______________________________ Business—_______
City ________________ State ________ Zip Code ________

____

Check One:

[ ] I am an Employer Representative

[ ] I am an Authorized Representative of, or an officer of the organization representing the employees for purposes of collective bargaining. State the name and address of your organization. ________

[ ] I am an employee of the employer and an Authorized Representative of two or more employees in the workplace where the substance is normally found. Signatures of authorizing employees are below:

Name ________________________ Phone __________

Name ________________________ Phone __________

[ ] I am one of three or less employees in the workplace where the substance is normally found.

Please indicate your desire: [ ] I do not want my name revealed to the employer.

[ ] My name may be revealed to the employer.

Authority:

Section (20) (a)(6) of the Occupational Safety and Health Act, (29) U.S.C. 669 (a)(6) provides as follows: The Secretary of Health and Human Services shall. . .determine following a written request by any employer or authorized representative of employees, specifying with reasonable particularity the grounds on which the request is made, whether any substance normally found in the place of employment has potentially toxic effects in such concentrations as used or found; and shall submit such determination both to employers and affected employees as soon as possible. If the Secretary of Health and Human Services determines that any substance is potentially toxic at the concentrations in which it is used or found in a place of employment, and such substance is not covered by an occupational safety or health standard promulgated under section 6, the Secretary of Health and Human Services shall immediately submit such determination to the Secretary of Labor, together with all pertinent criteria.

For further information:
Telephone: AC513-841-4382

Send the completed form to:

National Institute for Occupational Safety and Health
Hazard Evaluation and Technical Assistance Branch
4676 Columbia Parkway
Cincinnati, Ohio 45226

Chapter 6

Employee Screening: Employability Assessment

John E. Carnes, J.D.

In many instances, in order for an employer to make an intelligent, legal hiring decision, the services of professional medical personnel will be needed. These professionals will assist the employer in evaluating the applicant's physical or mental condition as it relates to job-related qualifications.

Generally, by statute and regulation, employer representatives may not make preemployment inquiries as to whether an applicant is handicapped or as to the nature or severity of a handicap. Inquiries may be made as to the applicant's ability to perform essential job functions. If an applicant indicates that he or she might have difficulty performing a particular job duty, discussion of possible accommodations would be appropriate.

As a general rule, preemployment physical examinations are prohibited by federal regulations promulgated in accordance with the Rehabilitation Act of 1973 (described later in this chapter). However, employers may condition an offer of employment on the successful completion of a physical examination.[1] This means that the employer should first evaluate the applicants' other qualifications, select those applicants to be offered employment, and then require a successful physical examination prior to entry on duty. Such an examination may be required only if all entering employees are subjected to it and if the information obtained is used only in accordance with the requirements of the statute.[2] The results of the examination must be kept confidential except that:

- Supervisors and managers may be informed regarding work restrictions and accommodations
- First-aid and safety personnel may be informed if a condition might require emergency treatment
- Government officials investigating compliance with the Rehabilitation Act shall be given relevant information upon their request[3]

Employers engaged in evaluating applicants for hire have legitimate concerns about the cost of compensation claims, the number of lost workdays resulting from injury, and the need to provide a safe environment for employees.[4] However, these legitimate concerns sometimes lead employers to establish policies permitting the hire of only "perfect physical specimens."[5] These policies have led some employers in the railroad and trucking industries, for example, to reject applicants based solely on the results of low-back X rays. In most of these cases, the employers have lost the handicap discrimination suits filed against them.[6] The problem for such employers and the physicians testifying on their behalf is that the courts have been convinced that low-back X rays, taken alone, do not have a high positive value for predicting future disability.[7]

In *Bozanski v. A.P.A. Transport, Inc.,* the Maine Supreme Judicial Court concluded that an assessment of ability to drive a truck based solely on a low-back X ray did not constitute the individualized evaluation required by state law.[8] The court faulted the selection process because the physicians advising the employer had not performed a clinical examination or taken a medical history of the job applicants. There was simply no factual basis to believe with a reasonable probability that the applicants' handicaps would prevent them from safely performing the duties of the job.[9]

An employer cannot escape liability under the handicap discrimination statutes merely by relying on the opinion of a physician. Employers must establish that they relied upon "competent medical advice that there exists a reasonably probable risk of serious harm."[10] Where the medical advice is based on substantial evidence, the employer's position should prevail. In *State of Minnesota v. Metropolitan Airport Commission,* the court ruled in favor of the employer despite the opinions of three physicians who testified on behalf of the plaintiff.[11] The question was whether an applicant with a back condition was physically capable of safely performing the duties of a maintenance worker. The opinion of the employer's physician was based on a medical history, a clinical examination, and an X ray showing disk-space narrowing and actual degenerative change. The information the physician gathered for the employer and his professional evaluation of it constituted the required factual basis to believe with a reasonable probability that the applicant could not perform the job safely.

Because employers cannot avoid liability by relying upon a physician's opinion or report unless that opinion or report is informed and reasonable, it is incumbent upon the employer to carefully inform the physician of the duties and requirements of employees' jobs.[12] It would be advisable for the employer to invite the physician to visit the job site so that he or she can observe the operation and speak with people who actually do the job. With this knowledge, the physician can make the proper comparison between the actual limitations of a disability, if any, and the work to be done. Employers who make the effort to adequately inform their medical advisors will reap the benefits at the other end of the process; they will avoid the risk of losing qualified workers who might otherwise be screened out, and they will not break the law.

The Impact of Civil Rights Legislation

In passing the civil rights statutes of the 1960s and 1970s, Congress and the states acted to ensure equal opportunities for individuals who are members of groups that had been discriminated against in the past. In 1972, the year before the enactment of the federal Rehabilitation Act of 1973,[13] Congress acknowledged that of the 14 million physically handicapped adults in the United States who were able and willing to work, only 800,000 were employed.[14] Determined to correct this waste of energy and talent, the federal government and the legislatures of all the states but one[15] have enacted statutes that prohibit employment discrimination on the basis of handicap. The purpose of this legislation is to "promote and expand employment opportunities to the public and private sectors for handicapped individuals."[16]

People with handicaps have not generally been faced with the kind of hatred and bigotry found in cases of discrimination on the basis of race, color, or national origin.[17] They have, however, been burdened with stereotyped assumptions about their abilities and with well-intentioned paternalism. The result is the same: the denial of equal employment opportunity.

From the multitude of state and federal laws and regulations that address handicap discrimination, three principles emerge:

- Employers must treat people with handicaps as individuals, not merely as members of a group with certain common characteristics.
- Employers must assess the individual's actual ability to perform the essential functions of the job.
- If the handicap impairs the person's ability to perform the duties of the job safely, the employer must make those reasonable accommodations that allow the individual to perform the job safely.

By using this approach, the employer not only will be in compliance with the law but also will be contributing to the goal of bringing handicapped persons into the mainstream of American life.[18]

Employers' Obligations under Laws Prohibiting Handicap Discrimination

The most significant legislation addressing handicap discrimination in employment is the Rehabilitation Act of 1973.[19] The act prohibits discrimination on the basis of handicap by federal employers (Section 501) and private employers with federal contracts of more than $2,500 (Section 503).

It also requires that these employers take affirmative action to hire and promote qualified handicapped persons. Section 504 of the act orders that employers funded by federal grants not discriminate against any "otherwise qualified handicapped individual."

Several federal agencies have promulgated regulations designed to carry out the statute's provisions. For example, employers are required to make a reasonable accommodation to the individual's handicap in order to place the person in the position, unless the accommodation would cause an undue burden on the employer's business.[20] Job qualifications that tend to screen out handicapped persons must be eliminated unless they can be shown to be job related.[21] In addition, limits have been placed on preemployment inquiries and examinations.[22] Employers who cannot remain in compliance with the requirements of the implementing regulations risk not only an expensive court-imposed remedy for the victim of the discrimination but also the loss of their federal contract or federal financial assistance.

The Rehabilitation Act applies to those who meet its definition of *handicapped individual.* A person is considered handicapped if he or she "has a physical or mental impairment which substantially limits one or more of such person's major life activities, has a record of such an impairment, or is regarded as having such an impairment."[23] The term *major life activities* is defined by regulation as "functions such as caring for one's self, performing manual tasks, walking, seeing, hearing, speaking, breathing, learning, and working."[24] The words *has a record of such an impairment* mean that the person has a history of disability or was misclassified as being handicapped in the past.[25] The words *is regarded as having an impairment* refer to those situations in which an employer treats the person as if he or she had a physical or mental impairment that substantially limits a major life activity when in fact the person has no such impairment.[26]

Handicapped applicants are entitled to the job for which they have applied if they are *otherwise qualified.* Applicants are otherwise qualified if they can perform the *essential functions of the job*[27] in spite of the limitations of their impairment.[28] Therefore, an employer may not disqualify a handicapped person simply because he or she may have difficulty performing job duties that are not essential. If the handicapped individual cannot perform the essential duties of the job because of the handicap, the employer must determine whether a reasonable accommodation can be made that will enable the individual to perform those functions. If a reasonable accommodation can be made, the employer must hire the handicapped applicant. To determine whether an accommodation can be made, the employer may need to consult with its medical advisor as well as with the applicant.

The types of accommodations that can be made are limited only by the ingenuity of the employer and the handicapped person and the state of technology. A reasonable accommodation might involve making interpreters or readers available or keeping work schedules flexible. The worksite itself might be altered to make work areas accessible to people in wheelchairs. Equipment can be modified, and other barriers can be eliminated.

However, an employer does not have to make an accommodation if doing so is unreasonable. An accommodation is not considered reasonable if it imposes an undue burden on the employer or if it requires a fundamental alteration in the nature of the business or program.[29] The burden of proving the hardship on the business rests with the employer.

Factors that may be considered when determining whether an accommodation creates an undue burden include the size of the business and its budget, the nature of the operation, and the cost of the accommodation. If a number of accommodations will enable the handicapped employee to perform the essential duties of the job, the employer may select the one that costs the least.

Although collective bargaining agreements do not supersede the requirements of employment discrimination laws, the provisions of such agreements may be considered when reviewing the reasonableness of a proposed accommodation.[30]

To avoid liability when they reject an applicant because of the presence of a physical handicap, employers must be able to show that their physical qualifications for the job are job related and that they had a factual basis to believe that the applicant's impairment creates a "reasonable probability of substantial harm."[31]

Before making such judgments, employers must make two inquiries:

- What is the nature of the potential risk; that is, what kind of harm might the handicap cause? If the potential injury is minor, employers cannot reject the applicant even if the probability is high that the injury will occur. If the potential injury is of a serious nature, employers cannot deny the person employment opportunity unless facts support a reasonable probability that substantial harm will occur. In other words, remote safety risks do not justify denying the handicapped individual the job.
- If there exists a reasonable probability of substantial harm, is there a reasonable accommodation that would allow the person to do the job without the risk?[32]

This type of analysis by employers requires that they and the medical professionals advising them engage in effective fact gathering. The employer's obligation to gather the relevant facts before making an employment decision is based on the Congressional intent expressed in the Rehabilitation Act to prohibit employers from denying employment to handicapped persons on the basis of *misinformed stereotypes.*[33]

Because a factual basis is required for the employer's hiring decisions, a good-faith or rational belief on the part of the employer that the handicap prevents safe performance is an insufficient defense.[34] Handicap discrimination is most often the result of ignorance; therefore, to allow a good-faith or rational-basis defense would undermine the basic purpose of the handicap discrimination statutes. Similarly, the employer's decision cannot be based on medical reports alone, except in cases where inability to function safely is readily apparent. The determination of whether employing the individual would create a reasonable probability of substantial harm must be made "in light of the individual's work history and medical history."[35]

Generally, handicapped individuals must be hired if they are able to safely perform the job's essential duties at the time of application. However, employers are permitted to consider injury that will probably occur at some future time.[36] If the evidence available indicates that the time of harm is remote or at some indefinite future time, the employer may not reject the individual.

How near in time to the date of application must the probable harm be in order to justify rejection of a handicapped applicant? Neither the statutes nor the courts have answered this question. One court has pondered the problem and provided some guidance, if not an answer. In *E. E. Black, Ltd. v. Marshall,* the federal district court acknowledged that the risk of future injury can be, in some cases, a basis for rejecting a presently qualified handicapped person. It then stated that an employer could lawfully reject a qualified applicant if it were determined that the person, once performing job duties, would have a 90 percent chance of suffering a heart attack within one month.[37] How the courts will address less extreme situations remains to be seen.

Summary

The goal of Congress and the various state legislatures is to ensure that handicapped persons who can work are given that opportunity. This goal cannot be realized as long as stereotyped assumptions and vague predictions about future ability remain the basis for employment decisions. It is for this reason that the statutes and the courts that interpret them require employers and the medical professionals who advise them to have a factual basis for their preplacement screening decisions.

In many instances, employers' decisions will be only as good as the quality of the advice they receive from the physicians. Physicians' recommendations will be valuable only if they have had the opportunity to educate themselves about the job's essential duties, to determine the actual physical abilities of the applicant, and to utilize tests that have a high positive value in predicting the risk of further injury.

References

1. 29 C.F.R. §1613.706.6(b); 41 C.F.R. §41.55.

2. *Id.*

3. 41 C.F.R. §60-741.6(c)(3).
4. Rockey, Fantel, and Omenn, Discriminatory aspects of pre-employment screening: low-back x-ray examinations in the railroad industry, 5 *Am. J. L. & Med.* 197 (1979); Center, Employment discrimination implications of genetic screening in the workplace under Title VII and the Rehabilitation Act, 10 *Am. J. L. & Med.* 323-47, Fall 1984.
5. Rockey and others, cited in reference 4.
6. *See, e.g.,* Rozanski v. A.P.A. Transport, Inc., 512 A.2d 335 (Me. 1986).
7. *Id.* at 340-41.
8. Rozanski v. A.P.A Transport, Inc., cited in reference 6.
9. *See also* Maine Human Rights Commission v. Canadian Pacific Railroad, 458 A.2d 1225, 31 FEP Cases 1028 (Me. 1983); Sterling Transit Co. v. Fair Employment Practice Commission, 121 Cal. App. 3d 791, 28 FEP Cases 1351 (1981).
10. Lewis v. Remmele Engineering, Inc., 314 N.W. 2d 1, 4, 29 FEP Cases 576 (Minn. 1981).
11. State of Minnesota v. Metropolitan Airport Commission, 44 FEP Cases 542 (Minn. Ct. App. 1984).
12. *See* Anderson v. Exxon Co., 43 FEP Cases 1763, 1770 (N.J. 1982).
13. 29 U.S.C. §701-794 (Supp. V 1975).
14. 118 *Cong. Rec.* 3320-21 (1972) (Statement of Senator Williams).
15. *Fair Employment Practices Manual,* BNA Labor Relations Reporter, State Law Chart, p. 451;102-104 (1986).
16. 29 U.S.C. §701(8) (1976).
17. Comment, Section 504 of the Rehabilitation Act: analyzing employment discrimination claims, 132 *U. Pa. L. Rev.* 867-99 Ap. 84; Alexander v. Choate, 469 U.S. 287, 295 (1985).
18. 42 *Fed. Reg.* 22, 676 (May 4, 1977).
19. 29 U.S.C. §701-794 (Supp. V 1975). Employers must also be aware of and in compliance with their state and local equal employment opportunity statutes. *See* Lab. Rel. Rep. (BNA), State FEP Laws (1986), for a one-volume collection of all state statutes and regulations relating to handicap discrimination in employment.
20. 29 C.F.R. §1613.704 (federal employers); 41 C.F.R. §60-741.6 (federal contractors); 28 C.F.R. §41.53 (programs).
21. 41 C.F.R. §60-741.6.
22. 29 C.F.R. §§1613.705 and .706; 28 C.F.R. §41.55.
23. 29 U.S.C. §706(7)(B) (1982).
24. 45 C.F.R. §84.3(j)(2)(ii) (1983).
25. 45 C.F.R. §84.3(j)(2)(iii) (1983).
26. 45 C.F.R. §84.3(j)(2)(iv) (1983).

27. 45 C.F.R. §84.3(k) (1985).
28. Southeastern Community College v. Davis, 442 U.S. 397 (1979).
29. *Id.*
30. Bay v. Bolger, 540 F. Supp. 910, 926-27, 32 FEP Cases 1652 (E.D. Pa. 1982).
31. Mantolete v. Bolger, 767 F.2d 1416, 38 FEP Cases 1081 (9th Cir. 1985); Mikucki v. U.S. Postal Service, 41 FEP Cases 1503 (D.C. Mass. 1986).
32. Adelman, Employment discrimination—Section 501 of the Rehabilitation Act of 1973; Finally, a legal standard—Mantolete v. Bolger, *Ariz. St. L. J.* 147-60, 1986.
33. Mantolete, at 1086.
34. Mantolete, at 1087.
35. Mantolete, at 1086.
36. E. E. Black, Ltd. v. Marshall, 497 F. Supp. 1088, 23 FEP Cases 1253 (D. Hawaii 1980).
37. E. E. Black, at 1104.

Chapter 7

Employee Screening: Drug Testing*

Mark A. Rothstein, J.D.

Introduction

The controversy surrounding drug testing in the workplace epitomizes many of the contemporary clashes between labor and management. Drug testing of employees is an effort to deal with the workplace effects of a larger societal problem of drug abuse; drug testing uses new technology in attempting to control a human problem; and drug testing creates conflicts between employee interests in autonomy and privacy and employer interests in health, safety, and productivity.

From a legal standpoint, drug testing also raises a wide range of recurring issues. There are the differing rights of public and private employees, the conflict between federal policy (requiring or encouraging testing) and state policy (increasingly restricting testing), and the efforts to expand the reach of various statutes (such as handicap discrimination laws) and the common law to challenge drug testing. Drug testing to protect public health and safety may be legitimate and justified, but only if certain enumerated prerequisites and safeguards are satisfied.

Determining the Reasonableness of Drug Testing

Although the specific legal criteria vary with the source of the legal protection, essentially the courts seek to determine whether a challenged drug

*This chapter is adapted from an article by Mark A. Rothstein originally published under the title "Drug testing in the workplace: the challenge to employment relations and employment law" in the *Chicago-Kent Law Review* [63(3):110–61, 1987]. Reprinted by special permission of IIT Chicago-Kent College of Law.

testing program is reasonable under the circumstances. One way of looking at the issue is to see whether reasonable grounds exist to suspect that the testing will turn up evidence of work-related drug use and whether the measures adopted are not excessively intrusive.[1] Another way is to focus upon the following four factors: who is tested, when is the testing performed, how is the testing performed, and what is done with test results.

Who Is Tested?

The starting point for determining whether any particular drug testing is reasonable is to look at the individual being tested. In other words, the job description and responsibilities of the person tested are very important. The courts have been more willing to sanction the use of drug testing where employees and co-workers may be endangered by drug impairment.[2] Drug testing in other job classifications is less likely to be upheld.[3]

When Is the Testing Performed?

Drug testing may be conducted at a variety of stages during the employment relationship, including preemployment, periodic, upon return to work following a leave of absence, after an accident, based on suspicion of drug use, and randomly. The timing or circumstances of the test often affect the legality of the test.

Preemployment testing is the most prevalent form of drug testing. It is also the most likely to be upheld. Applicants do not have any vested rights in their jobs and if they are denied a job because of a drug test they have only lost an expectancy as opposed to current employees whose loss probably would be considered more tangible.

Periodic testing, especially when used as part of an overall medical evaluation of fitness, also is likely to be upheld.[4] For other types of testing, without a particularized or individualized need for testing, the courts are more inclined to find that testing is unnecessary and therefore unreasonable. Random testing, particularly unsystematic random testing, where the individuals to be tested are selected subjectively, has been looked upon with distrust by the courts who are fearful of abuses in selection.[5] Similarly, surprise, mass testing has been held to be unlawful.[6]

With specific evidence of the need to test, the courts are more inclined to uphold the testing. Drug testing of certain employees who were identified in reports as drug users has been upheld.[7] Post-accident testing also has been upheld. In *Division 241, Amalgamated Transit Union v. Suscy,*[8] the Seventh Circuit upheld the Chicago Transit Authority's rule mandating drug testing for bus drivers involved in a serious accident or suspected of being intoxicated.

The courts have not required "probable cause" before upholding an individual drug test. "Reasonable suspicion," a lesser standard, has been widely adopted.[9] "The 'reasonable suspicion' test requires that to justify this intrusion, officials must point to specific, objective facts and rational inferences that they are entitled to draw from these facts in the light of their experience."[10]

Reasonable suspicion goes to individual drug testing. An unresolved issue is whether evidence of widespread drug abuse in the community or a problem within a group of workers is needed to justify wider testing. In *Lovvorn v. City of Chattanooga,*[11] the drug testing of fire fighters was struck down because of a lack of reasonable suspicion of the need to test:

> The City has not pointed to any objective facts concerning deficient job performance or physical or mental deficiencies on the part of its fire fighters, either in general or with respect to specific personnel, which might lead to a reasonable suspicion upon which tests could be based.[12]

How Is the Testing Performed?

The testing procedures used may affect the legality of the testing. In *Jones v. McKenzie,*[13] the court held that the use of an unconfirmed EMIT test, which violated a specific regulation mandating confirmation, was arbitrary and capricious.[14] Confirmatory testing, such as the use of gas chromatography/mass spectronomy to confirm an initial immunoassay, will increase the accuracy of the test and the likelihood of legality. In *National Treasury Employees Union v. von Raab,*[15] the Fifth Circuit upheld drug testing by the Customs Service in large part because of specific measures to ensure the reliability of test results. These measures included confirmatory testing, chain-of-custody procedures, allowing the employee to choose a laboratory for retesting, and a quality assurance program.

Safeguarding the chain-of-custody of the specimen is necessary to eliminate the possibility of confusion, mishandling, or sabotage. In addition, it may be necessary to retain the sample to allow for independent confirmation of the results. In *Banks v. FAA,*[16] the discharges of air traffic controllers were set aside because the urine samples had been destroyed before they could be retested by an independent laboratory.

A final issue relates to sample collection. The courts have recognized a substantial privacy interest in urination.

> There are few activities in our society more personal or private than the passing of urine. Most people describe it by euphemisms if they talk about it at all. It is a function traditionally performed without public observation; indeed, its performance in public is generally prohibited by law as well as social custom.[17]

Consequently, direct observation of urination is unlikely to be upheld. In *Caruso v. Ward,*[18] police officers were required to urinate in the presence of a superior officer of the same sex to ensure the regularity of the sample.

The court found this process especially troublesome. "[T]he subject officer would be required to perform before another person what is an otherwise very private bodily function which necessarily includes exposing one's private parts, an experience which even if courteously supervised can be humiliating and degrading. . . ."[19]

What Is Done with Test Results?

Workplace drug testing programs are more likely to be upheld if individuals who test positively are rehabilitated rather than discharged.[20] This often relates closely with the duty to make reasonable accommodation to handicapped workers. For example, in *Hazlett v. Martin Chevrolet, Inc.,*[21] an employer was found to have violated Ohio's handicap discrimination law by discharging an employee suffering from drug and alcohol addiction and refusing to grant a one month disability or sick leave so that the employee could obtain treatment. Employees with other illnesses previously had been given leaves.

The Elements of a Legal, Ethical, and Effective Drug Testing Program

If there is one general criticism that can be leveled at managers in the public and private sectors regarding drug testing, it is that they have too eagerly embraced drug testing as *the* solution to the problem of workplace drug abuse. Before drug testing is implemented there must be a detailed and thoughtful consideration of whether there is a workplace drug abuse problem, whether drug testing is essential to combat the problem, whether the benefits of drug testing outweigh the costs to employers and employees, and whether drug testing can be undertaken in a way that will ensure accuracy, fairness, and privacy.

While some people have recommended unrestricted drug testing or no drug testing at all, there is a growing consensus—from the AFL-CIO[22] to the AMA[23]—that limited drug testing is permissible. For example, the AMA's Council on Scientific Affairs recommended:

> That the AMA take the position that urine drug and alcohol testing of employees should be limited to: (a) preemployment examinations of those persons whose jobs affect the health and safety of others, (b) situations in which there is reasonable suspicion that an employee's job performance is impaired by drug and alcohol use, and (c) monitoring as part of a comprehensive program of treatment and rehabilitation of alcohol and drug abuse or dependence.[24]

Placing careful controls on drug testing is an attempt to accommodate the legitimate concerns about test accuracy and privacy with legitimate concerns about public health and safety. It is even more difficult to move beyond generalities to concrete guidelines on workplace drug testing. A legal, ethical, and effective drug testing program should satisfy each of the following requirements:

1. *Reasonable suspicion exists to believe that there is at least some class-wide problem of drug abuse among the relevant group of employees.* Drug testing is an extreme measure and it should not be undertaken lightly. The only compelling reason to test is to protect employee and public safety. Although drug testing should not be started only *after* a tragic accident, there are sound reasons why it should not be initiated unless there is at least some evidence of a drug abuse problem in the locality, in a particular profession or job classification, or at a particular employer.[25] One way of determining whether there is a problem at a particular workplace is for all employees to take a drug test anonymously. The results will indicate whether there is a problem and, if so, its nature and scope. This information also is valuable in designing education and rehabilitation programs.[26]
2. *There are no feasible alternatives to detecting impairment, including supervision and simulation.* The primary concern underlying drug testing is that drug-impaired employees will be impaired on the job. Drug testing, however, does not measure impairment. It measures prior exposure, which is used as a surrogate for impairment based on one of the two following theories. First, employees who use drugs off the job are more likely to use drugs on the job or to report to work under the influence of drugs.[27] Second, prior drug use may impede performance even though no impairment is noticeable.[28] If impairment or the effects of impairment are detectable, then there is no need for drug testing. One way to detect impairment is through regular, close supervision.[29] Another way is for the employee to demonstrate fitness via simulation.[30]
3. *The drug testing program is limited to workers who, if working while impaired, would pose a substantial danger to themselves, other persons, or property.* Among the numerous asserted justifications for employee drug testing are the following: (1) Drug use is illegal and therefore employers have a responsibility to discover employees who may be breaking the law; (2) Drug abusing employees often need substantial sums of money to buy drugs and these employees are likely to steal from their employer or to accept bribes on the job; (3) Employees using drugs are likely to have a reduction in their productivity; (4) Maintaining a drug-free workplace is essential to an employer's public image; and (5) Drug testing is essential to protect safety and health.

   First, as to illegality, it is clear that employers are not concerned about illegality per se. If they were concerned simply about law-breaking, measures other than drug testing are likely to be much more effective in detecting wrongdoing. For example, an employee (and management) federal income tax return screening every April 15th would undoubtedly be quite revealing. Of course, it is the province of the Internal Revenue Service and not the employer to detect tax irregularities. Similarly, it is the responsibility of law enforcement agencies and not employers to prevent illegal drug use.

Second, as to theft and bribery, the sudden need for more money to support a drug habit is only one reason why an employee might become dishonest. To be thorough, employers would need to know if an employee were gambling, suffering losses in the stock market, or even having an extra-marital affair. Preemployment background and reference checks and post-hiring supervision and auditing are much more effective in preventing theft and bribery than urine testing.

Third, productivity is a legitimate concern of an employer. Productivity, however, is directly measurable and is done so on a continual basis by employers. A decline in productivity is an end point and it is irrelevant whether the decline is caused by boredom, personal problems, or drug abuse. Lack of productivity is a better measure of possible drug use than urine testing.

Fourth, from a legal and policy standpoint, public image is a deeply troubling rationale for employment policies. Historically, many forms of employment discrimination have been defended on grounds such as "customer preference."[31] The law has correctly rejected such asserted defenses. Public image is not only so vague to justify nearly any action,[32] but in the case of drug testing, it is a two-edged sword. Drug abuse in the United States is a pervasive, intractable social problem and the fact that an employer has, among its employees, one or more individuals with a substance abuse problem is unlikely to generate public disdain. The way in which the employer deals with the problem, however, may directly affect a public image. Indiscriminate and heedless drug testing without regard for employee rights can influence the way in which the employer is regarded by current employees, potential employees, customers, and shareholders.

Fifth, safety is the only justifiable reason for employee drug testing. It is true that current drug tests do not measure impairment and only measure prior exposure. Nevertheless, there is ample evidence that individuals who use drugs often take them at work or report to work impaired.[33] For employees in safety-sensitive positions, prudence demands that public safety considerations outweigh even the legitimate concerns of employees.[34] For employees not in safety-sensitive positions, such as retail or clerical workers, there is no justification for drug testing. Reasonable supervision will ensure that satisfactory performance is not impeded for any reason, including drugs.

If safety is the only compelling reason for drug testing, the nature of this exception needs to be further defined. The danger posed by an impaired worker must be *substantial.* This is based on the severity of the consequences, the likelihood of danger, and the immediacy of the harm. To justify drug testing, the risk of harm from an impaired worker also must be otherwise unpreventable (as by supervision, quality control, and work review) and the consequences irreparable. Nuclear power, chemical plant, and transportation workers are the best examples.[35] Even as to these employees, however, the other elements still need to be satisfied.[36]

4. *Testing not based on individualized, reasonable suspicion is limited to preemployment and periodic testing.* Preemployment and periodic testing (especially as part of a preemployment or annual medical examination) are the least objectionable forms of testing. They permit the discovery of individuals who have a substance abuse problem within the context of a medical examination. There is no stigma attached to supplying a urine sample in this context. The medical setting also helps to encourage truthful disclosure by a substance-abusing employee, protects confidentiality, and facilitates treatment.

   The other acceptable time for testing is when there is reasonable suspicion of impairment. This is a closer case. If an employee in a safety-sensitive job is observed to be drowsy, dizzy, disoriented, or otherwise is suspected of being impaired, regardless of the results of a drug test, the employee should not be permitted to continue work and should be referred to a physician. Thus, the need for a drug test under these circumstances may be questioned because the behavior establishing reasonable cause also demands action immediately and cannot await the results of a drug test.[37] The other issue raised by reasonable cause testing is that clear guidelines must be established for determining reasonable cause. Without such guidelines there is a danger of arbitrariness in selecting the employee for testing.[38]

   Despite the drawbacks of reasonable cause testing, employers should be provided with some basis for aperiodic or unprogrammed testing. Recreational as well as compulsive drug users may be able to forego the use of drugs for a short period of time each year to test negatively. In those job categories where drug testing is acceptable, it ought to be effective. Reasonable cause testing, including post-accident testing, should be permissible.

   Some people have suggested (and some statutes have used the approach)[39] that the *only* permissible drug testing is for reasonable cause. For employees working alone (such as truck drivers), it is hard to imagine that there ever would be reasonable cause until after a tragic accident occurred. Thus, reasonable cause testing should not be the only basis for drug testing.

   Random testing and surprise, round-up testing are unacceptable. As noted earlier, these tests have been struck down in several public sector cases on constitutional grounds.

5. *State of the art screening and confirmatory test procedures are performed by trained professionals, off-site, under laboratory conditions.* Employers that use "do-it-yourself" drug testing kits and unconfirmed screening tests are engaged in a false economy. Unless the best technology is used, drug test results are unreliable and likely to be challenged in court. Even the best analytical techniques are only as good as the people performing the tests. Careful laboratory selection and ongoing quality review are essential.
6. *Specimen collection is not observed.* With the growth of employee drug testing there have been numerous reports of employees attempting to substitute "clean urine"[40] or otherwise tampering with specimens.[41] Some employers, in response, have taken to observing employees in the act of urination. For many employees, this aspect of drug testing is the most objectionable, degrading, and insensitive element. It is highly unlikely that the benefits of observation (preventing tampering by a few individuals whose drug problems were not otherwise detectable) outweigh the human relations, employment relations, and public relations costs of observation.
7. *Testing is performed for the presence of prescription drugs and alcohol as well as illicit drugs.* If the underlying purpose of drug testing is safety, there is no reason why drug testing should be limited to illicit drugs. In terms of the number of people who abuse them and the fatalities, injuries, and property damage caused by their effects in the workplace, alcohol and prescription drugs (often in combination) pose a much greater threat than illicit drugs.[42]
8. *There is valid employee consent before the testing and an opportunity to explain a positive test result.* An argument could be made that consent to drug testing is never voluntary (or valid) when employees are likely to be discharged or applicants not hired if they refuse. Nevertheless, if drug testing is essential to protect public safety in the face of a drug abuse problem by certain employees, and if the other criteria for testing are met, an employer ought to be able to make consent to drug testing a condition of employment. Employers, however, should not perform drug testing surreptitiously, such as by simply testing all urine samples obtained as part of a preemployment or periodic medical examination.[43]

A related issue is whether applicants and employees should be given advance notice that a preemployment or periodic drug test will be performed. Some federal[44] and state[45] laws specifically mandate advance notice, but there is generally no such legal requirement. The obvious drawback to notice is that it permits individuals to abstain before being tested and then to resume drug use after the test. This drawback, however, may be outweighed by the following considerations. First, providing employees with notice improves employee acceptability of the program. It indicates that the purpose of the testing is to promote public safety and not to "catch" employees. Second, as to applicants, company resources will be saved because habitual drug users will not proceed further with their application. Third, individuals genuinely interested in obtaining or retaining employment may cease using drugs before the test, and surveillance, supervision, and retesting may ensure that they do not resume drug use.

Finally, individuals should be given an opportunity to explain a positive test result. Even state of the art confirmatory testing may produce false positive results due to laboratory error or cross-reactivity with some medicines and foods.

9. *Test results are kept confidential.* Drug test results should be regarded in the same way as other medical records. Specifically, the data should be stored in the medical department (assuming there is one) and access should be limited to medical personnel. Supervisory and managerial employees should only be notified of the consequences of the results (e.g., employee A is medically unfit for work), but not the specific results.[46] Other information essential to personnel actions should be provided only on a "need-to-know" basis. When an initial drug screen is positive and a confirmatory test is scheduled, no results should be released until after the confirmatory test. The failure to maintain confidentiality may lead to liability based on invasion of privacy, defamation, intentional infliction of emotional distress, or other torts.
10. *The test procedures or resulting personnel actions do not violate applicable legal rights of applicants and employees.* A wide range of constitutional, statutory, and common law doctrines may be implicated by drug testing. Both the testing itself and any personnel actions based on the testing must be in accordance with these legal requirements.
11. *Drug testing is only part of an overall drug abuse program, including education and rehabilitation.* Drug testing should be only one part, and indeed should be the least important part, of a comprehensive drug abuse program. The other two components of the program should be drug awareness and employee assistance.

    Drug awareness programs are educational activities aimed at supervisors and employees. Supervisors need to be trained to recognize some of the "suspect changes in employee job performance and behavior that may portend a drug abuse problem."[47] They also need to be trained in how to respond to employees suspected of having a drug abuse problem.

    Employees also should be involved in a separate drug education program. Although there are several different models of programs, all programs teach employees to recognize the signs of drug abuse in themselves, family, friends, and co-workers. All programs also discuss the dangers of drug abuse and describe company and community services available for dealing with drug abuse.[48]

The other essential part of a drug abuse program is an employee assistance program (EAP). There are 8,000[49] to 10,000[50] EAPs today, giving about twenty percent of the work force access to such a program.[51] Most of the EAPs are in large companies.[52] Some of the programs are run in-house, others are run on a contract basis. Both types of EAPs work the same way. An employee may voluntarily enter the program or may be referred by a supervisor. The employee contacts the EAP and works out an individual treatment program. Participation in an EAP is kept confidential. In some instances, employer discipline is waived on the condition that the employee complete the EAP.

Conclusion

Drug abuse in America and drug abuse in American workplaces are complicated problems. Drug abuse will not be eliminated or even brought under control simply through law enforcement, military action, public relations campaigns, rehabilitation, legalization of certain drugs, or prohibiting any current drug user from obtaining private or public employment. Similarly, a facile solution to the problem of workplace drug abuse will not be found in a specimen jar or a million specimen jars.

At best, drug testing is a sometimes-necessary evil that is part of a comprehensive program to ensure the public health and safety. At worst, it is an unholy alliance of politics, profiteering, unrestrained technology, and heedless personnel policies.

The efficacy and desirability of drug testing in the workplace will continue to be weighed by judges, legislators, and policy makers in the public and private sectors. In making these decisions, it is essential to consider the limits of technology, the inability of drug testing to resolve the underlying problem of drug abuse, and the human and organizational costs of implementing drug testing programs. Drug testing must be considered in the light of established employment law principles, such as equal opportunity, job-related decisionmaking, and reasonable accommodation. Drug testing also must be viewed in the larger context of a society that is built on values of autonomy, privacy, and dignity.

References

1. *See* Everett v. Napper, 825 F.2d 341, 345 (11th Cir. 1987); *Lovvorn,* 647 F. Supp. at 882.
2. *See* Skinner v. Railway Labor Executives Ass'n, 109. S. Ct. _____ (1989).

3. *See, e.g.,* Bostic v. McClendon, 650 F. Supp. 245 (N.D. Ga. 1986).
4. *See* Curry v. New York City Transit Authority, 86 A.D.2d 857, 450 N.Y.S.2d 399 (App. Div.), *aff'd,* 56 N.Y.2d 798, 437 N.E.2d 1158, 452 N.Y.S. 2d 401 (1982).
5. *See* Feliciano v. City of Cleveland, 661 F. Supp. 578 (N.D. Ohio 1987).
6. Capua v. City of Plainfield, 643 F. Supp. 1507 (D.N.J. 1986).
7. *Allen,* 601 F. Supp. 482, *Turner,* 500 A.2d 1005; King v. McMickens, 120 A.D.2d 351, 501 N.Y.S.2d 679.
8. 538 F.2d 1264 (7th Cir), *cert. denied,* 429 U.S. 1029 (1976).
9. *See, e.g., City of Palm Bay,* 475 So. 2d 1322; *Caruso,* 133 Misc. 2d 544.
10. *City of Palm Bay,* 475 So. 2d at 1326.
11. 647 F. Supp. 875 (E.D. Tenn. 1986).
12. *Id.* at 882.
13. 628 F. Supp. 1500 (D.D.C. 1986), rev'd in part on other grounds, 833 F.2d 335 (D.C. Cir. 1987).
14. *But see* Satterfield v. Lockhead Missiles & Space Co., 617 F. Supp. 1359 (D.S.C. 1985); *Turner,* 500 A.2d 1005.
15. 816 F.2d 170 (5th Cir. 1987), *aff'd,* 109 S. Ct. ______ (1989).
16. 687 F.2d 92 (5th Cir. 1982).
17. *National Treasury Employees Union,* 816 F.2d at 175.
18. 133 Misc. 2d 544, 506 N.Y.S. 2d 789 (S. Ct. 1986).
19. *Id.* at 548, 506 N.Y.S.2d at 793.
20. *See* Exec. Order No. 12564, 51 Fed. Reg. 32,889 (1986).
21. 25 Ohio St. 3d 279, 496 N.E.2d 478 (1986).
22. *See* Ellenberger, *AFL-CIO Urges Privacy Protection, Treatment in Drug Abuse Testing.* BUS. & HEALTH, Oct. 1987, at 58.
23. Council on Scientific Affairs, American Medical Association, *Issues in Employee Drug Testing,* 258 J.A.M.A. 2089 (1987).
24. *Id.* at 2095. In the interest of disclosure, it should be noted that the author was the legal consultant to the American Medical Association in the drafting of this recommendation.
25. This information may come in many forms, such as drug-related arrests of employees, direct observation of drug use or discovery of drugs in the workplace, drug-related accidents, reliable reports by employees and supervisors, and published studies.
26. I am indebted to Dr. E. Carroll Curtis, Corporate Medical Director of Westinghouse Electric Corporation, for this suggestion.
27. *See* Bureau of National Affairs, *Alcohol and Drugs in the Workplace* 15 (1986) (cocaine hotline survey showed 83% of callers used some drug on the job); Note, *Employee Drug Testing—Issues Facing Private Sector Employees,* 65 N.C.L. REV. 832 (1987) (citing National Institute of Drug Abuse survey showing 10-23% of all workers use drugs at work, 90% of cocaine users use it during work hours).

28. One controversial study of airline pilots showed that impairment from marijuana continued for 24 hours after exposure. *Alcohol and Drugs in the Workplace, supra* note 27, at 17. This study has been attacked on methodological grounds and seems to contradict prior studies. Glasser, *Why Indiscriminate Urine Testing is a Bad Idea,* 1 SEMINARS IN OCCUP. MED. 253, 256 (Dec. 1986).

29. Supervision would not necessarily detect *drug* impairment, but would detect reduced efficiency. From an employer's perspective it should not matter whether the reduced efficiency is caused by drugs, lack of sleep, personal problems, or other factors. Only the treatment of the problem will be affected.

30. It has been suggested, for example, that rather than performing drug testing on airline pilots, the pilots should be required to demonstrate their fitness on a flight simulator periodically. Although the feasibility of such an approach may be questioned, the theory cannot be assailed.

31. For example, the policy of many airlines in hiring only female flight attendants was based in large part on the airlines' assessment that its mostly male business travelers would prefer female flight attendants. *See* Diaz v. Pan Am. World Airways, 442 F.2d 385 (5th Cir.), *cert. denied,* 404 U.S. 950 (1971) (rejecting defense).

32. The American Occupational Medical Association's (now known as the American College of Occupational Medicine) *Guidelines on Drug Screening* includes the following:

    > Any requirement for screening for drugs should be based on reasonable business necessity. Such necessity might involve safety for the individual, other employees, or the public, security needs, requirements related to job performance, or requirement for a particular public image.

    American Occupational Association, *Drug Screening in the Workplace: Ethical Guidelines,* 28 OCCUP. MED. 1240 (1986). The "public image" language is so open-ended as to render the guidelines meaningless. For an opposite view from the medical community, opposing drug testing, *see* Lundberg, *Mandatory Unindicated Urine Drug Screening: Still Chemical McCarthyism,* 256 J.A.M.A. 3003 (1986).

33. *See supra* note 27.

34. Some people have suggested that if any employees are tested, all employees be tested. I disagree. Drug testing is a sometimes-necessary evil that should be restricted to the fewest number of workers possible.

35. It is difficult to imagine a job in which there is a substantial risk to property but not to at least some person, where the employee is unsupervised, and where all of the other criteria set out in this article are met. Nevertheless, in such an event, a substantial danger to property would justify drug testing.

36. Testing airline pilots for illicit drug usage is widely recommended, but the testing probably will be valuable only in serving to reassure anxious passengers. According to the National Transportation Safety Board, since 1964 not a single pilot involved in the crash of a U.S. commercial aircraft tested positive for alcohol. Presumably, this would extend to other drugs as well. Accordingly, the American Medical Association does not recommend the testing of civilian flight crews. *See* Engleberg, Gibbons, & Doege, *Review of the Medical Standards for Civilian Airmen: Synopsis of a Two-Year Study,* 255 J.A.M.A. 1589 (1986).

37. A common justification for drug testing under these circumstances is to obtain proof of drug usage in order to have a discharge sustained by an arbitrator in the event of employee challenge. Most collective bargaining agreements, however, prohibit intoxication or impairment and a drug test would not prove anything except prior exposure. Thus, the best evidence to support a discharge would be the careful documentation of the employee's behavior.
38. An employee who worked where there was reasonable cause testing recently sought my help with the following problem. He and his supervisor did not get along and on numerous occasions the supervisor made him submit to a drug test. Each time the test was negative. The employee was concerned, however, that his chances for promotion would be adversely affected if his personnel file showed numerous for-cause drug tests, even though they were all negative. Certainly, the possibility exists for even more invidious forms of discrimination besides personal animosity.
39. SAN FRANCISCO POLICE CODE art. 33A, §§ 3300A.1 to 11 (1985); Glasser, *supra* note 28, at 258; Joseph, *Fourth Amendment Implications of Public Sector Work Place Drug Testing,* 11 NOVA L. REV. 605, 641 (1987); Panner & Christakis, *The Limits of Science in On-the-Job Drug Screening, Hastings Center Rep.,* Dec. 1986, 11; Russo & Sparadeo, *supra* note 18, at 302.
40. *See* Zeese, *Drug Hysteria Causing Use of Useless Urine Tests,* 11 NOVA L. REV. 815-819 (1987); Note, *Jar Wars: Drug Testing in the Workplace,* 23 WILLAMETTE L. REV. 529, 546 (1987).
41. *Id.*
42. *See* McBay, *Efficient Drug Testing: Addressing the Basic Issues,* 11 NOVA L. REV. 647, 650-51 (1987); Ross & Walsh, *supra* note 6.
43. There is no physician-patient relationship established between an applicant or employee and an employer-retained physician who is merely assessing fitness to work. M. Rothstein, *Medical Screening of Workers* 4-8 (1984). Therefore, there is no legal duty to inform test subjects what laboratory procedures will be performed on specimens, the results of the tests, or the effect of test results on employability. Consequently, some individuals could be denied employment on the basis of a drug test when they were unaware they were being tested for drugs.
44. Exec. Order No. 12564, 51 Fed. Reg. 32,889, 32,890 (1986), requires federal agencies to give employees 60 days notice before implementing a drug testing program, but individual notice before testing is not required.
45. Iowa H.F. 469 (1987) (30 days notice for regular physical examinations); MONT. CODE ANN. §39-2-304 (1987) (two weeks notice before annual physical examination); VT. STAT. ANN. tit. 21, ch. 5, § 512(b)(2)(1987) (10 days notice to applicants).
46. The Code of Ethical Conduct of the American College of Occupational Medicine (ACOM) provides that "[p]physicians . . . should recognize that employers are entitled to counsel about the medical fitness of individuals in relation to work, but are not entitled to diagnoses or details of a specific nature." AMERICAN COLLEGE OF OCCUPATIONAL MEDICINE CODE OF ETHICAL CONDUCT, 1988 (reprinted as the appendix to chapter 21).

47. Nelson, *Drug Abusers on the Job,* 23 J. OCCUP. MED 403 (1981).
48. *See* McLatchie, Grey, Johns, & Lomp, *A Component Analysis of an Alcohol and Drug Program: Employee Education,* 23 J. OCCUP. MED. 477 (1981).
49. Masi, *Employee Assistance Program,* 1 OCCUP. MED. STATE OF THE ART REVS. 653 (1986).
50. Bureau of National Affairs, *supra* note 27, at 39.
51. *Id.* at 40.
52. *Id.*

Chapter 8

*Employee Screening: AIDS Testing**

Mark A. Rothstein, J.D.

Americans have virtually limitless confidence in the ability of new technology to solve problems. In some instances, however, this confidence has been misplaced, either because the new technology was deficient or because it was introduced without a thorough consideration of its legal, ethical, and social consequences. The medical screening of workers for AIDS and AIDS-related conditions presents a case in point of the benefits and dangers of technological responses to new problems.

In part, that is because medical screening of workers brings together two fields—health care and personnel management—each of which has a propensity to apply new technology to problems that have significant non-technological dimensions. For example, in the health-care field, new technologies such as the artificial heart, in vitro reproductive techniques, and heroic life support systems all raise important social issues. Similarly, many personnel managers have waded into controversy by too casually using polygraphs to combat pilferage, psychological testing to screen out applicants with behavioral problems, and urinalysis to counter drug abuse.

Given these inclinations, it was predictable that one response to the threat of AIDS in the workplace would be a call for massive blood screening of applicants and employees, leading to the rejection or dismissal of all whose test results appear to reveal infection by the Human Immunodeficiency Virus (HIV), the virus associated with AIDS. But while the development of the HIV antibody test was an important step in combatting the spread of AIDS through donated blood, its use in employment screening is both medically

*This chapter is reprinted, with permission, from "Screening Workers for AIDS" by Mark A. Rothstein, which appeared in *AIDS and the Law: A Guide for the Public,* edited by Harlon L. Dalton, Scott Burris, and the Yale AIDS Law Project (New Haven: Yale University Press, 1987, pp. 126–41).

and legally problematic. The most widely used test, ELISA, is not reliable when used for large-scale screening of people. Further, because HIV infection in itself neither endangers coworkers nor affects their ability to work, an employer has little need to know a worker's antibody status. Indeed, because antibody status is generally not relevant to employment decisions, its use by employers may violate laws prohibiting discrimination against the handicapped. Finally, even when properly used, the test generates information that must be kept confidential; any careless use could be very damaging to the worker and costly to the employer.

The first part of this chapter presents a framework for analyzing medical screening questions in general and AIDS-related screening in particular. The second section examines the HIV antibody test, explaining what information the test was designed to yield, and how accurately it does so. The third part describes the limitations placed on the screening of employees by local, state, and federal law. Finally, the chapter concludes that use of the test in employment screening, even if legal, creates serious practical and ethical problems that outweigh any possible benefits.

Medical Screening of Workers

General Principles

Unlike employee-initiated check-ups, medical screening of workers by employers is usually tied to an actual or potential employment action. For instance, medical screening at the hiring stage determines in part whether an applicant will be employed. Once an employee is on board, screening may be used to determine job assignment. Later, medical screening may be used periodically to determine continuing fitness for the job and, in the event of injury or illness, to find out when or whether the employee is fit to return to work. Thus, it is an integral part of employers' ongoing efforts to maintain a healthy, safe, and productive workforce, and to minimize the costs associated with accidents and illness.[1]

It is helpful to divide medical screening into the assessment of current health status and the assessment of future health status ("predictive screening"). An employer's appraisal of current health status involves determining whether an individual, with reasonable accommodation (such as adding ramps for workers unable to use stairs), can safely and efficiently perform the requirements of the job. Predictive screening, on the other hand, involves determining whether an individual who is currently capable of performing the job has an unacceptably high risk of developing future health problems that would preclude safe and efficient job performance. From a medical standpoint, it is sometimes difficult to distinguish between the two. From a legal standpoint, however, the distinction is often critical, because predictive screening is more likely to run afoul of laws prohibiting discrimination in employment on the basis of handicap.

Medical assessments of workers' *current* physical abilities and limitations have been used widely since the turn of the century and are relatively uncontroversial. Indisputably, certain jobs require good vision, hearing, reflexes, balance, strength, coordination, or other attributes, the presence of which can be determined by means of medical questionnaires, examinations, and laboratory procedures. (There is, of course, inevitable debate about which jobs require which attributes.)

Predictive screening, however, focuses not on current ability or capacity, but on the likelihood that the capacities of particular employees will be substantially diminished in the foreseeable future. This is a highly speculative enterprise because individuals vary markedly in their susceptibility to illness and impairment, for reasons scientists do not fully understand. Increasingly, however, certain genetic, biochemical, physiological, and behavioral factors have been correlated with increased risk of future health problems. The key to predictive screening is identifying these factors.

The list of predictive screening factors is long and varied, ranging from genetic make-up, through ethnic background, to lifestyle and occupational history. For some factors, such as cigarette smoking (especially in combination with certain occupational exposures, such as asbestos), there is overwhelming evidence of an increased risk of serious illness. For other factors, such as psychological make-up, the evidence of increased risk is only suggestive or theoretical.

Numerous considerations play a part in determining whether an employer is legally, medically, and ethically justified in restricting an individual's employment opportunities based on a finding of "increased risk." These considerations include relative risk, absolute risk, severity of consequences, reversibility of illness, latency of illness, risk acceptability, and risk management. For example, the longer the time until the health problem is expected to materialize, the more speculative the prediction is from a scientific standpoint. In turn, the weaker the scientific basis for predictive screening, the more problematic the screening is from a legal, ethical, and policy standpoint.

AIDS Screening

An employer's assessment of the current health status of persons with AIDS or ARC involves several inquiries. The first issue that usually arises is whether an individual with AIDS, ARC, or a related condition is too ill to perform a job safely and efficiently. This is a legitimate area of inquiry, so long as AIDS-related conditions are evaluated in the same manner as are other medical conditions. The employer's focus should not be on the condition itself, but rather on its effects. Exposure to HIV (and the consequent development of antibodies to it) does *not* in itself impair job performance. Persons with AIDS or ARC, however, must be evaluated on a case-by-case basis. Many persons with ARC have only intermittent or mild symptoms. Even individuals with clinical or "full-blown" AIDS may have periods of remission during which they are physically well enough to work and would benefit psychologically and financially from being allowed to do so.

Whenever an employee's or applicant's ability to work is impaired, a second question arises: would a reasonable adjustment in working conditions eliminate the problem? "Reasonable accommodation" to the special needs of workers with AIDS or ARC may be required by laws protecting the handicapped. (Workers who are seropositive and asymptomatic will normally not need special accommodations.) Adjustments that could help a person with AIDS or ARC remain on the job include flexible work schedules (to allow visits to the doctor) and transfers to less strenuous tasks.

A third question that often arises is whether working conditions pose a significant health risk to immunosuppressed employees. It is possible, though unlikely in most settings, that the risk of exposure to infections in the workplace is greater for a person with AIDS or ARC than is the risk elsewhere. Such decisions, however, should be made on an individual basis by a physician familiar with the worker's medical record.

A final question is whether a seropositive person, or one who has AIDS or ARC, poses a health risk to coworkers or the public. According to the Centers for Disease Control, there is no medical justification for refusing to employ health-care, personal-service, food-service, or other workers who have AIDS or ARC, or who have been exposed to the virus. To be sure, in the unlikely event a person with AIDS contracted an opportunistic infection that proved to be readily transmissible, the individual should be excluded from the workplace if less drastic means of protecting against transmission are not available. Such decisions, however, should be made case-by-case, and should be based on sound, first-hand medical opinion.

In contrast to these attempts to assess the current employability of persons with AIDS or ARC, HIV antibody testing of applicants and employees is a form of *predictive screening* that could lead to rejection or firing of currently fit individuals because they are deemed to pose a *future* health risk. As the following discussion will show, this use of the test is not medically justified at the present time. The most commonly used test and test format produce a large number of incorrect results when employed as a general screening tool. Furthermore, even a true positive test result does not tell us whether the tested individual actually has AIDS or ARC or is certain to develop either condition. Even if it were shown that all or substantially all seropositive persons eventually develop clinical AIDS, the inquiry would shift rather than end, and the question would arise whether a given individual was *currently* well enough to perform the job.

The HIV Test and What It Measures

In 1982, it was established that AIDS was being spread through the transfusion of blood and Factor VIII, a blood plasma product used by hemophiliacs. Although only two percent of reported AIDS cases had been traced to transfusion,[2] the Public Health Service and the Food and Drug Administration (FDA) issued guidelines on March 4, 1983, designed to ensure the safety of the nation's blood supply.[3] The guidelines asked blood-collection centers: (1) to provide information about AIDS to donors; (2) to ask donors specific questions regarding signs and symptoms of AIDS; and (3) to advise donors in high-risk groups that they should not donate blood.

The discovery of HIV at the end of 1984 paved the way for the development of tests to screen the nation's supply of blood and plasma. The National Cancer Institute (NCI) developed the initial technology, then awarded nonexclusive, royalty-bearing licenses to five private firms to produce commercial antibody tests.[4]

The ELISA test is relatively inexpensive, costing between two and three dollars a test.[5] To be accurate, however, an ELISA test with a positive result should be repeated and then confirmed by another test procedure. The most commonly used confirmation test, the Western Blot, is much more expensive (about a hundred dollars), difficult, and time-consuming to perform.[6]

It is important to note what the HIV antibody test does and does not measure. First, the test does *not* identify individuals with AIDS. The Centers for Disease Control defines AIDS by its clinical symptoms (such as the presence of opportunistic infections or Kaposi's sarcoma). While a positive antibody test may help support a diagnosis, the test is not a primary diagnostic tool.[7] Further, a positive test does not necessarily mean that a person will get AIDS in the future. Although estimates have been revised upward several times, it is projected that only from 25 to 50 percent of seropositive persons will develop AIDS within five to ten years of seroconversion.[8]

Second, the test does not identify individuals with ARC, whose definition is also based on clinical features (for instance, fever, weight loss, lymphadenopathy, diarrhea, fatigue, night sweats) and by laboratory abnormalities indicative of immunodeficiency. The test does not necessarily predict ARC, either. According to most estimates, only a quarter of seropositive persons who do not develop AIDS will develop ARC.[9]

Third, the test does not identify all blood containing the AIDS virus. Since it was designed to detect only nonneutralizing antibodies stimulated by the virus, the test would not identify an individual as positive during the period of time between exposure to the virus and seroconversion—the development of antibodies—which usually takes from six to eight weeks but may take a year or more.[10] It also would not identify as positive individuals whose immune systems were so severely damaged by the virus that they were not producing antibodies.[11] (To be sure, such seriously ill people are unlikely to be present in the employment setting.) On the other hand, a *false* positive result may be caused by contamination, technician error, or confounding medical conditions.[12]

Legal Issues

When the HIV antibody test was approved in March 1985, some observers expressed concern that the test might be used not just to screen donated blood but to screen people for employment and insurance.[13] Some of these fears have been borne out. Insurers have shown an increasing interest in the test;[14] private employers generally have not,[15] although AIDS-based employment discrimination reportedly is widespread.[16]

The federal government has sent mixed signals on the issue of testing. The CDC's *Guidelines on AIDS in the Workplace*[17] rejected the use of antibody testing for health care, personal-service, food-service, and other workers. "Because AIDS is a bloodborne, sexually transmitted disease that is not spread by casual contact, this document does *not* recommend routine HIV antibody screening for the groups addressed."[18] On March 13, 1986, however, the Public Health Service recommended that all individuals in high-risk groups be tested for HIV antibodies.[19] Although this latter recommendation is not directed at the workplace, it may serve inappropriately to focus employers' attention onto the sexual orientation of applicants and employees. Moreover, the federal government itself has extended its testing program to include all military personnel, participants in the Job Corps, and foreign-service employees of the State Department.[20]

The legality of various approaches to testing is no more settled than is their medical necessity. In a few states and municipalities, new laws specifically limit antibody testing and discrimination based on HIV status. In the rest of the country, the principal check on antibody screening is likely to be state and federal laws forbidding discrimination on the basis of handicap. Furthermore, some testing programs could possibly violate race- and sex-discrimination laws. Finally, prudent employers should be aware that the very collection and possession of such sensitive medical data imposes on them a duty of confidentiality and that breaches could result in costly liability.

State and Local AIDS Testing and Discrimination Statutes

California, Delaware, Florida, Iowa, Massachusetts, Rhode Island, Texas, Vermont, Washington, and Wisconsin have enacted laws regulating the use of HIV antibody tests by employers. Wisconsin's law is one of the most explicit, prohibiting both testing itself and the use of test results. As amended, the law provides that *unless* the state epidemiologist and the Secretary of Health and Social Services declare "that individuals who have [HIV] infections may, through employment, provide a significant risk of transmitting [HIV] to other individuals," employers are prohibited from: (1) soliciting or requiring as a condition of employment that any employee or applicant take an antibody test; (2) affecting the terms, conditions, or privileges of employment or terminating the employment of any employee who obtains an antibody test; and (3) entering into an agreement with an employee or applicant offering employment or any pay or benefit in return for taking an antibody test.[21]

A number of California cities, including Los Angeles[22] and San Francisco,[23] as well as Austin[24] and Philadelphia,[25] have enacted ordinances prohibiting discrimination in employment based on AIDS. These laws also extend protection to people who have ARC, carry HIV, or are merely believed to be in a high-risk group. San Francisco specifically prohibits AIDS testing unless the employer can show that the absence of AIDS is a bona fide occupational qualification.

Federal and State Handicap Discrimination Statutes

The federal Vocational Rehabilitation Act and similar laws in virtually every state prohibit discrimination in employment on the basis of handicap. These may provide the best sources of protection against AIDS-based discrimination. In addition to probably prohibiting discrimination (in hiring and firing, and in the terms and conditions of employment) directed against persons having or believed to have AIDS or related medical conditions, handicap-discrimination laws also may prohibit employers from requiring or using the results of HIV antibody tests under most circumstances. The applicability of these laws to AIDS has been the subject of controversy.

In *School Board of Nassau County v. Arline,* the Supreme Court reserved for another day the question of what constitutes a "handicap" with regard to AIDS. However, in deciding that the Rehabilitation Act covered contagious diseases, the Court stressed that "society's accumulated myths and fears about disability and disease are as handicapping as are the physical limitations that flow from actual impairment."[26]

In 1988, Congress passed the Civil Rights Restoration Act over the veto of President Reagan. One provision of that law, section 9, amends the Rehabilitation Act to clarify the coverage of individuals with contagious diseases.

> (C) For the purpose of sections 503 and 504, as such sections relate to employment, such term does not include an individual who has a currently contagious disease or infection and who, by reason of such disease or infection, would constitute a direct threat to the health or safety of other individuals or who, by reason of the currently contagious disease or infection, is unable to perform the duties of the job.

Based on this amendment, an individual with a contagious disease is covered by sections 503 and 504 so long as the individual does not pose a direct threat to the health or safety of others and is able to perform the duties of the job. Furthermore, the legislative history of this provision, sponsored by Senators Tom Harkin of Iowa and Gordon Humphrey of New Hampshire, makes it clear that the amendment "does nothing to change the current laws regarding reasonable accommodation."

The several sections of the Rehabilitation Act regulate different types of employers, ranging from the federal government itself to organizations that receive federal funding. The specific provisions vary in the kinds of testing programs allowed, but the act generally prohibits covered employers from making preemployment inquiries about or testing to determine whether an applicant is handicapped, unless the inquiry or test is relevant to the applicant's ability to perform job-related functions.[27]

Department of Health and Human Services regulations implementing Section 504 of the Rehabilitation Act (the provision that applies to recipients of federal funds) preclude recipients of federal financial assistance from singling out individuals for medical screening:

> Nothing in this section shall prohibit a recipient from conditioning an offer of employment on the results of a medical examination conducted prior to the employee's entrance on duty, *Provided,* That: (1) All entering employees are subjected to such an examination regardless of handicap. . . .[28]

While requiring that medical examinations be given universally or not at all, the regulation quite sensibly does not insist that the medical procedures used on each individual be identical. Obviously, an individual's sex, medical history, and health status might alter the specifics of an examination. Nevertheless, another regulation implementing Section 504 provides that "a recipient may not make use of any employment test or selection criterion that screens out or tends to screen out handicapped persons or any class of handicapped persons" unless the test or criterion is shown to be job-related.[29] "Class of handicapped persons" is not defined but could be interpreted to include individuals who have been exposed to HIV and consequently are perceived to be handicapped. Identical regulations apply to Section 501 (the provision that covers federal agencies in their capacity as employers).[30]

The regulations implementing Section 503 (the provision that governs entities that enter into contracts with the federal government) permit preemployment medical examinations of handicapped applicants even if an examination is not required of the nonhandicapped. The regulations also provide, however, that if such examinations "tend to screen out qualified handicapped individuals," they may not be used unless they are "related to the specific job or jobs for which the individual is being considered and [are] consistent with business necessity and the safe performance of the job."[31]

Many state handicap-discrimination laws are worded quite generally and have not yet been interpreted judicially or administratively. Thus, it is not clear whether testing itself is generally illegal, though it is widely believed that the *use* of antibody test results in employment decision making is illegal absent a showing of job-relatedness.[32] A notable exception to the lack of clarity of state laws on this issue is California's Fair Employment Practice Law.[33] Regulations implementing that law specifically limit preemployment inquiries, medical examinations, and selection practice to job-related criteria.

In general, the standards that apply to job applicants apply to current employees as well. Thus, performing an HIV antibody test or inquiring into test results during a routine periodic medical examination may not violate handicap-discrimination laws, but the *use* of this information to deny employment opportunities (for example, promotions or desirable transfers) or as a basis for dismissal would most likely be prohibited.

For the most part, handicap-discrimination laws were not enacted with much consideration of their effect upon individuals at risk of *future* illness. Although high-risk individuals (as well as persons perceived to be at high risk) are probably covered by the law,[34] the courts are less clear about when the increased risk of illness will justify a refusal to employ. Speculation about future medical conditions will not justify an adverse employment decision,[35] but a *well-founded* concern about an employee's future health may permit an employer to screen out the individual.[36] Among the factors that a court would probably consider in deciding whether an employer may base a hiring decision on risk of future illness are the likelihood the illness will develop, its severity, the probable time period before the onset of the illness, the individual's risk relative to the employee norm, whether the employer has made an individualized determination of fitness, and whether reasonable accommodation is possible.[37]

Employers may, of course, have good-faith concerns about absenteeism, turnover, health-insurance costs, coworker preference, and customer preference. These defenses, however, usually have been rejected in handicap-discrimination cases involving other medical conditions. They are also likely to be rejected in AIDS cases in which the individual is currently able to perform the job. It is clear that these laws impose certain very real costs upon employers. They provide, however, in effect, that the policy in favor of equal employment opportunity for the handicapped takes precedence over productivity.

Other Antidiscrimination Laws

A single ELISA test has an acceptable level of accuracy only when performed on selected populations with a high prevalence of seropositivity. Thus, there is a sounder medical basis for testing in high-risk groups than in the general population. Selective testing, however, may raise legal problems. Employers may violate certain employment discrimination laws if they engage in selective AIDS antibody testing. For example, Wisconsin,[38] the District of Columbia,[39] and about fifty cities, including New York[40] and Philadelphia,[41] have laws prohibiting discrimination in employment based on sexual orientation. An employer who tests only known or suspected homosexuals would probably violate these laws.[42]

By engaging in *selective* HIV antibody testing, an employer also might run afoul of Title VII of the Civil Rights Act of 1964, which prohibits discrimination in employment on the basis of race, color, religion, sex, or national origin. For example, testing only Haitians would probably constitute discrimination on the basis of national origin. Testing only males, or only single males, would probably constitute sex discrimination. Finally, because black and Hispanic Americans are more likely than whites to contract AIDS,[43] it could be argued that use by employers of the HIV antibody test to screen out high-risk persons disproportionately excludes blacks and Hispanics from employment. If a Title VII case were brought, and if the court determined that the claim fell within the scope of the statute, the burden would shift to the employer to prove that seronegativity was a bona fide occupational qualification or was otherwise job-related, or that the HIV antibody test was justified by business necessity. Failure to satisfy this burden would result in victory for the applicant or employee.[44]

Disclosure of Test Results

An individual's HIV antibody test result is extremely personal, and disclosure of it could well lead to embarrassment and discrimination. Therefore, employers who require or otherwise obtain this information may be risking tort liability under a variety of legal theories. For example, actions might be brought for invasion of privacy based on inappropriate publication of the results; for defamation based on inaccurate disclosure of accurate results or accurate disclosure of inaccurate results; for negligence based on negligent maintenance of records, negligent reporting of results, or the failure to maintain the security of records; and for intentional infliction of emotional distress if an individual were subjected to harassment or ridicule by supervisors, coworkers, or customers after test results were disclosed.

Tort actions have already been brought based on the wrongful disclosure of analogous, highly personal information. For instance, in *Houston Belt & Terminal Railway v. Wherry,*[45] a railroad employee was tested for drugs when he fainted following an accident on the job. The initial test result showed a "trace" of methadone, but a follow-up test showed the presence of a normal compound whose characteristics resemble methadone. The employee was later discharged for failure to report his accident in a timely manner. The railroad wrote a letter to the Department of Labor stating that the employee "passed out and fell" and that "traces of methadone" were present in his system. The Texas Court of Civil Appeals affirmed an award of one hundred fifty thousand dollars in compensatory damages and fifty thousand dollars in punitive damages based on the railroad's libelous statements.

In another case, a Texaco employee sued his employer and supervisor for the tort of outrage and invasion of privacy based on his supervisor's alleged disclosure to other refinery employees that the plaintiff was undergoing psychiatric treatment.[46] The Supreme Court of Oklahoma denied the claim, stating that no action for invasion of privacy would lie where *"only a small group* of coworkers were made privy to Eddy's private affairs. . . ."[47] If an employer discloses private facts about an employee to the general public, however, it *would* constitute an invasion of privacy.

The first AIDS-related tort actions have already been filed. According to the complaint in one such case, the county health commissioner in Fayette County, Ohio, received an anonymous note stating than an employee of a local restaurant had AIDS. The commissioner then forwarded the note to the owner of the restaurant, who read it aloud at a meeting of restaurant employees. The employee, with twenty-two years of service, was fired. An action based on wrongful discharge and defamation against the county health commissioner and restaurant owner was brought in March, 1986, seeking $1.5 million in damages.[48] In another case, a Massachusetts court recognized a tort action for invasion of privacy where a supervisor failed to keep an employee's diagnosis of AIDS confidential.[49] Other tort actions undoubtedly loom on the horizon.

Some Final Thoughts on Testing

Like quarantine, testing has considerable appeal to many people who wish to "do something" about the spread of AIDS. Closer examination shows that worker screening is not a panacea, and, in fact, that its costs may exceed its benefits. Although some components of the situation, such as the accuracy of the test, may be expected to change, universal testing is now an expensive way for employers to generate information that they do not need and may not be allowed to use. Before embarking upon an extensive testing program of doubtful medical efficacy and legality, it is important to inquire into the motivation for the testing.

There are three possible motivations behind an HIV antibody testing program. First, there is a desire to protect the health of coworkers and customers. This does not justify use of the test. The overwhelming weight of medical evidence demonstrates that exclusion of even persons with clinical AIDS is unnecessary to protect the health of other people. Screening is more likely to be used to mollify coworkers and customers or to reduce health insurance and other perceived costs. Most people are in fact terribly afraid of AIDS, but a testing program may increase fear of the illness in the workforce without enhancing understanding; indeed, given the fear, an error-prone testing program could result in considerable resentment and panic.

Second, employers may expect economic benefits from HIV testing. But while some employees who have AIDS or ARC will generate considerable costs in benefit claims and reduced productivity, the test is not an effective way to address this problem. The use of the test in appraising current health status is unnecessary; seropositivity does not substantially affect the current ability to work and does not increase current costs for the employer; AIDS and ARC can be detected by the very symptoms that reduce the ability to perform on the job. Predictive screening might be used as a way to identify those people who at some time in the future may develop AIDS or ARC, but such a use, in addition to being imprecise, is probably illegal. If an employer may not *use* the results, why should employee relations be undermined and tort liability risked in obtaining and retaining such sensitive information?

Third, testing may be seen as a way to further public health generally and specifically the health of seropositive individuals. So far, federal health officials have not called for universal testing or nonvoluntary testing of high-risk individuals. But even if they eventually do, employers are badly suited to play this role. So long as employers can discriminate against persons with AIDS-related conditions, there is a basic conflict between the employer as surrogate public health official and the employer as employer. Furthermore, considerations of medical ethics strongly suggest that a medical test should not be performed unless some useful social purpose could be achieved. For asymptomatic seropositive individuals, however, there is nothing doctors can do. The same medical advice—in particular, avoidance of high-risk activities[50]—should be given to both seropositive and seronegative individuals. Being tested may be beneficial for some people, but it may also be very harmful, and the decision (certainly with regard to employment) should rest with the individual.[51]

New medical screening technology should not be introduced to the workplace setting without a thorough consideration of the relevant medical, legal, and social consequences.[52] This is particularly so when, as with AIDS, the effects of the test results are so crucial and wide-ranging.

References

1. M. Rothstein, Medical Screening of Workers 9 (1984).
2. *AIDS Antibody Screening Test,* 57 Analytical Chemistry 773A (1985).
3. 32 MMWR 101 (1983).
4. Petricciani, *Licensed Tests for Antibody to Human T-Lymphotropic Virus Type III,* 103 Annals Internal Med. 726, 727 (1985).
5. Levine & Bayer, *Screening Blood: Public Health and Medical Uncertainty,* Hastings Center Rep., Aug. 1985, at 8, 9.
6. For a technical discussion of how the ELISA test works, see Council on Scientific Affairs, American Medical Association, *Status Report on the Acquired Immunodeficiency Syndrome—Human T-Cell Lymphotropic Virus Type III Testing,* 254 J.A.M.A. 1343 (1985); *see Puzzling Western Blot Results Worry Nation's Blood Bankers,* Med. World News, Dec. 22, 1986, at 69.
7. *See Acquired Immune Deficiency Syndrome (AIDS) Update—United States,* 32 MMWR 309 (1983) (AIDS diagnosis requires underlying immunodeficiency and

presence of unexplained opportunistic infection or Kaposi's sarcoma in patient under sixty years of age); *AIDS Antibody Screening Test,* note 2 above ("Because the ELISA screening test detects only antibodies to the AIDS virus, it is not a test for AIDS virus and is not intended to diagnose AIDS").

8. Institute of Medicine, National Academy of Sciences, Confronting AIDS 91 (1986) [hereinafter *Confronting AIDS*]; *see also* Goedert, Biggar, Weiss, *et al., Three Year Incidence of AIDS in Five Cohorts of HTLV-III Infected Risk Group Members,* 231 Science 992 (1986).

9. Landesman, Ginzburg & Weiss, *Special Report—The AIDS Epidemic,* 312 New Eng. J. Med. 521, 522 (1985).

10. *Confronting AIDS,* note 8 above, at 45; Curran, *et al., The Epidemiology of AIDS: Current Status and Future Prospects,* 229 Science 1352, 1354 (1985); *see also* Marlink, *et al.,* 315 New Eng. J. Med. 1549 (1987) (letter) (low sensitivity of ELISA testing in early HIV infection).

11. Leeson, *HTLV-III Antibody Tests and Health Education,* 1 Lancet 911 (1986).

12. *See, e.g.,* Biggar, 315 New Eng. J. Med. 457 (1986) (letter) (possible nonspecific associations between malaria and HTLVIIILAV); Hunter, 2 Lancet 397 (1985) (letter) (persons with HLADR and HLADQW may test positive on ELISA; follow-up with Western Blot eliminates problem); Merianon, 1 Lancet 678 (1986) (letter) (persons with thalassemia may test positive on ELISA); Mortimer, Parry & Mortimer, *Which Anti-HTLV-III LAV Assays for Screening and Confirmatory Testing?* 2 Lancet 873 (1985) (persons with malaria may test positive on Western Blot); Mendenhal, *et al.,* 313 New Eng. J. Med 921 (1986) (letter) (persons with hepatitis may test positive on ELISA).

13. Bayer & Oppenheimer, *AIDS in the Workplace: The Ethical Ramifications,* Business & Health, Jan.–Feb. 1986, at 30, Levine & Bayer, note 5 above.

14. *See, e.g.,* Blaine, Iuculano & Clifford, Insurance Issues Related to AIDS (1986); Health Insurance Association of America. The Acquired Immunodeficiency Syndrome & HTLV-III Antibody Testing (Draft Position Statement, 1985); Kristof, *More Insurers Screen Applicants for AIDS,* N.Y. Times, Dec. 22, 1985, at 5.

15. *See, e.g., Companies Taking Low-Key Approach to AIDS in Workplace, Survey Finds,* 4 Empl. Rel. Weekly (BNA) 291 (1986); Lewin, *AIDS and Job Discrimination,* N.Y. Times, Apr. 15, 1986, at 30. But at least one private employer has been screening workers for HIV since spring 1986. *Newspaper Gives AIDS Tests,* N.Y. Times, Oct. 31, 1986, at A17.

16. *See, e.g.,* McCormack, *AIDS-Phobia Creates Discrimination in the Workplace,* Houston Post, Feb. 7, 1986; at 18E; Roth, *Many Firms Fire AIDS Victims Citing Health Risk to Coworkers,* Wall St. J., Aug. 12, 1985, at 19.

17. *Guidelines on AIDS in the Workplace,* 34 MMWR 682 (1985).

18. *Id.* (emphasis in original).

19. Altman, *U.S. Urges Blood Test for Millions With High Risk of AIDS Infection,* N.Y. Times, Mar. 14, 1986, at 1.

20. *See* Bayer & Levine, *Risks of Federal Screening,* N.Y. Times, Jan. 12, 1987, at A21; Bayer, Levine & Wolf, *HIV Antibody Screening: An Ethical Framework*

for Evaluating Proposed Programs, 256 J.A.M.A. 1768 (1986). The testing of foreign service employees has been challenged. Local 1812, American Fed. of Gov. Employees v. United States Dep't of State, No. 87-012) (D.D.C., filed Jan. 20, 1987) (reported in 2 AIDS Policy & Law (BNA), Jan. 28, 1987, at 1).

21. Wis. Stat. Ann. §103.15(2)(a), (2)(b), (3) (West Supp. 1985).
22. Los Angeles Code art. 5.8 §§45.80-45.93 (1985).
23. San Francisco Police Code §§3801-3816 (1985).
24. Austin Ord. No. 861211-V (Dec. 11, 1986).
25. Phila. Exec. Order No. 4-86 (Apr. 15, 1986).
26. 107 S. Ct. 1123, 1128 n.7, 1129 (1987).
27. 29 C.F.R. §1613.706 (1986); C.F.R. §60-741.6 (1986); 45 C.F.R. §84.14 (1986).
28. 45 C.F.R. §84.14(c) (1986).
29. *Id.* §84.13(a).
30. 29 C.F.R. §§1613.705-706 (1986).
31. 41 C.F.R. §60-741.6 (1986).
32. *See, e.g.,* Cecere, *AIDS Presents Many Legal Issues for Workplace,* Legal Times, Dec. 2, 1985; Leonard, *AIDS and Employment Law Revisited,* 14 Hofstra L. Rev. 11 (1985); Leonard, *Employment Discrimination Against Persons with AIDS,* 10 U. Dayton L. Rev. 681 (1985).
33. Cal. Admin. Code §§7293.5-7294.2 (1985).
34. *See, e.g.,* E. E. Black, Ltd. v. Donovan, 497 F. Supp. 1088 (D. Hawaii 1980).
35. *See, e.g.,* Bentivegna v. United States, 694 F. 2d 619 (9th Cir. 1982); Bucyrus-Erie Co. v. Department of Industry, Labor & Human Relations, 90 Wis.2d 408, 280 N.W.2d 142 (1979).
36. *See Donovan,* 497 F. Supp. 1088; *In re* State Div. of Human Rights, 118 A.D. 2d 3, 504 N.Y.S. 2d 92 (App. Div. 1986); *see also* Cal. Lab. Code §7293.8(d) (West Supp. 1986).
37. *See* M. Rothstein, note 1 above, at 121-29.
38. Wis. Stat. Ann. §111.36 (West Supp. 1985).
39. D.C. Human Rights Act §1-2512 (1986).
40. N.Y. (City) Admin. Code §§8-107-108.1 (1986).
41. Philadelphia Code §9-1103a(1) (1985).
42. In jurisdictions without sexual-orientation discrimination laws it would not be illegal to refuse to employ a homosexual because of animosity toward homosexuals. It may violate a handicap discrimination law, however, to refuse to employ a homosexual because of a belief that this person is more likely to contract AIDS.
43. *See* 35 MMWR 757, 758 (1986).
44. Testing only former drug users might violate the 1978 amendment to the Rehabilitation Act, which protects current and former drug abusers whose current abuse does not constitute a direct threat to the safety or property of others. 29 U.S.C. §706(7)(B) (1982).

45. 548 S.W. 2d 743 (Tex. App.), *cert. denied,* 434 U.S. 962 (1977).
46. Eddy v. Brown, 715 P.2d 74 (Ok. 1986).
47. *Id.* at 78 (emphasis in original).
48. Saxton v. Vanzant, No. 86-CIV-59 (Fayette Cty., Ohio Ct. C.P., filed Mar. 7, 1986) (reported in 1 AIDS Policy & Law (BNA), Apr. 23, 1986, at 3).
49. Cronan v. New England Tel. Co., 41 Fair Emp. Prac. Cas. (BNA) 1273 (Mass. Super. Ct. Aug. 15, 1986).
50. *See* Council of Scientific Affairs, note 6 above, at 1344.
51. *See* Bayer, Levine & Wolf, note 20 above.
52. *See generally* M. Rothstein, note 1 above, at 191-207.

Chapter 9

Occupational Health Nursing and Worksite Programs

Lisa B. Chace, M.S.N.
Richard D. Tucker, J.D., M.H.A.
Richard J. Torraco, B.S.N., M.S.
Patricia van Horne, R.N.

Familiarity with the worksite is a critical factor in developing successful occupational health services programs. Certain program components are impossible to correctly implement without understanding an employee's work demands. Preplacement screening, for example, requires tests and conclusions to be job-specific. Work-hardening programs, which prepare an injured worker for reintroduction into the workplace, require a simulation of jobsite demands. Medical diagnosis and treatment, particularly relating to arm pain, require a careful ergonomic evaluation of the injured worker's job. Tasks for these program elements and many others cannot be performed correctly solely from the hospital or clinic—they require worksite involvement.

Coordinating Injury Management with Worksite Involvement

When health care providers manage employee injuries, they must obtain many kinds of information from the employer in order to make appropriate recommendations. The importance of understanding employees' jobs and interacting with staff at their worksites is best illustrated by examining what could happen if injury management did not consider the worksite. An employee who experienced arm pain while doing assembly work, for example, would first go to the in-hospital program, where a medical history would be taken, an examination would be performed, and a diagnosis of possible carpal tunnel syndrome would be made. Without a detailed understanding of the employee's work, the physician treating this patient might take the employee out of work or prescribe "light duty" for two weeks. The employee then would either remain out of work or return to work with no direction to the employer from the health care provider other than an assignment of "light duty."

Unless the employee worked for a company that had a relatively sophisticated occupational health program of its own, the result might be that the employee would be placed in an inappropriate job that leads to further aggravation of the injury and possible long-term disability. This situation could create animosity between the employee and the employer if the employee believed the injury had been exacerbated as a result of the ignorance of the employer. Further, the health care provider might lose confidence in the employer's ability to handle cases such as this one and might be less likely to return the employee to work in the future.

The preceding example shows inefficient use of resources by the provider, a potentially harmful situation for the employee, and a costly solution for the employer. The employer would have to pay for both the injured employee's lost wages (in the form of disability or workers' compensation benefits) and the ongoing medical care. The employer also would have to replace the injured worker for an indefinite period of time. These are only some of the problems that result from an approach to injury management that is not intimately involved with the worksite.

An occupational health program that is more involved with the worksite might handle the same case as follows: After the injured employee had been seen in the hospital's program, the hospital's administrative or nursing personnel would contact the employer with information about the employee's injury assessment. A written report detailing the nature and extent of the injury, the treatment necessary, and a discussion of the employee's work capacity would then be submitted. The employee would return to work with specific, detailed restrictions on what he or she could and could not do (for example, an employee might need to avoid repetitive use of the right arm, pushing and pulling more than five pounds, and lifting more than five pounds). A worksite visit would be scheduled as soon as possible after the employee returned to work, and the provider, through an occupational health nurse, would review the alternative job placement, make any necessary modifications in the work being done, and review the original job to see how it might be modified to allow the employee to return to his or her original job.

As part of this on-site evaluation, the provider could educate both the employee and employer as to which specific activities in the employee's job caused the injury and what could be done to avoid these problems in the future. If in-hospital follow-up services were necessary, they would be scheduled according to the employee's work schedule and communicated to both the employee and the employer. If the employee were unable to work, the employer would be told how long the employee would be out so that other arrangements could be made. The provider could also continue to monitor the injured employee while he or she was working and could reschedule an evaluation with the physician if necessary.

The Role of the Occupational Health Nurse

The most important hospital staff member who routinely interacts with the worksite staff often is the occupational health nurse. The occupational health nurse can function as a cost-efficient extension of the physician and the hospital. The occupational health nurse serves as the liaison between the health care provider and the company and its employees in addition to providing assessment and monitoring skills at the worksite. The nurse's role requires a thorough understanding of the worksite and of the pressure facing the employee and the employer, as well as an ability to make practical and realistic recommendations based on the nature of the injury and the work being done.

To be an effective liaison, the nurse must be able to communicate with the most appropriate manager at the facility, be it a supervisor, a safety director, or a personnel representative. Because most employers are not accustomed to a hospital-based nurse visiting their facility as a part of patient care, the initial contact with the employer needs to be handled carefully. The employer, the employee, and the occupational health clinic should engage in a thorough discussion of the benefits of the nurse's on-site visit, emphasizing the mutual goal of returning injured employees to work.

A plant tour is valuable during the nurse's initial visit so that the nurse can get a general sense of the work environment, the types of jobs being performed, and the employee emphasis on safety. In some cases, however, employers will not permit the nurse to visit their facility or observe their employees. Some, fearing that employees' knowledge of the rehabilitation program may lead to an increase in the number of injuries, may allow the nurse to tour the facility with the stipulation that he or she not speak with employees.

The frequency of workplace visits by occupational health nurses varies depending on the number of employees being treated for work-related problems and the severity of their injuries. Visits may be on a weekly or monthly basis. Prior notification of the site visit should be given to the appropriate company contact. The visits should be an educational experience for both the employer and the clinic. One goal is to orient an employer toward thinking about effective methods of injury prevention for current jobs as well as for new jobs. Another goal is to make the provider aware of the production, ergonomic, and possible toxic exposure issues facing the industry.

One of the primary roles the occupational health nurse plays is to help an injured employee return to work either at full or modified capacity. This role often involves finding or creating a job that accommodates the injured employee's physical limitations rather than totally removing an employee from work after an injury. To do this, the nurse must frequently assess the workplace as an integral part of the worker reintegration process. The nurse becomes the first line of communication among the physician, the employee, and the immediate supervisor at the workplace.

It is important for the nurse to focus on the alternative employment opportunities available to a specific injured employee. A great deal of time can be saved if the injured employee and his or her supervisor are with the nurse when possible jobs are considered. This can help to eliminate misunderstandings regarding how the job is to be performed. The nurse can also assist in facilitating communication between an employee and his or her supervisor.

Listening to the employee is vital. The employee who has input in determining the work he or she performs during the rehabilitation period is more likely to be satisfied with the job and will be better prepared to cooperate physically with the program.

The occupational health nurse is in an excellent position to demonstrate to the employer and the employee how a job might be performed to prevent further injury. It is wise to suggest inexpensive or easily implemented modifications in order to increase the likelihood of their implementation. Basic principles of ergonomics are applied when assessing a potential workstation or job. For example, a person with a back injury may have restrictions that limit lifting, bending, and twisting. Changes in a workstation may be recommended to ensure that an employee's neck, arms, or back remain in a neutral position. Most jobs can be modified to eliminate twisting and bending by changing the height of the workstation and by relocating essential tools and materials. In addition, the nurse can demonstrate to the employee and the supervisor how to move about to avoid back strain. Hyperextension exercises can be taught at the workstation if the job requires back flexion. Suggesting that employees stand on rubber mats placed on the cement floor is an inexpensive modification. Steel-toed shoes or boots with added support and cushioning may also be recommended for employees whose jobs involve walking or standing on cement floors.

It is also important for the nurse to point out that if recommended procedures for an injured employee are implemented for the entire work force, they will aid in the prevention of future injuries and overuse syndromes among healthy employees. As the nurse works with an employer over a period of time, he or she will become familiar with factors that contribute to work-related injuries, such as each employer's production schedule, overtime policies, and pace of work. Knowledge of these factors is also important when designing limitations for any injured employee.

Occupational Nursing Delivery Models

Hospitals follow one of two models in their use of occupational health nurses. In one model, the nurse works out of the hospital's occupational health clinic and serves as a liaison to employers. In the other, the nurse works directly at one or more worksites providing a variety of services that the employers buy from the hospital.

Utilizing the clinic-based occupational health nurse in the reintegration of injured workers into the work force can be highly beneficial for both employers and the hospital. Employers should see their compensation costs decline when they establish a solid relationship with the local hospital through consistent medical contact. The hospital strengthens its relationships with employers through the worksite reintegration process and also increases the likelihood that it will be sought as a resource for additional health-related services.

Larger employers of 400 employees or more have traditionally provided in-house occupational medical clinics to maximize productivity while minimizing lost–work time and reducing workers' compensation costs. The small-to-medium-sized employer has needs similar to the large employer but often is unable to invest in the resources and capital equipment necessary to operate an in-house occupational medical department.

Hospitals have responded to the needs of these employers by providing qualified nurses to deliver a comprehensive system of occupational health services at the worksite with prevention as the primary focus. The major benefit of this "contract" service to the smaller employer is that hospitals provide only the number of weekly on-site nursing hours the employer actually needs, thereby limiting the employer's financial investment. The employer delegates the occupational health administrative and clinical responsibilities to the hospital-based program.

Both the smaller employer who contracts for 6 hours of nursing time each week as well as the larger employer who contracts for 40 hours of service each week can benefit from the hospital's systematic approach to the delivery of occupational health care, the hospital-based resources behind the program, the access to continuing education afforded the nurses, and above all, the assurance that qualified occupational health professionals are managing the entire system.

The occupational health nursing service can work equally well in both manufacturing environments and service-oriented business settings if the programs are flexible in adapting to the existing characteristics of the companies in which they function. Minor changes can be made to tailor the nursing service to company size, mission, and health service needs.

Essential Clinical Components of an On-Site Program

The most common services provided to both types of employers include return-to-work interventions, workers' compensation consultations, worksite clinical health management services, first-aid services, safety assessments, health screenings, and training services. These clinical components are essential to a successful workplace nursing program but are not necessarily all-inclusive. On-site nursing programs and their components should be specifically tailored to individual employers' needs.

Employers do not want their capital and human resources distracted and tied up by injuries, illnesses, workers' compensation premiums, and employee time away from work. An on-site nursing program addresses these concerns in several ways but does so most directly through return-to-work services.

Return-to-Work Services

If an employee is absent from work because of an illness or injury, and if there is no regular contact between the employee and the employee's supervisor or personnel representative, he or she can easily get "lost" in the course of medical care. Employees may know when they are scheduled for a medical appointment, but they may not know how and when this relates to when they can return to work.

The employee's physician is responsible for the medical aspects of an employee's treatment and recovery, but the physician generally is unfamiliar with the work tolerance and production aspects of various jobs. Will the physical restrictions necessary for the employee's recovery be compatible with the performance requirements of the employee's job when he or she returns to work? Is light- or limited-duty work that is compatible with the employee's physical restrictions available to the returning employee? Although supervisors or company representatives can respond to these workplace issues, they are unfamiliar with the medical aspects of the employee's case.

The on-site occupational health nurse is in the unique position of knowing the employee and his or her medical condition as well as the details of department work schedules and job requirements. The nurse's return-to-work intervention involves keeping in touch with ill or injured employees who are absent from work by providing employees with helpful advice and health guidance; letting them know what to expect before, during, and after a surgical procedure or medical treatment; and calling them during their absence to assure them that the company is concerned about their situation and is already preparing for their safe return to work. The nurse can also ensure that light- or limited-duty work is available and can communicate this information to the treating physician so that early return to work can be achieved.

Workers' Compensation Consultations

In addition to the substantial savings to the company that can be realized through nursing interventions to prevent lost-work time, nursing input can assist in the resolution of problematic workers' compensation cases. A company's human resources or benefits administration department can readily handle straightforward claims for injuries that are clearly work related. However, if the workers' compensation case is complicated by a claim resulting from a lengthy illness, a reinjury, or a case where malingering may be a factor, the assistance of the on-site occupational health nurse is needed to expedite the claim. Workers' compensation claims that are processed quickly result in cost savings to the company through insurance premium reductions.

Worksite Clinical Health Management Services

On-site health management is extremely popular with employers because it is responsive to their individual needs and is conveniently available at their workplaces. Individual employee medical records can be maintained on-site by the nursing program so that primary care can be delivered and documented. Nurses can then provide individual employee health services such as blood pressure monitoring, dressing changes, suture removal, health counseling, diet and nutrition counseling, and other types of assistance for health-related concerns. However, follow-up care for treatment initiated by the employee's physician is provided only after contacting the physician and obtaining necessary permission. If referrals to other health care providers are needed, the occupational health nurse screens the provider on the basis of such criteria as quality of care, payment provisions, and geographical location.

First-Aid Services

All employers, especially those engaged in potentially hazardous industries such as manufacturing and construction, should provide on-site first aid in the event of accident or injury. The Occupational Safety and Health Administration's general industry standards require that some form of first aid be available at the worksite. A part-time on-site nursing program can provide first-aid coverage during regularly scheduled hours each week. To provide coverage during other shifts and when the occupational health nurse is not on-site, first aid can be provided by a trained and certified employee team. In addition to initially training the first-aid team, the nurse can provide periodic refresher training and recertification. This team approach to providing first aid, which is directed by the nurse and supported by management, leads to a dynamic, responsive program of enthusiastic team members responsible for first aid who are an asset to the company.

Safety Assessments

The recognition of unsafe conditions on the job and the evaluation of unhealthful work practices are the goals of the "safety assessment," in which the occupational health nurse periodically tours all work areas to identify unsafe conditions and promote workplace health. If an occupational health program is to be truly effective in meeting its goals of promoting the safety and health of its work force, its operation cannot be limited to the four walls of the nurse's office. The program should be highly visible in all areas of the workplace and sensitive to individual employees' needs.

By conducting frequent walk-through assessments of all company work areas, the occupational health nurse can evaluate unsafe conditions and work behaviors and can conduct follow-up visits with individual employees to monitor their care at the work area. With each walk-through assessment, the nurse learns more about overall company operations, individual processes, and each employee's job. This information is vital to accurately assessing an employee's fitness for duty. Finally, having a health professional frequently present and available to employees in and of itself increases the general level of safety awareness among employees.

Health Screenings

Health screenings at the workplace can be divided into two groups:

- Health screenings of employees required by government, industry, or other regulations
- Health screenings of employees done for health promotion purposes

Both kinds of health screenings involve testing large numbers of employees for one or more bioassay, sensory, or other health parameters, such as blood pressure or hearing levels, for the purpose of identifying employees whose results may be normal, abnormal, or borderline. For health promotion screenings such as a serum glucose screening for diabetes, follow-up of employees whose results are borderline or abnormal includes employee education, counseling, and medical referral to an appropriate health provider. For health screenings required by regulatory agencies, such as pulmonary function testing of employees whose work activities require that they wear a respirator under certain job conditions, the follow-up of employees with abnormal screening results may also involve a temporary change in work status until the underlying health condition is resolved.

Most health screening programs can be provided on company premises to reduce or eliminate lost-work time involved in having each employee go off-site for testing.

Training Services

The training component of an on-site nursing program should address a variety of commonly expressed health and safety education needs. For example, individual health education programs can include back care and back injury prevention, stress management, cardiopulmonary resuscitation (CPR), nutrition and weight reduction, and AIDS education. Educational programs should be conducted during normal working hours and, if necessary, be rescheduled for employees unable to attend during regular work hours.

Evaluation of Program Effectiveness

To evaluate a workplace occupational health nursing program, the hospital must periodically assess its performance against predetermined goals and objectives. In addition to hospital performance evaluations, workplace nursing programs must also work with client companies to assess the effectiveness of the program as a contracted service. Evaluation of the workplace nursing program from the perspective of both the hospital and the client provides vital feedback on the quality of the service and the overall viability of the program.

The Hospital's Perspective

Hospital-based occupational health nursing programs provided on company premises can deliver a valued service to employers in an economical and convenient fashion. One of many benefits is the increased goodwill between employers and hospitals that results from tailoring health services to meet employers' specific needs.

If an on-site nursing program is well managed, the consistent presence of a hospital-employed occupational health nurse at client companies will strengthen the hospital's relationship with these organizations. The nurse will become the employer's "health expert" and will be consulted regarding health issues as well as future health service needs.

The on-site occupational health nurse is called upon to make many health referrals for employees. Successful workplace occupational health nursing programs provide employee health referrals based on a number of considerations such as medical specialty, quality of care, geographical location of the health care provider, and insurance and payment provisions. Referrals are made primarily with the employee's interests in mind, and they may not consistently go to health care providers employed by or on the medical staff of the hospital. Yet the hospital and its medical staff expect some increased utilization of their services from a regional network of workplace occupational health nursing programs. A summary of the referrals made by the program's nurses can be compiled periodically to document the program's impact in this area.

Since the on-site nursing program need not be limited geographically, the program can establish important relationships with employers beyond the hospital's traditional service area. If necessary, the program can refer employees to hospitals, clinics, and other medical facilities and primary care providers outside the hospital's service area.

The Employer's Perspective

The further removed a resource is from a manager's direct control, the more important communication becomes in assessing the value of that resource. A hospital-based workplace nursing program is an example of a resource that is not under the direct control of the management of the program's clients (the employers who use its services). Thus, a program's self-evaluation of the effectiveness of the nursing program and its communication of the resulting information to an employer becomes critical to maintaining the employer's support.

Employers investing in contracted occupational health programs expect to know how the program is being utilized. What activities and accomplishments has the program achieved, and what are the overall patterns of employee utilization? If the program projected cost savings for an employer, how much did the program save the employer during a specified period of service? These questions are best answered for clients through periodic written reports. Written reports can provide such details as what programs were conducted and when they were held, rates of employee utilization of program services, and cost savings attributable to the program.

Of primary importance is that reports be written with the nonmedical reader in mind and that they address all program benefits important to the employer, such as whether lost-work time has been reduced through occupational health nursing interventions. Reports should provide the management team of the client with as much detail as possible about impact on health care costs without revealing confidential medical information. Reports should provide information on overall patterns of employee utilization, such as the percentage of the total employee population using the program during a given time period and a ranking of the most frequent versus the least utilized types of care provided by the occupational health nurse.

To be effective, the evaluation process should function as a dialogue between the nursing program staff and the management team of the client. Information should be shared and constructive feedback elicited. A report focused on the program's specific activities is most effective. The process of reviewing the entire program should involve a description of each activity (for example, a companywide serum cholesterol screening), how it was utilized and received by employees, and how the activity might be conducted more effectively in the future. New or future expanded activities that the nursing program is planning should be detailed in the report so that the management team of the client can offer suggestions and grant approval.

Key personnel from both the occupational health nursing program and the client company should be involved in the program evaluation, including the occupational health nurse and his or her supervisor, top managers of the client company (especially the company executive who originally gave final approval to purchase the program), and company employees, who serve as day-to-day liaisons between the occupational health nursing program and the employer. The frequency of program evaluation can be mutually determined. If a thoroughgoing evaluation is conducted with the objectives of all parties in mind, everybody wins—the hospital, the employer, and the employee.

Chapter 10

Health Promotion Services

Roy K. Gerber, M.B.A.

About 75 percent of all community hospitals now have some type of health promotion program, which is composed of services that can be successfully integrated into an occupational health services product line to benefit both the hospital and the employers it serves. There is, however, some overlap, confusion, and interchangeable use of terminology within the health promotion field. *Health promotion services* are traditionally defined as "... programs, policies, and services which are primarily directed at maintaining or increasing levels of health among those who are not ill."[1] Similarly, *wellness* focuses on apparently healthy people and attempts to move them to higher or optimum levels of mental, physical, emotional, and social functioning. *Disease prevention* targets populations at risk for disease and then attempts to bring about a reduction of risk factors. In contrast, *medical care* generally focuses on sick people and their restoration to a condition characterized by the absence of disease. *Health education* provides information on health to a wide variety of populations.[2]

For a broad operational working definition in this chapter, *occupational health promotion* will be defined as services targeting essentially functioning (employed) healthy populations at the workplace. These services generally motivate employees to take responsibility for enhancing their own well-being, reducing their risk factors for illness, or seeking care for any medical problems they face. The services include programs that help to identify potential health risks or precursors of disease; to teach information, options, and skills to modify behaviors linked to health risks; and to create supportive environments for sustained changes in health behaviors.

Health Promotion Services at the Worksite

Health promotion programs at the worksite can differ greatly in their desired impact, intensity, and duration.[3] The programs fall into three categories:

awareness and motivation programs, behavior change programs, and corporate culture change programs.

Awareness and Motivation Programs

Awareness and motivation programs such as brown bag luncheons on various health information topics generally serve to hook or motivate employees to seek additional information or to consider making life-style modifications. Also included in this group would be newsletters, paycheck stuffers, screening programs without follow-up (health fairs), and health-risk assessments without feedback sessions. These types of programs are generally low in cost, and yet they provide high visibility at the worksite. They seldom bring about changes in health behavior, but they can be an effective means of challenging employees' assumptions about their health and laying the groundwork for more intensive behavior change programs.

Behavior Change Programs

Behavior change programs are designed to facilitate changes in employees' health behaviors and include topics such as stress management, physical fitness, weight control, back care, low-fat/low-cholesterol diets, smoking cessation, and health-risk assessments with feedback and follow-up. Because these types of programs have participant life-style changes as their goals, they potentially can facilitate long-term change with attendant payoffs to both employers and employees.

Corporate Culture Change Programs

Corporate culture change programs focus on bringing about long-term sustained changes in health behavior within an organization. Using his Normative Systems approach in a model called Lifegain, Robert F. Allen postulated the need for organizations to actively support positive health behavior changes made by individuals within the organization in order to sustain those changes.[4] Programs within this category include those on developing fitness centers, changing corporate policies such as flexible work hours to permit attendance at programs, offering health-food alternatives in cafeterias and vending machines, adopting nonsmoking policies, changing benefit design to encourage prevention and early detection of disease, adopting broadbrush employee assistance programs, and implementing other ongoing long-term changes demonstrated by company management.

Benefits of Occupational Health Promotion Programs to Hospitals

As part of their efforts to seek out new business opportunities, many hospitals have turned to delivering health promotion services to companies.

Hospitals expect many benefits in providing such services: generating new revenue and profit sources, increasing patient referrals and hospital utilization, developing relationships with business and industry, enhancing the hospital's image, and fulfilling the hospital's mission statement.

New Revenue or Profit Sources

Generally speaking, traditional occupational health services tend to be more profitable than occupational health promotion programs. There are probably several reasons. Many occupational health services other than health promotion are covered by insurance or mandated by workers' compensation because they are medical or clinical in nature. If neither is the case, chances are that employers are in the habit of paying for these types of services anyway. According to a *Hospitals* magazine Hamilton/KSA survey of 623 hospitals conducted in late 1988, 12.4 percent of the hospitals surveyed reported making a profit in health promotion. About 37 percent of the hospitals were breaking even, and 51 percent were losing money.[5]

On the basis of these data, a hospital should not expect that its occupational health promotion program will inevitably be profitable. Many experts feel that because of the difficulty that health promotion programs have in becoming financially viable on their own, hospitals will end up integrating health promotion as a product into various product lines.[6] On the other hand, many programs do generate a profit even after full allocation of indirect expenses.

There is an interesting side note to a consideration of the potential of health promotion for enhancing hospital revenue. Against the backdrop of efforts to reduce or lessen health care expenditures, occupational health promotion programs stand alone in that they focus on reducing the *demand* for medical services rather than seeking to alter the access or *supply* side of the equation. Simply stated, over the long run, the key to reducing the demand for medical services is for employees to stay healthy.

If occupational health promotion programs actually succeed in reducing the demand for medical services, hospitals will face an interesting dilemma. Hospitals are diversifying into occupational health services to generate new revenue and profit, increase referrals and utilization, develop new and better relationships with business and industry, enhance their image, and fulfill their mission as health care providers. Decreasing the demand for hospital services through health promotion will certainly build improved relationships with business and industry, enhance the hospital's image, and fulfill its mission. These are positive results. Decreasing demand, however, is likely to decrease new revenue and profit and decrease referrals and utilization. This can place a hospital's immediate financial needs in conflict with the hospital's business relationships, image, and mission. It will be interesting to see how hospitals resolve this dilemma.

Increased Referrals and Hospital Utilization

Occupational health promotion programs can generate referrals for the hospital and members of the medical staff. Examples of these types of opportunities include identification and referral of employees at high risk for illness who are discovered through fitness assessments or health-risk assessments, referral to a hospital's alcohol/drug treatment program or psychiatric program from an employee assistance program, and generation of laboratory, pulmonary, and other ancillary charges from screening programs.

Occupational health promotion differs from occupational health services such as preemployment physicals, executive physicals, substance abuse screening, on-the-job injury treatment, and return-to-work examinations because the revenues from health promotion are more difficult to track in terms of generating referrals to inpatient, ancillary, or physician resources. Although referrals from routine occupational health services are usually direct and immediate, referrals from health promotion services (excluding employee assistance programs) are generally indirect and difficult to document at the time of admission. Health promotion participants who have been referred may take weeks or months to follow up on suggested referrals and may fail to indicate the source of the referral during the admission process.[7] There have been some instances in which referrals from health promotion programs have been tracked via social security numbers, but it is still difficult to establish causal relationships; some of these patients might have sought medical help regardless of their exposure to health promotion programs.

Relationships with Industry

The introduction of health promotion programs in occupational settings can help establish long-term relationships with business and industry. Beginning relationships with companies through health promotion is also a proven way to get a foot in the door with relatively low-priced programs. These efforts establish a foundation for future services: "The marketing battleground of the 1990s will not be in generating new customers; instead, the challenge will be to enhance relationships with existing customers, evolving them into being your clients."[8] In other words, when a hospital successfully demonstrates its competency in solving health care problems related to employee health habits, client companies are grateful and interested in learning what other health services are available from the hospital. Successful relationships with companies can therefore create a marketing information conduit for hospitals, an excellent opportunity to learn which other health care needs are going unmet. This "relationship marketing" approach provides the tactical sales advantage of having the hospital seen as not just another vendor but rather as a proven problem solver that may be able to help further.

Enhanced Hospital Image

Providing occupational health promotion services also helps a hospital enhance and maintain its image with the employees of the client company. These services were once considered a soft benefit used by hospital-based health promotion programs as justification for their existence even though they lost money. However, some market research has shown that these types of programs can be an effective marketing service exchange in which the client company employee forms opinions and beliefs about the health care provider. In one study, employees who had participated in occupational health promotion programs not only rated the provider hospital as their preferred hospital in the event inpatient treatment was needed, but they also rated the provider hospital's medical staff, nurses, physical plant, and equipment higher than a control group.[9] This "halo effect" was particularly interesting in that the health promotion programs were delivered on-site at the company and there was no interaction with the hospital's medical staff, nurses, physical plant, or equipment.

Fulfillment of Hospital Mission

Finally, occupational health programs can help a hospital fulfill its mission statement because most mission statements include meeting the health care needs of the community. The workplace is the site of greatest impact on the adult community population.

Benefits of Occupational Health Promotion to Industry

Industries perceive a variety of direct and indirect benefits resulting from occupational health promotion programs. These benefits fit into two general categories: economic benefits and enhancement of corporate culture and image.[10] *Tracking the Impact of Health Promotion on Organizations* phrased these same categories in terms of four major organizational goals:

- To improve the image of the organization that sponsors health promotion programs
- To improve the organization's financial operations
- To maximize appropriate utilization of health care services
- To improve the quality of the work environment and the quality of health care[11]

Economic Benefits

Companies perceive that occupational health promotion programs improve productivity levels and reduce benefits and human resources development costs. Companies make the following assumptions:

- Improvement in productivity levels will result because healthier employees are absent from work less, therefore decreasing the amount of sick time paid to employees and employee replacement costs. Healthier employees potentially can contribute up to their maximum abilities while they are on the job because of their physical, mental, and emotional well-being.
- Reduction in benefits costs will result from healthier employees using less health, disability, and workers' compensation insurance.
- Reduction of human resources development costs will result from having healthier workers who will have lower turnover rates. Companies therefore will have to recruit and retrain employees less often.

These three economic benefits are based on companies' perceptions. Hospitals often market occupational health promotion programs on the premise that the programs do, in effect, produce these benefits. Research to support this claim is lacking, however. Although the connection between personal life-style and health status has been well documented,[12] it is more difficult for a health promotion program to track or evaluate its direct benefits to business and industry than it is for the other occupational health services. Effective occupational health promotion programs help employees adopt healthy life-styles, and there are numerous studies that show that employees with healthy life-style habits utilize the health care system less than those without healthy habits.[13,14,15] At this time, however, a definitive study using randomized experimental and control group samples, controlling for exogenous factors, and demonstrating cause and effect does not exist. It is unclear when these cost/benefit ratios will be established.

At present, health promotion professionals must rely on common-sense justification for health promotion services. For example, in 1982 Bethesda Healthcare Inc. in Cincinnati conducted a pilot program for physical fitness/ life-style education at a medium-sized employer (300 employees). At the end of the program, the data collected on each participant included eight biometric measurements (for example, cardiovascular endurance, muscular strength and endurance, body fat, and flexibility) along with eight measurements of participant-perceived well-being (for example, ability to manage stress, energy levels, and morale).

Fairly dramatic statistically significant changes were reported in all of the measures. To sell additional programs, Bethesda Healthcare planned on presenting the findings and extrapolating their results to existing studies that showed the cost/benefit ratio. After the client company's vice-president of human resources learned of the results, he asked, "How soon can you do another program for us?" Bethesda Healthcare offered to show the company representatives additional evaluation data before they made a hasty decision. The company's vice-president replied, "Look, all I know is my employees love the program. They tell me they look better, feel better, and have more energy. That's good enough for me."

The implications are that cost/benefit data are needed to document the efficiency of health promotion services, and this is particularly true in the workplace, where decisions are determined by financial considerations. However, decisions on the benefits of perceived improvements in quality of life, morale, and health resulting from health promotion programs sometimes are made simply on the basis of employees' recommendations.

Improvement in Corporate Culture and Image

Improvement in the community image and in the national image of a company is a benefit to be derived from occupational health promotion. Many factors determine how a company is perceived by its employees and how it is positioned in the eyes of its community (customers). Health promotion programs generally make for good media coverage, and the association of healthy employees with a company's product or service is often an image not generally achievable without paid advertising. Similarly, health promotion programs usually can convey a message of caring to employees throughout an organization, regardless of whether or not the employee actually participated. This "halo effect" is similar to the aforementioned impact that occupational health promotion programs can have on the employees' perception of the hospital provider.

References

1. Goodstadt, M. S., Simpson, R. I., and Loranger, P. O. Health promotion: a conceptual integration. *American Journal of Health Promotion* 1(3):60, Winter 1987.
2. U.S. Department of Health, Education, and Welfare. *Healthy People: The Surgeon General's Report on Health Promotion and Disease Prevention.* Washington, DC: U.S. DHEW, Publication No. 79-55071, 1979, p. 119.
3. O'Donnell, M. Definition of health promotion. Part II: levels of program. *American Journal of Health Promotion* 1(2):3–7, Winter 1986.
4. Allen, R. F., and Judd, A. Achieving health promotion objectives through cultural change systems. *American Journal of Health Promotion* 1(1):45–46, Summer 1986.
5. Sabatino, F. G. The diversification success story continues: survey. *Hospitals* 63(1):27, Jan. 5, 1989.
6. Health promotion in ambulatory care. *Optimal Health* 4(3):18–20, Jan.-Feb. 1988.
7. Sol, N. Tracking the elusive patient accrual data. *Optimal Health* 3(5):15, May–June 1987.
8. Brown, S. W. The health care marketing professional in 1990. Presentation given at the Eighth Annual Symposium for Health Care Marketing, Academy of Health Services Marketing of the American Marketing Association, New Orleans, Feb. 1988.

9. Unpublished market research performed for Bethesda Hospitals, Inc., Cincinnati, 1984.
10. O'Donnell, M. P., and Ainsworth, T. H. *Health Promotion in the Workplace.* New York City: John Wiley & Sons, 1984, pp. 11–14.
11. Kernaghan, S. G., and Giloth, B. E. *Tracking the Impact of Health Promotion on Organizations: A Key to Program Survival.* Chicago: American Hospital Publishing, Inc., 1988.
12. Iverson, D. Making the case for health promotion: a summary of the scientific evidence. In: Bellingham, R., and Cohen, B. *The Corporate Wellness Sourcebook.* Amherst, MA: Human Resource Development Press, 1987, pp. 60–64.
13. Bly, J. L., Jones, R. C., and Richardson, J. E. Impact of worksite health promotion on health care costs and utilization. *Journal of the American Medical Association* 256(23):3235–40, Dec. 1986.
14. Health Research Institute. Corporate wellness programs: 1987 biennial survey results. *Health Action Managers* 2(7), Apr. 10, 1988.
15. Herzlinger, R. E., and Calkins, D. How companies tackle health care costs: part III. *Harvard Business Review* Jan.–Feb. 1986, pp. 70–80.

Chapter 11

Employee Assistance Programs

Rob Ryder

Over the past 40 years, employee assistance programs (EAPs) have gradually become a widespread and common part of employee health and employee relations strategies for corporate America. The rise of EAPs is attributable in part to an increasing public awareness of the relationship between good mental health and good physical health and to an increasing corporate awareness of the relationship between good employee mental health and good corporate fiscal health. In the past 10 years, many hospitals have embraced the role of EAP provider as part of their health care mission. Only a few, however, have made the logical formal connection between EAPs and occupational health services programs.

The EAP Model

Employee assistance programs vary widely from provider to provider in terms of structure and services provided. The following description provides an overview of the most common EAP delivery model.

Employee assistance programs are counseling programs designed to help a company's employees and their dependents cope with or overcome various problems that periodically arise at work and at home. The typical EAP incorporates a broadbrush approach to confidential employee/dependent counseling and is equipped to deal with all types of employee problems, including alcohol/drug abuse, family/marital difficulties, and psychological, financial, and legal problems.

The EAP model is based on centralized intake by a counselor/case manager who assesses the problems of employees or their dependents, performs short-term problem solving or therapy for a specified number of sessions (as allowed by the EAP's contract with the employer), refers employees/dependents to appropriate community resources when more in-depth or specialized therapy is indicated, and provides follow-up support after treatment or referral. Employees can use EAP services in two ways:

- An employee may recognize the need for assistance and contact the EAP counselor independently (self-referral).
- A supervisor may refer an employee when the supervisor feels that an employee's job performance or work status is being negatively affected by the employee's personal problems (management referral).

Program Components

In addition to counseling, most EAPs also provide their corporate clients with the following services:

- Consultation on the development of a strong company EAP policy that is consistent with existing organizational policies
- Comprehensive supervisory training on effective utilization of the EAP, including management skills for recognizing and helping troubled employees, orientation to EAP policies and procedures, and specialized training for recognizing and working with substance abuse at the workplace
- Promotion programs designed to inform employees and dependents about the EAP resources, including on-site orientations, program brochures, posters, and newsletters
- Educational workshops for the entire employee population that deal with mental and physical health and quality-of-life issues
- Record-keeping systems that comply with existing laws and sound clinical practice and include regular review by a quality assurance team
- Periodic utilization reports for corporate management, which aggregate services rendered to employees, including the total number of employees served, with professional classifications and types of problems addressed

Other services offered by some EAPs that are not as common include:

- Trauma intervention teams trained to intervene with groups of employees in the event of a critical event or disruption at the work-site (such as employee deaths or layoffs)
- Substance abuse case management for chronic cases
- Case management and review of all psychiatric claims made on a company's health insurance plan
- Individualized wellness counseling for life-style and health-risk behaviors such as weight control, smoking cessation, and fitness

Staffing

Most commonly, EAPs are staffed with master's-degree-level or doctorate-degree-level counselors who are licensed or certified mental health professionals experienced in problem assessment, crisis intervention, and primary therapy. All EAP counselors should work under direct medical/clinical supervision and participate regularly in case reviews. In addition to clinical work, counselors also serve as "account executives" to the corporate client and must therefore also possess excellent public relations skills. The role of account executive includes scheduling workshops and training, preparing utilization reports, and facilitating general communication with corporate management for EAP-related issues.

Management staff for EAPs usually consists of a person who is clinically prepared (that is, meets licensed counselor qualifications) and who is capable of providing clinical supervision. In addition, the EAP program manager is responsible for day-to-day operations including management of the budget, staff scheduling, corporate client relations and contract negotiations, program marketing, and development of new services.

The responsibilities of the EAP support staff are to receive clients at the EAP office, answer phones, schedule appointments, and provide clerical support for clinical staff. Occasionally, EAPs will hire staff to fill special functions such as training or substance abuse counseling. As a rule, however, having a staff of generalists is more flexible and economical.

Business Operations

Employee assistance programs are usually sold to corporate clients on a capitated basis, with prices ranging anywhere from $10 to $80 per employee per year, depending on the number of sessions contracted for and the number of program components included in the EAP coverage. An average price for comprehensive three- to six-session coverage would range between $20 and $40 per employee per year.

The primary EAP market consists of companies of 100 or more employees. Although smaller companies have many of the same needs as larger employers, they usually are more difficult to sell on the concept of offering an EAP to their employees. Because the labor requirements of implementing an EAP are the same regardless of company size, per-capita costs are higher for smaller companies. Because small companies often have limited resources, implementing an EAP may not make financial sense for them.

Personal marketing strategies are the most effective approach for selling EAPs. However, these strategies must focus on identifying clients' needs and connecting them with EAP resources as opposed to simply presenting (selling) the EAP product. A particularly effective marketing tool for the EAP is the focus group. *Focus groups* bring together small groups of corporate representatives to discuss their needs with regard to EAP-related employee problems. The groups can then be followed up through personal visits by EAP staff to discuss how focus-group input is being integrated into the EAP and to explore possible applications of the EAP with that specific company. This type of marketing can be accomplished effectively by EAP management and clinical staff in conjunction with existing marketing resources.

Motivating Factors for Hospital Sponsorship of EAPs

Although some hospitals have been involved in the EAP business for almost 15 years, the majority of hospital-sponsored EAPs have developed more recently. Driven by changes in reimbursement, economic climate, consumer demand, and inpatient emphasis, hospitals have become alert to nontraditional means of delivering traditional services. Employee assistance programs represent one of those means. There are five primary motivations for hospitals to become involved in the EAP field: filling beds and creating referrals for the hospital medical staff, improving corporate relations, improving community relations, gaining a profit, and providing EAP services to hospital employees.

Referral Generation

The desire to fill beds and create referrals is probably the most common misguided reason for a hospital to enter the EAP field. Hospitals often believe that an EAP will create a captive distribution system for filling chemical dependency and psychiatric beds. In reality, the majority of employee problems that manifest themselves through an EAP are handled most efficiently and cost-effectively (for the employee and the corporate client) on an outpatient basis by master's-degree-level counselors who are not necessarily on the hospital's medical staff. In fact, in our experience, more than 70 percent of all client problems seen in a three-session model can be resolved by the EAP with no outside referral at all.

When a referral is indicated, the referral resource used is often dictated by the employee's insurance carrier, and that resource may not be the EAP's base hospital. Exclusive referral to one's own hospital or medical staff will soon be viewed by corporate clients as a conflict of interest and will jeopardize long-term survival of the EAP. This is not to say that hospital/medical staff referrals will not come from the EAP. They will! However, as a primary motivator for entering the EAP field, referral generation is flawed.

Corporate Relations

As a motivator for entering the EAP field, the establishment of relations with the corporate community is one of the most valid. Except through health maintenance organizations and preferred provider organization arrangements, hospitals do not often have the opportunity to enter into long-term contractual relationships. It is through these types of relationships that feelings of trust and loyalty (that is, informal partnerships) are developed between hospitals and corporations. The corporate sector is playing an increasingly important role in the control of the health care dollar. It is therefore important that hospitals find as many ways as possible to enter into protracted relationships with corporations now in order to create corporate partnerships that will pay dividends in the future.

An effective EAP is a good way to gain significant influence in a corporation. It assists the corporation with employee relations, is a relatively inexpensive benefit, and has the potential to save the corporation health-related labor costs. We have found that once a relationship with a corporation is established through an EAP, inevitably doors will open for other types of hospital or hospital-based services.

Community Relations

In any community there are far more "well people" who might need a hospital's services in the future than there are "sick people" who need the hospital's services now. An employee assistance program is really a "well-patient" service. Unlike traditional health insurance, it is a benefit that companies want their employees to use as much as possible. Therein lies the benefit for the company. Therefore, most companies will give an EAP constant exposure through brochures, posters, newsletters, and the like. Most people who use an EAP are "well people" who need help in coping with problems in their lives. Because an EAP is marketed and available to the "well" population (that is, all employees), it gives the hospital constant exposure to a market segment that would not even think about care otherwise. If an EAP's services are expanded to cover things such as wellness counseling or sick-child care, then this "well" market is expanded even further.

A hospital provides services for significant health problems that come and go. Because the hospital's role and involvement with the public is episodic, public awareness of the hospital also comes and goes. An EAP provides a way for the hospital to help people with the little problems of everyday life that are always there. Through the EAP, exposure to and awareness of the hospital is constant.

Profit

Although the EAP is capable of carrying its own weight financially, it is not by any means a cash cow. It takes time to establish an EAP and develop its credibility. As with many businesses, building a critical mass is the key to profitability. In our experience, the program needs approximately one EAP counselor for each 10,000 employee sessions (the number of eligible employees multiplied by the number of sessions contracted for). In the early stages of an EAP, it is likely that the program will have more counselor time than necessary; however, it is not advisable to start an EAP with part-time staff. Consistency and credibility, which are the keys to long-term success in an EAP, can only be built with a full-time, committed staff. For example, it took Interstate Health Services, Inc., two years after the initial marketing effort to the corporate community to become profitable. This EAP now realizes a return on revenue of approximately 10 percent. This success notwithstanding, if short-term or long-term profit is the only motive for starting a hospital-based EAP, there are probably better investments than entry into the competitive EAP market.

EAP Services for Hospital Employees

There is no better reason for a hospital to start an EAP than to provide service to its own employees. Offering an EAP to the hospital's own employees as the first client group can mitigate much of the expense in program development and much of the potential embarrassment if the program needs to be refined. Moreover, if a hospital is unwilling to provide an EAP for its own employees, it has no business trying to sell the service to other corporations.

There are, however, some liabilities to starting an internal EAP for hospital employees. The greatest is confidentiality. The EAP needs to be supported by a strong hospital policy that guarantees confidentiality. In addition, it is preferable that the EAP office be located outside the hospital and that the EAP staff not be associated with any internal hospital department other than the EAP (especially the personnel or human resources department, which may be viewed by employees as a direct agent of the employer and thus discourage self-referral to the program). If possible, it is also advantageous for the EAP to be placed in a corporation that is separate from the hospital corporation.

The EAP should contract with and be paid by the hospital for services as though it were any other corporate client. This in fact allows the hospital to be the "first pill out of the bottle," a client base from which to create the critical mass that will allow for more rapid development of the EAP product and market. In addition, providing EAP services for hospital employees on an in-kind basis (that is, with no contract and no exchange of funds) can lead to short-term program failure if hospital employees eat up EAP resources.

Pros and Cons of Hospital-Sponsored EAPs

As institutions committed to the provision of health care, it seems logical that hospitals should excel as EAP providers. Clearly, there are advantages that hospital-sponsored EAPs may have. The first is availability of resources. A good EAP must be clinically sound. If a hospital has psychiatric, chemical dependency, or behavioral medicine programs, they can be invaluable in providing assistance in the areas of psychiatric supervision, in-service education, and clinical programming for EAP staff at a cost that is far less than would be paid to outside consultants for the same services. In addition, services inherent to hospital operations (such as printing and audiovisual services, library resources, and 24-hour phone coverage) can be invaluable in the initiation and maintenance of a high-quality EAP program.

The reputation and credibility of a hospital should reasonably enhance the image of the EAP; however, this assumption may not always hold true. In 1985, Interstate Health Services, Inc., of Colorado Springs, Colorado, commissioned a blind market study of the 42 largest employers in its area. The most significant finding of this study was that 52 percent of those companies surveyed indicated a distrust for hospitals and the health care system in general. Fifty-four percent of the companies also indicated that although they think hospitals provide high-quality care, they do not believe that they do it as economically as possible.[1] The greatest liability of hospital-sponsored EAPs, then, is the fear on the part of the corporate client that the EAP exists only to fill hospital beds or to create physician referrals or that a hospital-sponsored EAP may not be the most economical way to get EAP services.

The best way to combat employer distrust of hospital-sponsored EAPs is to maintain fastidious records of referrals made for and chosen by EAP clients. A hospital that has built such a record from offering its EAP program to hospital employees before attempting to sell the program to employers is in a much better position than a hospital with no record on which to stand. Hospital employee experience with the EAP can be used to show referral patterns and establish credibility. The price concern can be rapidly resolved through the competitive bidding process in communities where there are nonhospital EAP providers. Where there is no competition, there is no substitute for sound market research to determine what price the market will bear for EAP services.

Physically locating an EAP in the hospital can also be a liability. Employers generally do not want to send their employees "to the hospital" to get help for job or life problems. This stigma can be overcome simply by locating the EAP away from the hospital.

The trend in the EAP field toward national providership of services may pose both a problem and an opportunity. Large health care providers may maintain toll-free phone numbers and provide initial intake and triage of cases over the telephone. Most hospitals are unable to cope with the geographical scope of such competitors. Excellent service and personalization of services can be used to effectively combat this national approach to a regional market.

The EAP as an Occupational Health Services Product

Hospital-sponsored employee assistance programs may be associated with a myriad of hospital departments or programs ranging from wellness to chemical dependency. In its purest form, however, the EAP is probably as bona fide an occupational health service as one could hope to find. Traditionally, occupational health services have often been limited to the treatment and prevention of job-related illness and injury, with the major goal of helping employers control the costs of workers' compensation. Historically, American management practice has also attempted to separate employees' occupational health problems from their personal health. Increasing evidence indicates that this notion is not only inaccurate but also counterproductive when it comes to managing occupational injuries and illnesses and the labor costs that stem from these conditions.[2,3,4,5] Employee assistance programs can and should form the link between traditional occupational health concerns and personal health and life issues. Although EAPs and traditional occupational health services programs have their similarities and differences, the symbiosis that is inherent in the two is undeniable.

Program Similarities

The primary market for both EAPs and traditional occupational health services is the corporate community. By law, occupational health services should be available to all employees who have a need for intervention or treatment. This need is usually manifested as job-related physical illness and injury. By policy, an EAP is usually also available to all employees. Its use may also be indicated through job-related problems (usually job performance) or simply by a feeling of need on the part of the employee. Like traditional occupational health programs, the EAP is available to employees at no personal expense, with the employer paying a fee or premium to ensure that the service is available.

Case management and support of the employee for the earliest possible recovery and return to normalcy are integral parts of high-quality EAP and traditional occupational health programs. With both programs, cost containment and prevention through education and intervention are the key components to long-term survival in the corporate marketplace.

Program Differences

Although the emphasis is slowly changing in both occupational health services and EAPs, it is still safe to say that the primary difference between the two programs is that EAPs focus on mental and emotional well-being whereas occupational health services focus more on physical well-being. Occupational health program expenses to the employer are usually variable based on utilization rates and are paid through workers' compensation insurance, while EAP expenses are generally fixed on a per-capita basis and paid directly by the employer.

Opportunities for Overlap

More and more, the medical field is recognizing the importance of good mental/emotional health in the recovery process for illness and injury. However, workers' compensation carriers scrutinize psychological referrals to determine whether there is a clear and undeniable connection between an employee's work-related condition and his or her mental or emotional state before they will reimburse such a referral. Ironically, from the perspectives of early recovery, cost containment, and preventive medicine, the referral that is made prior to the "undeniable connection" stage may ultimately be most effective.[6]

An employer with an EAP has the capability to effect early intervention without having to worry about increased workers' compensation expense or carrier approval. In effect, an EAP increases the value of a cooperating occupational health services program because it gives the occupational health physician an additional resource that has already been paid for and approved under a capitated arrangement. In addition, assuming that the occupational health services program and the EAP are both part of the same system, case management for both programs is enhanced through consistency of philosophy, communication, and purpose (that is, getting the patient back to work and out of treatment as soon as possible).

The resources inherent in a good EAP form a perfect match for meeting many of the occupational health needs of most companies. With EAP staff as part of the occupational health services team, new connections and mutually beneficial uses of the service will constantly be found. Employee assistance programs and occupational health services together create a provider network with limitless scope. However, the relationship between the two programs must be clearly defined and structured. For example, the EAP and the occupational health services program, working cooperatively, can offer increased value and effectiveness in a number of difficult occupational health areas: family intervention, drug testing, problem assessment, trauma intervention, and life change adjustment.

Family Intervention

An employee who is injured or disabled at work will need the support of his or her family to maximize recovery and minimize the time needed to recover. Similarly, the family of an injured employee will need new coping skills and strategies for dealing with the recovery process as well as the life situation created by the injury or illness. An EAP can provide the resources necessary to treat the entire family system, thus increasing the effectiveness of the occupational health services intervention.

Drug Testing

Employers are increasingly instituting drug-testing policies at the workplace. Often, occupational health programs are charged with carrying out these policies (see chapter 7). An EAP provides a qualified resource for constructively intervening with employees who test positively for drugs. Occupational health services programs without EAP support are often left in the awkward position of having to deal with positive results only through the termination or disciplinary process of the company involved. This situation may compromise the integrity of the occupational health services department with employees and raise serious ethical questions about the necessity of treatment once a problem is identified. Even if an employee is terminated for drug use, an employer may have extended liability for knowing of a hazardous situation but not acting on it. Intervention through the EAP can mitigate this liability.

Employee assistance program involvement in drug testing is, however, not without its risks. An EAP's effectiveness and approachability can quickly become contaminated if it is perceived to be the enforcement arm of a drug-testing program. In order to keep the integrity of an EAP untarnished, some EAPs have created affiliated yet separate products (programs) to deal exclusively with occupational drug and alcohol issues.

The EAP's role in drug testing should be to provide help to those "positive-test" employees who want it. This help should be offered through the occupational health services program, accepted by the employee, provided by the EAP, and supported by the employer (through policy and practice). To ensure confidentiality, all EAP information-release procedures should be the same as for any other type of EAP referral, and the EAP should not participate in management decisions regarding an employee's employment status.

Problem Assessment

Employee assistance programs can be an invaluable tool for the occupational physician in assessing an employee's mental state and motivation for recovery. Programs with properly credentialed counselors can also provide psychometric support to the treatment plan.

Trauma Intervention

Occupational injury many times is accompanied by a traumatic event at the worksite. In these cases, both victims and their colleagues may need assistance in responding to the event. Trauma intervention not only improves recovery for the victims but also may prevent future stress-related injuries among the "survivors."

Life Change Adjustment

As with the families of patients, the patients themselves often need coping skills for dealing with life changes, such as marital/family problems, career changes, or behavior changes. This type of counseling is consistent with the majority of EAP work.

Future Directions

In a troubled economy, one cannot expect business and industry to pay for an EAP based on a blind faith that it will ultimately produce labor cost savings. More rigorous evaluation of the cost-effectiveness of the stand-alone EAP will be required to solidify its place in the benefits packages of the future.[7] Unfortunately, this type of evaluation is very difficult and expensive to obtain given the number of variables that must be controlled for when evaluating the cost savings that could possibly be associated with an EAP. Cost containment associated with traditional occupational health services, on the other hand, is relatively easy to identify and evaluate (for example, number of injuries, average lost-work time, and medical costs). The EAP as an integral part of an occupational health services approach can contribute to the savings generated by a successful occupational health services program. This partnership will not only improve the effectiveness of the occupational health services program but will also ensure that the EAP is available to employees for all types of problems, both work-related and personal.

References

1. Research Consulting Group, Inc. Consumer research: industrial medicine clinics. Colorado Springs, CO: RCGI, 1985.
2. Ryder, R., and Mauer, G. The relationship between health risk populations and health-related labor costs. In: *Proceedings of the 19th Annual Meeting of the Society of Prospective Medicine,* vol. 2. Indianapolis: Society of Prospective Medicine, 1984.
3. Murphy, J., et al. The relationship between personal/mental health problems and health-related labor costs. In: *Proceedings of the 19th Annual Meeting of the Society of Prospective Medicine,* vol. 1. Indianapolis: Society of Prospective Medicine, 1984.
4. Berry, C. *Good Health for Employees and Reduced Health Care Costs for Industry.* Washington, DC: Health Insurance Institute, 1981.
5. Kernaghan, S. G., and Giloth, B. E. *Tracking the Impact of Health Promotion on Organizations: A Key to Program Survival.* Chicago: American Hospital Publishing, Inc., 1988.
6. Kaminer, A. Role of the medical department. *Occupational Medicine State of the Art Reviews: The Troubled Employee* 1(4):545, Oct.–Dec. 1986.
7. Masi, D. Employee assistance programs. *Occupational Medicine State of the Art Reviews: The Troubled Employee* 1(4):653–65, Oct.–Dec. 1986.

Chapter 12

Occupational Rehabilitation Services

Sandra Figler, D.P.H., M.B.A.

Occupational rehabilitation services represent unique business development opportunities both as extensions of hospital-based and freestanding injury management programs and as diversification efforts of rehabilitation programs. Included under the umbrella of occupational rehabilitation services are evaluation, medical management, physical restoration, education/prevention, and related case management services—all of which are designed to control long-term economic loss to employers and employees and to reintegrate injured workers into the work force.

Many existing occupational health services programs are focused on the high-volume market of injured employees who will experience relatively little time away from work. An average of 60 percent of work injuries involve four weeks or less of lost-work time.[1] Employees with such injuries require limited if any physical restoration services involving major rehabilitation therapy (usually physical therapy).

Although the provision of urgent care and acute injury treatment addresses the high-volume market for occupational health services, occupational rehabilitation services offer the health care provider the opportunity to enhance existing market penetration and to identify significant new customers and markets. Successful business development is tied to the rehabilitation provider's ability to demonstrate to potential clients that these services can reduce or control long-term costs, maximize the injured worker's functional abilities, and expedite an employee's return to work.

Occupational rehabilitation providers serve those workers with injuries that will result in extended periods of lost-work time, especially those who will lose at least two to six months of work time. Such workers will generally have more severe disabling musculoskeletal or cumulative trauma injuries, often affecting the back, upper extremity, or hand. A timely return to work for these employees may translate to a return to a modified or alternative job or retraining for related gainful employment. Moreover, the longer an injured employee is off work (even three to five weeks), the more likely that psychological, vocational, and financial issues and problems must also be resolved for the returning injured worker to achieve and maintain acceptable work performance levels.

Services of Occupational Rehabilitation Programs

Figure 12-1 illustrates the range of occupational rehabilitation product offerings designed to meet the needs of various customer bases.[2] Probably the most sought-after evaluation and restoration services by all customer segments are work tolerance screening, work capacity evaluation, and work hardening.

Work tolerance screening is a two- to four-hour assessment of the injured worker's physical, psychological, and functional tolerance to critical demands of a given job and is conducted by a physical or occupational therapist. During the evaluation process, the employee demonstrates his or her ability to respond to simulated work task demands.

Work tolerance screening also is offered as a key component of *work capacity evaluation.* Work capacity evaluation is a dynamic multistep four- to eight-hour process that measures a person's capacity to sustain dependable job-specific work performance. In addition to work tolerance, the employee's work history, physical/medical condition, pertinent psychological factors, and employment capability are integrated into the assessment process. A vocational counselor may assist the physical or occupational therapist by providing an analysis of the physical demands of the specific job.

One variation on the work capacity evaluation process is a *functional capacities assessment* (FCA). An FCA is a five- to eight-hour evaluation of the employee's physical and psychological abilities at a given point in time. Although it is less job focused than a work capacity evaluation and is not dynamic, an FCA is attractive to those referral sources seeking information comparable to standardized test results.

A work tolerance screening or comprehensive work capacity evaluation may result in a recommendation that the employee be enrolled in a *work hardening* program. Work hardening is a four- to six-week program of structured, graded physical reconditioning and work simulation to build motivation and improve work, specific job tolerance, and employment feasibility. Ideally, the program is jointly conducted by a physical therapist and an occupational therapist under the supervision of a physician. Typically, the employee begins with three to four hours a day of programming for four days per week, later expanded to five to six hours per day by the end of the first week.

As insurance carriers and employers increasingly seek to predict the level of performance that can be expected from employees returning to work after

Figure 12-1. Customer–Product Mix for Occupational Rehabilitation Services

CUSTOMERS

▲ Employers
Personnel director
Safety director
Occupational MD/RN
Benefits manager
Company physician

■ Private Rehab Firms
Case managers
Rehab RN

● Insurance Carriers
Claims managers
Rehab RN

* Other
State workers' comp.
Attorneys
Dept. voc. rehab
Private physicians

PRODUCTS

Employers	Ins. Carriers	Pvt. Rehab	Other	**Acute Injury Treatment**
▲	●	■	*	Medical case management
▲	●	■		Return-to-work examinations
▲				Urgent care/ancillaries
▲				Basic PT
▲	●	■		Referral consultation
▲	●	■	*	Disability evaluation
▲				Occupational nursing
				Physical Rehabilitation
▲	●	■		PT treatment
▲	●	■	*	Work capacity evaluation
▲	●	■	*	Work hardening
▲	●		*	Job modification/analysis
▲	●	■	*	Independent medical evaluations
▲	●	■	*	Back/pain clinics
▲	●		*	Job development
▲	●		*	Case management

Source: Adapted from Figler, S. Integrating and marketing injury prevention and rehabilitation services. *Journal of Ambulatory Care Marketing* 2:69–77, June 1988.

an injury as well as to limit economic loss, work capacity evaluation and work hardening have become competitive and "hot" service offerings. This competition has resulted in a plethora of new programs that are labeled as work hardening but that lack the critical component of job simulation. True job simulation attempts to replicate the tasks, tools, physical exercise and motions, and conditions involved in a specific job. For example, to represent the materials, tools, and apparatus necessary to simulate the repetitive operations found in construction and distribution industries, one might use a loading bay for lifting boxes; height-adjustable wooden beams for nailing and drilling; and pipes, fittings, and wrenches for plumbing.

Because there has been incredible growth in the number of both true and imitation work hardening programs, the primary accrediting body for rehabilitation services and programs, the Commission on Accreditation of Rehabilitation Facilities (CARF), has moved to initiate an accreditation process for work hardening programs. However, until accreditation is accepted and valued by consumers, the provider must recognize the need for educating referral sources regarding the "value-added" benefits of true work hardening.

In addition to the foregoing services, programs may provide a broad range of services aimed at prevention and education, such as a "back school" or an ergonomic worksite evaluation. A back-school program developed by a physical or occupational therapist usually consists of an evaluation of company problems followed by two to four hours of small-group sessions involving 15–20 employees at a time. The ideal on-site back-school program involves observing and videotaping employees performing their job functions so that specific problems and concerns, including the videotapes, can be incorporated within class training sessions on anatomy, posture, and injury prevention.[3]

In addition to worksite back programs, progressive employers have begun to accept the value of ergonomic evaluation with the objective of identifying any need to modify tools or the workplace to match the general physiological and psychological limitations of workers.

Independent medical or disability evaluations (second opinions), the major "hot" physician-conducted rehabilitation service, are yet another product that can be added to the services provided by a program's therapists and vocational counselors. Given the shortage of physicians experienced in workers' compensation, there continues to be a tremendous demand for physicians able to provide definitive, concise diagnoses/prognoses. Moreover, the physicians involved in providing independent medical examinations represent a potentially significant referral source for work evaluations and work hardening.

Finally, although not a billable service in many settings, case management—by which is meant the coordination and control of the appropriateness and dollars involved in provider services—is nonetheless a critical service for program management and success.

Referral Sources for Occupational Rehabilitation Programs

The ability to successfully enhance or expand an occupational health services product line is at least in part determined by a provider's understanding of and response to the customers who refer employers for rehabilitation services. The provision of rehabilitation services broadens the customer or referral source base beyond physicians and employers to include insurance carriers, disability management firms, attorneys, and state-operated workers' compensation units. In fact, for injury cases that involve extended lost-work time of six months or more, these new customers tend to dominate the customer base and often become critical and even primary referral sources.

The rehabilitation referral network is composed of individuals holding a wide range of position titles and responsibilities. A critical referral source for rehabilitation services is the rehabilitation nurse or case manager/supervisor employed by insurance carriers or state-operated workers' compensation units. Employers and insurance carriers also contract with disability management firms (also called "rehab firms") to manage complex cases and control economic liability. For the sake of convenience, the following text will refer to these individuals as case managers, although their actual titles will vary.

Case managers monitor and coordinate the use of services for each individual case, often to the point of recommending or referring the client to specific physicians or hospital-based and freestanding providers. In fact, it is not unusual for case managers (particularly those employed by a carrier) to refer 200 or more patients per year for independent medical or disability evaluations as well as for physical rehabilitation services. Even in states in which the selection of occupational providers is, according to law, a matter of patient choice, the case manager may steer patients to selected providers.

The role and influence of the case manager vary depending on the size of a firm's compensation business and the firm's philosophy, as well as whether the case manager is part of a disability management firm under contract to an employer or insurance carrier. Typically, case managers will cover a preassigned geographical territory, with the size of that territory determined by population and caseload concentration. The degree of specialization of the case manager will also depend on the manager's caseload. A case manager with a smaller caseload (20–40 cases) often services severe trauma cases (such as head or spinal cord injuries) as well as complex musculoskeletal problems.

The case manager's role will also depend on the philosophy of the firm that employs the case manager. Many employers and insurance carriers do not fully recognize the positive cost-benefit of external case management for all cases regardless of length of treatment. For example, individuals employed by disability management firms often handle only those cases that involve postinjury care of six months or more. Major national and regional workers' compensation carriers, such as Liberty Mutual, Aetna, and Hartford, tend to employ rehabilitation nurses to manage the more complex and higher-dollar-cost cases. These case managers thus often require more extensive rehabilitation resources for a comparatively smaller caseload.

Nurses employed by state-operated workers' compensation units, private attorneys, and case managers comprise the other key rehabilitation customers, although they represent much smaller referral volumes. Of more than 40 states with workers' compensation units, 22 states provide for direct referral of more complex cases to external rehabilitation providers. Attorneys will also get involved and recommend providers (particularly for evaluation services) in extended lost-work time cases.

Business Potential of Occupational Rehabilitation

The business development potential and market demand for evaluation and treatment services is significant. Functional capacities assessments, work capacity evaluations, and work hardening typically comprise more than 75 percent of the product mix of occupational rehabilitation programs. Work capacity evaluations and functional capacities assessments alone may represent 25–40 percent and work hardening up to 50 percent of the overall services. Back schools are already the third most popular promotion/prevention program in industry, behind only smoking cessation and weight loss. Generally, traditional physical therapy modalities, work tolerance screening, worksite evaluation, case management, and vocational services make up the remaining product mix.[4]

In addition to its emphasis on services that are not provided by physicians, other operational and financial characteristics of occupational rehabilitation differentiate this business segment from urgent care and acute injury treatment. Providers of injury treatment services enjoy higher patient volume but comparatively lower dollar revenue per visit and per case. With an average charge of $60 per injury visit, the provider of injury treatment services seeks to enroll several hundred companies while significantly supplementing basic injury visit revenue with revenue from physical assessment and ancillary examinations.

In contrast to urgent care and acute injury treatment, occupational rehabilitation programs have a lower volume but a higher revenue per case. The greatest revenue per case derives from work hardening, followed by work capacity evaluations and functional capacities assessments. Revenues for a typical work hardening case average about $2,400 ($150 per day for an average program of four days per week for four weeks) as compared to an average charge of $300 to $500 or more per case for an acute injury treatment program. Each work capacity or functional capacity evaluation provides average revenue of $250 to $350 for about four to six hours of therapy staff involvement. Screening revenues range from $100 to $300 per evaluation depending on length and intensity.

Given these distinctive operating and financial conditions, it is not surprising that financial break-even for an occupational rehabilitation program may occur as early as 6 months to a year in contrast to the 18 months to 2 years typical of acute injury treatment programs. For freestanding and hospital-based programs, break-even timing will depend on the extent of cost allocations or overhead pass-throughs levied by the sponsoring hospital.

With careful planning, even prevention and education services such as worksite evaluation and ergonomics can be structured as financial break-even or moderately profitable services. Often, a company will become interested in these services as a result of reduced employer benefits costs deriving from successful employee rehabilitation care.

Critical Success Factors

Most often, rehabilitation services are developed to complement and broaden a provider's existing range of occupational health services. However, with thorough internal and external market analysis and careful business planning, providers with limited or no acute injury treatment services can create successful occupational health programs focused exclusively on rehabilitation services. Factors critical to program success include:

- Identifying and linking with orthopedists, physiatrists, and other treatment professionals with strong workers' compensation track records
- Recruiting and training appropriate staff and establishing a strong customer service orientation
- Establishing strong program management
- Linking with acute injury management and other feeder systems
- Meeting basic equipment and dedicated space needs
- Establishing sound case management practices, including development of case protocols and tracking systems
- Implementing effective marketing and sales strategies

Linkage with the Treatment Community

Physicians and therapists act both as referral sources and major distribution channels for occupational rehabilitation programs. Therapists and physicians who have established strong track records in occupational health care often receive referrals directly from employers and insurance carriers. Hospital-based or freestanding programs can benefit if they have already established relationships with these members of the treatment community for the provision of such program services as medical management and work hardening.

Orthopedists, neurosurgeons, neurologists, and physiatrists are the specialists most commonly involved in the medical management and direction of occupational rehabilitation programs. Orthopedists remain the dominant specialty chosen by insurance carriers, disability management firms, and employers for the bulk of musculoskeletal rehabilitation cases, particularly back injuries. Such clients are increasingly recognizing the importance of comprehensive diagnostic and treatment approaches and the benefits of conservative, nonsurgical treatment approaches.

The preferred linkage for occupational rehabilitation providers might be with a strong multispecialty group with a track record in occupational rehabilitation. In those markets in which single-specialty groups dominate, the critical physician link is to an orthopedic group that has its own linkages with other specialists that can broaden the range of offered services.

The hospital-based provider without in-house occupational rehabilitation expertise should consider joint ventures or less formal linkages with freestanding occupational and physical therapy practices. In some markets, an offer of financial resources or improved access to distribution channels may serve as an inducement for private-practice therapy clinics. A provider could also establish a strong negotiating position by offering an enhanced physician referral base because carriers in most states still require a physician's prescription for reimbursement of work evaluation and work hardening services.

Providers must be aware of already-existing physician/therapist relationships if they are to select and develop successful distribution linkages and create a strong market position. Formal ties may exist in those states in which orthopedists can buy in to private therapy practices. Less formal ties may exist when physicians own the office buildings in which therapists are housed.

Therapist Recruitment and Training

An occupational rehabilitation program should not be initiated without in-house therapists who understand and are responsive to the unique needs of industry. Recruitment of at least one primary therapist, especially a physical therapist, with an existing track record in occupational health care programming is a critical first step. Other highly motivated therapists can learn a great deal about industry's needs by visiting other programs, attending training seminars, and visiting local companies.

Probably the most significant issue in successful program positioning and long-term growth is the entrepreneurial or customer-oriented mind-set of the therapy staff and their understanding of referral source needs. Even traditional inpatient rehabilitation providers are setting time-limited and measurable return-to-work goals.

Both the key physicians (especially the medical director) and primary therapists must be flexible and motivated enough to be willing to visit the worksite to gain firsthand knowledge of specific job demands and industry needs. As the program develops, willingness to provide worksite services will be essential to program growth and differentiation. Once a provider has made some inroads in returning specific employees back to work, the employer is likely to seek additional programs for reducing long-term injury and rehabilitation costs.

Although industry expertise is ideal, therapists should at least have a strong track record of work with lower back and musculoskeletal injuries. Should therapists have little experience with work-related injuries, they must be motivated to obtain training prior to program start-up and continually seek to upgrade their industry knowledge base.

Because physical therapists function as the lead discipline for work evaluations, it is important that the physical therapist have substantial prior exposure to industry. The physical therapist's familiarity with the impact of work conditions and job demands on musculoskeletal conditions becomes particularly significant because work evaluation often is the entry or feeder point to work hardening. In this time of shortages of skilled physical therapists, attracting an experienced physical therapist may require developing creative financial-incentive packages or joint venturing with experienced private practitioners.

Because occupational therapists are trained to educate and are often trained in job analysis, the occupational therapist is likely to be the lead therapist for work simulation. The occupational therapist is more likely to have a shorter learning curve to understand how to simulate specific job conditions and tasks for clients. Nonetheless, the occupational therapist and the physical therapist (along with the physician, the rehabilitation counselor, and the consulting psychologist) must operate as members of a multidisciplinary effort for treatment planning and work evaluation and work hardening programming to achieve timely return-to-work results.

Although hard-and-fast rules for staffing do not exist, generally a ratio of one licensed therapist to every six full-time patients is a useful guideline for work hardening. Generally, one licensed therapist will be supplemented with at least a 0.5 to 1 full-time equivalent (FTE) aide depending upon whether a simulation or evaluation function is involved. Because work evaluation requires musculoskeletal and job assessment components, both licensed occupational therapy and physical therapy staff time will be required for this service. Careful projection of likely product/service mix and adjustment to meet actual demand will determine the optimal staffing pattern over time.

Program operations should also allow staff enough time for creative development and use of equipment and space. Although basic workset and workstations are now available for job simulation, therapists must have adequate time to adjust existing equipment and create makeshift resources to respond to specific patient job needs.

Computerized equipment cannot begin to cover the wide range of job demands in major urban markets, nor can the provider afford this costly alternative. The time and resource investment in allowing staff to develop creative solutions of their own for one specific job may only require a few hours and yet result in high payback in terms of staff learning and retention. The right blend among computerized evaluation equipment, purchased workstations, and creative in-house simulation tools demonstrates to the customer the provider's concern for the client's unique needs.

The Program Management Team

Where management resources are particularly limited, a provider offering both acute injury treatment and occupational rehabilitation programs should recruit two managers—a manager responsible for the overall product line and a manager for the rehabilitation program. Because the rehabilitation program involves distinctive consumers, referral sources, and services, a manager responsible for acute injury treatment services is not likely to have the depth of knowledge and time available to devote to successfully managing both programs. By segmenting the management of the rehabilitation program, the product line manager can devote additional attention to acute injury treatment services in addition to overall product line coordination.

A strong business manager is needed to operate the rehabilitation program—a manager who is also well versed in clinical issues and workers' compensation reimbursement issues. This manager must also be able to complement the skills of the manager responsible for the larger occupational health program of which the occupational rehabilitation program is a part.

Linkage with Feeder Systems

Although it may be financially feasible to start up a rehabilitation program without an initial (and ongoing) flow of referrals from acute injury feeder programs and facilities, achieving desirable profit margins by year 2 will prove increasingly difficult without such a network. Whether injury treatment programs, hospitals, employers, or physicians become the primary referral sources, it is dangerous to rest program success on a high volume of referrals from only one or two primary sources, particularly one or two lead orthopedists.

Nurturing and expanding feeder relationships is also critical to long-term success. The provider without strong in-house acute injury treatment programs can nonetheless use this apparent weakness as a basis for networking with freestanding urgent care providers. This can be done by offering to supplement urgent care providers with strong rehabilitation services rather than by competing within the acute injury management market.

Because occupational rehabilitation programs are still only in the growth phase of the product maturity cycle, lead physicians (and to a lesser extent, therapists) will be subject to temptation from varied sources of competition, including other hospitals and proprietary firms. In some instances, joint venturing with key physicians can serve to head off the financing or development of competitive programs by physicians.

Space and Equipment

Starting up a successful occupational rehabilitation program requires a commitment to meeting at least minimum dedicated space and equipment needs. A bare minimum of 1,600 to 2,000 square feet should be available for physical restoration and exercise, work evaluation, and job simulation needs. Of this, a minimum of 600 to 800 square feet should be devoted to job simulation and should not be shared by other therapy services.

Even state industrial commissions have begun to recognize the importance of dedicated space for work simulation. The Rehabilitation Division of the Industrial Commission of Ohio, which approves vendor claims, now requires that work hardening programs devote a minimum of 100 square feet per claimant to work simulation. A preferred total program allocation of 2,500 or more square feet will build in the ability to effectively respond to a growth in volume or programming needs.

Many hospitals now face continuing shortages of adequate space even for general outpatient therapy treatment. Often, inpatients and outpatients with physical rehabilitation needs are treated in the same areas because of ongoing space considerations. Although it may be necessary to begin the work evaluation and restoration/exercise components in shared space, even those components will not be able to respond to program growth needs without dedicated space. Increasingly, potential providers are looking to nonhospital or off-campus locations to resolve therapy space shortages for occupational rehabilitation and other growth programs.

Because therapy services represent the essence of the occupational rehabilitation product line, work evaluation and work hardening must not be mixed with nonoccupational services in existing occupational therapist and physical therapist departments that serve both inpatients and outpatients. Unique space demonstrates unique identity and can be the basis for success comparable to this activity.

If a provider has outpatient therapy space devoted to a program with somewhat comparable resource/equipment needs—particularly sports medicine—it may be possible (and cost-effective during the start-up phase) to share space and exercise equipment and some equipment for evaluation or physical therapist treatment. Patients suffering from extensive deconditioning will require basic exercise and a physical therapist before they will be ready for job simulation.

A potential rehabilitation provider should also plan for a bare minimum of $75,000 to $100,000 in treatment-related equipment costs during year 1 of the program. At least one major piece of computerized evaluation equipment, workstations for simulation, and exercise equipment will be included within equipment needs.[5]

Only one piece of computerized equipment, a personal computer, is actually necessary to start up a program. Computerization allows for:

- Objective measurement of the possible ramifications of an injury

- Collection of normative data
- Comparison of preprogram, ongoing, and postprogram gains
- Preparation of reports of objective findings that need to be available to meet legal reimbursement and workers' compensation commission requirements

The BTE Work Simulator, which is manufactured by Baltimore Therapeutic and comes with a personal computer, is probably the most common piece of equipment used for both evaluation and job simulation. Recently, some therapists have indicated a preference for the Lido Workset as an alternative to the BTE. With the swift entry of the Cybex back systems into the market, many programs have bought the three major Cybex machines ($130,000), while others have been more conservative and have purchased only the Cybex trunk extension/flexion testing machine (which costs $40,000 or more) or comparable machines.

Case Management

Case management is essential to (1) facilitate coordination and delivery of services among the multiple disciplines and departments involved, (2) monitor referral source satisfaction and obtain appropriate external resources, and (3) ensure timely attainment of case objectives. Inadequate and ineffective communication and patient tracking is the most common complaint against providers. Poor patient tracking and coordination is believed to lead to duplication of resources, fragmented care, and high costs for payers.

Providers can differentiate themselves from competitors through the availability of formal communication and tracking systems with designated case coordinators or managers. The successful program will select at least one staff member to function as a case manager or service assurance coordinator and resource developer. The provider offering a full range of occupational health services should allocate at least one FTE to this function who focuses on both the acute injury and rehabilitation components.

Protocols for work evaluation and work hardening can also help serve as an internal case management as well as a quality control tool. Protocols and procedures should stress acceptance and discharge criteria, job-specific goals, frequency and duration of treatment, clue points for related psychological and vocational services, and measurable levels of functional skill improvement. However, formal procedures and protocols should not be allowed to become a substitute for staff creativity in meeting patient job simulation and treatment needs.

Marketing and Sales

In addition to internal operational issues, direct sales and marketing should be considered a key element in ongoing program growth. Although rehabilitation does represent new customer segments, sales personnel versed in other occupational health services can learn to market the unique benefits and features of occupational rehabilitation.

As in marketing acute injury treatment services, clinical staff should not be assigned a primary direct sales role unless they have prior successful occupational sales experience. The role of the primary sales representative is to identify and confirm prospects and to close the sale. Clinical staff can selectively assist with the sales function by providing technical information to strong prospects to help the salesperson close the sale.

Market education and staff recruitment/training are key in determining the optimal point at which to launch a program. Potential referral sources often must be educated as to the value of these services, and this education must begin at least three to four months prior to program start-up. In addition, staff training and recruitment must be planned so that both the work evaluation and work hardening/job simulation components can be initiated concurrently. Although it is possible to begin (and many facilities do) with a few work hardening patients prior to the start-up of a formal program, patients will be lost to the system if work evaluation (a significant feeder or entry point) cannot be offered along with work hardening/job simulation.

References

1. National Council on Compensation Insurance. *Workers' Compensation Claim Characteristics.* New York City: NCCI, 1985, pp. 54–55.
2. Figler, S. Integrating and marketing injury prevention and rehabilitation services. *Journal of Ambulatory Care Marketing* 2:69–77, June 1988.
3. Morris, A., and Randolph, J. Back rehabilitation programs speed recovery of injured workers. *Occupational Health and Safety,* 53(7), pp. 53–55, July–Aug. 1984.
4. Matheson, L. *Work Capacity Evaluation: A Systematic Approach to Industrial Rehabilitation.* Anaheim, CA: Employment and Rehabilitation Institute of California, 1986.
5. Bettencourt, C., Charlstrom, P., Brown, S., Lindau, K., and Long, C. Using work simulation to treat adults with back injuries. *American Journal of Occupational Therapy* 40:12–18, Jan. 1986.

Part 2

Operational Issues

Chapter 13

The Marketing Plan

Frank H. Leone, M.P.H., M.B.A.

During the 1980s, a striking trend has been developing in workplace health and safety. To meet their work force's health care needs, employers have increasingly turned away from in-house personnel and internal programs and have begun contracting with external providers.

This externalization of occupational health services has occurred at a most fortuitous time for hospitals and other providers. The occupational health market represents an opportunity for providers facing economic uncertainties. In the short term, providers can benefit from an occupational health program's relatively lucrative payer mix (for example, employer-paid and workers' compensation) as well as new contractual revenue opportunities. In the long term, strong relationships with business and industry establish a foundation for subsequent employer–provider endeavors.

Ten Basic Marketing Requirements

Hundreds of provider-based programs have rushed to capitalize on opportunities to market occupational health services to employers. The marketing of these programs, however, is an art that has yet to come of age. Systematic market research and market planning are the exception rather than the rule. Many "programs" merely package a loose set of preexisting hospital services and "market" them to industry under the guise of an occupational health program. To be successful in developing an occupational health marketing plan, a hospital should follow ten basic marketing requirements:

- *Listen to the consumer.* Occupational health programs should respond to consumers' needs rather than simply selling a package of preexisting services. It is wise to assess employer needs through periodic formal market research and other informal mechanisms.

- *Market to a select target audience.* In a typical program service area, the "actual" market consists of approximately 100–150 key individuals who possess the authority to make occupational health purchasing decisions. A program must identify these individuals, assess their companies' individual needs, and determine which companies are priority targets for individual sales efforts. If possible, the program should develop personal relationships with these individuals.
- *Differentiate clearly from other programs.* Genuine innovation in hospital-based occupational health programs is rare. Programs frequently offer the same breadth of services, the same unsubstantiated rationale for these services (for example, "lower health care costs and increased productivity"), and a familiar, undistinguished promotional approach. Successful programs generally offer something more with a sense of excitement and enthusiasm.
- *Professionally assess the market.* It is difficult to imagine the consumer product industry launching a new product without first commissioning a market assessment. Yet few occupational health programs assess their prospective consumers before establishing or refining a program. Effective market research provides critical competitor intelligence; a measure of employer wants, needs, and perceptions; precise demographic data; and priority sales prospects.
- *Forecast future change.* Even when programs complete consumer research and devise marketing plans, they rarely consider the implications of potential future trends. The health care world changes rapidly, necessitating best estimates for future changes in consumer demand and the competition and the possible directions for product line development that would result from such changes.
- *Make internal marketing a priority.* Occupational health programs require the involvement of many departments and individuals. Programs must therefore be aggressively marketed internally as well as externally by proactively dealing with physicians and other key personnel and openly discussing the mutual benefits of a successful program. These individuals must feel that they are part of the program.
- *Thoroughly assess the competition.* An occupational health program normally does not operate in a vacuum without competition. Consequently, a program must assess its competitors to identify their existence, services and prices, strengths and weaknesses by service, and approximate market penetration.
- *Promise only what you can deliver.* It is tempting for an occupational health program to be "all things to all people." Yet programmatic diversification is very difficult, diffuses valuable resources, and can ultimately result in ineffective services. Programs should add new product line components only as market research identifies a clear marketplace need for a service that can be provided professionally.

- *Continually measure consumer satisfaction.* Episodic, one-time market research is insufficient to monitor changing marketplace trends. An effective assessment plan requires annual formal market research, periodic (for example, quarterly) calls to current clients, and daily feedback via patient satisfaction surveys.
- *Market your accomplishments.* Consumers, including employers, flock to a winner. Programs must take full advantage of their track record through testimonials, data summaries, or summary client lists.

Assessing Internal Capabilities

Market assessment begins with an evaluation of the hospital's internal capabilities and limitations in providing occupational health services. A questionnaire can be a useful tool to investigate the availability of personnel. The questionnaire should be distributed to key medical staff members, ancillary departments, and heads of other departments likely to have services to contribute to the program (for example, audiology and respiratory, physical, and occupational therapy).

Questions should elicit such information as when staff is available, what limitations they may have, and what kind of turnaround time the program should expect on referrals, laboratory tests, and the like. Such a survey is good public relations and serves to minimize surprises once a program is functioning.

Program planners should also conduct interviews with upper management, key medical staff, and other current or potential in-house providers of occupational health services. These interviews should be designed to identify strengths and weaknesses for each potential service offering, explore the competitive environment, and establish a basis for good long-term relationships.

Any existing program uncovered in the internal assessment should be converted into benefits that can be used in marketing the occupational health program. Perceived weaknesses or limitations require immediate attention. Common occupational health program limitations include inadequate building space or parking facilities, an antiquated hospital-based billing system, poor patient tracking and case management, and insufficient personnel. Solutions for any potential problems or limitations must be devised before proceeding further.

Assessing the Competition

Assessing the competition is not as difficult as it may seem because, in most circumstances, there are initially only a few significant competitors. In the competitive assessment, program planners should identify the following for each significant competitor:

- Institutional strengths and weaknesses
- Breadth of services
- Pricing structure
- Strengths and limitations of each service
- Market penetration
  - Nature and degree
  - Level of consumer satisfaction

Gathering intelligence about the competition is an ongoing process. Helpful sources of information include the hospital staff; formal consumer research; and networking with current and prospective clients, insurers, and the community at large. If the program has a sales staff, they can serve as the "eyes and ears" of the program and can learn a great deal about what the competition is offering. After the program has gathered and summarized information about its competitors, it can identify its own market opportunities, fee structures, and likely competitive advantages.

Assessing the Consumer

There are three primary ways to assess consumer wants and needs: focus group interviews, survey research, and in-depth interviews with key individuals.

Focus Group Interviews

Focus group interviews are a highly effective technique for quickly learning about the marketplace, assessing the competitive environment, and test marketing ideas and marketing strategies. The following principles should be kept in mind when conducting or contracting for focus groups:

- *Conduct a pair of focus groups.* Conducting only a single focus group session poses a risk that some dynamic may occur that would invalidate the session. For example, a participant may be overly dominant or negative, thus intimidating other participants. Conducting a second session not only significantly minimizes this risk but also gives prospective attendees an alternative session date.
- *Use an experienced moderator.* An experienced moderator knows what questions to ask, when and how to interrupt or probe, and how to make participants comfortable and willing to share their feelings. Moderators should also have knowledge in occupational health and experience with occupational health focus groups.
- *Conduct focus groups at a neutral location.* A neutral location, such as a restaurant or hotel, that is easily accessible for most participants should be used. Representatives from the hospital should not be

present. Hospital staff can subsequently study focus group findings through formal transcripts of each session.

- *Recruit carefully.* In general, focus group attendees should be drawn from prospective client organizations based on the following pool in order to get the most direct and knowledgeable input concerning occupational health issues:
  - Business of fewer than 100 employees: president
  - Business of 100–400 employees: director of personnel
  - Business of 400 or more employees: benefits manager

  Recruitment should begin two to three weeks before the sessions and involve an honorarium ($50 to $100 depending on location) and a complimentary meal.

The optimal size for a focus group is six or seven individuals. The optimal length of a session is 90 to 120 minutes. Invitations should mirror the industrial mix of the service area and include individuals from companies most likely to use external occupational health services because of location or injury incidence.

Crucial issues that can be addressed during the focus group sessions include:

- Primary health and safety problems at the workplace
- The current solutions to these problems
- Priority health and safety needs
- Current providers, services, and fees
- Satisfaction with these providers
- Perceptions of the client hospital
- Potential marketing approaches
- Identity and involvement of the company's insurers

Survey Research

Survey research is the next step in a comprehensive marketplace assessment. A survey sample of approximately 150 key employers is normally sufficient, with the majority of the sample drawn from companies with 100–400 employees.

Although a mail survey is the least costly option, it traditionally generates a response rate no higher than 20 percent. A telephone survey is more costly ($25 to $50 per completed interview) but usually produces a better response rate. The ideal option is a one-time mail survey (generally yielding about a 20 percent response rate) with a follow-up telephone survey to nonrespondents.

The survey should be based upon information obtained in the internal assessment, competitor assessment, and focus group sessions. At a minimum, the survey should address employer needs, use and evaluation of current providers, priority health and safety issues, injury and illness incidence rates, and basic demographic data.

Figure 13-1 is a prototype of a questionnaire intended to assess what services an employer may be interested in and how intensely the employer may be interested in the service. This relatively simple questionnaire provides a considerable amount of valuable information. Responses can be rated on a scale of 7 to 1 to rank order all services by overall preference. Employers who express a high degree of interest in a service (for example, a 6 or 7) can be targeted as potential purchasers of that service.

Figure 13-1. Prototype of an Employer Interest Questionnaire

How interested would your company be in each of the following health care services if they were reasonably priced? (Circle one choice for each service.)

	Very Interested		Somewhat Interested			Not Interested	
At Workplace							
Hearing testing/follow-up	7	6	5	4	3	2	1
Physician at/available to workplace	7	6	5	4	3	2	1
Nurse placement at worksite	7	6	5	4	3	2	1
Back injury prevention	7	6	5	4	3	2	1
Stress reduction	7	6	5	4	3	2	1
Employee assistance (EAP)	7	6	5	4	3	2	1
Blood pressure screening	7	6	5	4	3	2	1
At Nonworkplace Location							
Workers' comp evaluations	7	6	5	4	3	2	1
Preemployment physicals	7	6	5	4	3	2	1
Other physical examinations	7	6	5	4	3	2	1
Back injury rehabilitation	7	6	5	4	3	2	1
Emergent/urgent care	7	6	5	4	3	2	1
Drug testing	7	6	5	4	3	2	1
Work hardening programs	7	6	5	4	3	2	1
Occupational health seminars	7	6	5	4	3	2	1

Survey research should also identify services employers are currently offering to their employees, the provider of each service, and employers' degree of satisfaction with each provider. Figure 13-2 illustrates a prototype

Figure 13-2. Prototype of a Current Service Satisfaction Questionnaire

Which of the following services has your company either received or provided during the preceding 12 months?

	Yes	No	If Yes, Name Provider (include in-house)	Degree of Satisfaction (Circle one) High	Medium	Low
At Workplace						
Hearing testing/follow-up	___	___	___________	3	2	1
Physician at/available to workplace	___	___	___________	3	2	1
Nurse placement at worksite	___	___	___________	3	2	1
Back injury prevention	___	___	___________	3	2	1
Stress reduction	___	___	___________	3	2	1
Employee assistance (EAP)	___	___	___________	3	2	1
Blood pressure screening	___	___	___________	3	2	1
At Nonworkplace Location						
Workers' comp evaluations	___	___	___________	3	2	1
Preemployment physicals	___	___	___________	3	2	1
Other physical examinations	___	___	___________	3	2	1
Back injury rehabilitation	___	___	___________	3	2	1
Emergent/urgent care	___	___	___________	3	2	1
Drug testing	___	___	___________	3	2	1
Work hardening programs	___	___	___________	3	2	1
Occupational health seminars	___	___	___________	3	2	1

of a questionnaire intended to capture this information. Note that the list of services is identical to the list portrayed in figure 13-1.

Survey research can also be used to prioritize workplace health and safety problems. Such information can help a program design marketing campaigns in response to the most commonly cited problems and to develop background information on individual employers. Figure 13-3 is a prototype of a questionnaire used to obtain this type of information.

Beyond gathering information on attitudes and preferences, surveys should be designed to directly request information on basic incidence rates and medical practices, including:

- Annual number of preemployment physical examinations
- Annual lost workdays due to workplace injuries
- Total lost workdays per year
- Total number of workers' compensation claims
- Types of required medical surveillance examinations

Finally, surveys should identify the following demographic information:

- Number of employees (this information can differ markedly from published accounts)
- Miles (or driving time) to the closest medical facility
- Self-insured or not self-insured
- Type of company

Figure 13-3. Prototype of an Employer Health and Safety Concern Questionnaire

At the present time, how serious do you consider each of these health and safety problems at your workplace?

	Very Serious		Somewhat Serious			Not Serious	
Low productivity	7	6	5	4	3	2	1
High absenteeism	7	6	5	4	3	2	1
Unsafe working conditions	7	6	5	4	3	2	1
Environmental contaminants	7	6	5	4	3	2	1
High health care premiums	7	6	5	4	3	2	1
Employee morale	7	6	5	4	3	2	1
Workplace injuries	7	6	5	4	3	2	1
Workers' comp claims	7	6	5	4	3	2	1

Some researchers use employers' standard industrial classification (SIC) codes obtained from state departments of labor to categorize local employers; however, the use of these codes may result in too many narrowly defined categories to be useful. More practical data can be acquired by asking each employer to define its company type (that is, service industry, heavy manufacturing, and so forth).

Survey results in the aggregate can be interesting but often are misleading. Researchers can help clarify results by segmenting the results in three ways:

- *Company size.* Employers responding to the survey can be sorted as small companies (either fewer than 50 or fewer than 100 employees, depending on the area), mid-sized companies (100–400 employees), and larger companies (more than 400 employees). Although there are notable exceptions, mid-sized companies will be the prime targets for most hospital-based programs because, as a general rule, they have higher injury incidence rates and are unlikely to have in-house medical services.
- *Distance from provider.* Given the critical importance of proximity of service in occupational health, it is useful to segment survey respondents by distance from the workplace to the provider (for example, less than 1 mile, 1 to 3 miles, and so forth). All other things being equal, programs should target the closest firms first.
- *Company type.* Depending on the industry mix in a given service area, results should be aggregated by company type. Common types include heavy manufacturers, light manufacturers, and transportation, chemical, and service companies.

In-Depth Interviews

The third source of consumer information involves in-depth interviews with likely program constituents. Examples include major insurers, key employers, and active business and safety groups or coalitions, although client bases will vary depending on the nature and scope of offered services.

Designing the Marketing Plan

Few hospital-based occupational health programs produce a strategic plan to serve as a program guide. Such plans are crucial; a strategic plan for a program is the equivalent of a blueprint for a new home. A successful plan requires several things:

- *Clearly defined goals.* In occupational health, goals can be expressed in terms of volume of patient visits, revenue, or break-even periods.

- *Organizational consensus.* Hospital management and staff must have input and must buy in to the plan.
- *Specified action.* The plan should include an "action appendix" that specifies activities, responsibilities, and implementation dates.
- *Sound market research basis.* The soundness of research behind the plan will be substantiated once it has been established.

The plan must become a central part of day-to-day operations. Successfully implementing the plan requires that the program develop strategies for each of the four classic Ps of marketing (price, product, place, and promotion) for each service.

Price

In occupational health, price is usually quite inelastic, meaning that reductions in price are not likely to increase market share. Pricing strategy involves identifying the going market rates for each service and establishing price at that level ("market pricing") or at a defined percentage of a competitor's price ("shadow pricing").

Unlike many other segments of the health care market, employers are generally aware of specific charges. Consequently, cost-based charges hold little or no relevance when pricing for employers.

Naturally, pricing decisions vary greatly by service, the existence and market penetration of the competition, and the geographical area. A service new to the marketplace, for example, may require a special discount in order to get a foot in the door and establish a track record.

Product

Product differentiation is the key factor in the second classic P of marketing. Market research should identify the limitations of competitors' offerings or specific needs in the marketplace. The astute program planner should then address these weaknesses or marketplace needs as opportunities. For example, if the primary competitor is a clinic that provides quality service and feedback, but is open only 12 hours per day, a hospital-based program should match the clinic's convenience while operating during hours more responsive to the client's needs.

As a rule, employers look for the following five product attributes:

- *Leadership.* Programs need a single, strong individual who can serve as the liaison between the employer and the provider's program.
- *Continuity of care.* Employers require effective case management of their employees in order to get injured workers back to work in the shortest possible time period. A program should have the ability to provide long-term case management for these workers and not lose track of patients somewhere in the system.

- *Operational efficiency.* Employers require that the injured or ill worker be absent from the workplace for the shortest possible time period. Operational efficiency, including easy access, short waiting periods, and efficient follow-up communication, is vital.
- *Bedside manner.* Employers constantly cite the clinician's bedside manner as the key measure of program quality. This translates to the general principle that marketing is the responsibility of the entire program staff.
- *Sharing of data.* Employers generally like to see reports, data, and some basic accounting of cost savings such as lost workdays attributable to employee injuries.

Ultimately, the most effective marketing tool of all is simply good performance. Highly competent programs staffed by professional, friendly, and enthusiastic individuals maintain a considerable competitive advantage.

Place

Employers rate location as their first prerequisite of an occupational health program. In choosing a location for the provision of clinical services, a hospital should consider the following locations in priority order:

1. A freestanding facility on the hospital campus (this provides the best of both worlds: a cliniclike setting that is immediately accessible to the hospital)
2. A freestanding satellite facility associated with the hospital
3. A hospital-based program with a dedicated entrance
4. A program that operates out of the emergency department

Examples of these approaches to service locations are provided in various chapters of this publication; see especially chapter 16 for the merits of freestanding facilities.

Ultimately, a program should make every effort to provide as many services as possible directly at the worksite. On-site programs can forge a strong bond with employers and provide the hospital with a considerable competitive advantage. It seems likely that on-site delivery of physician and nursing services as well as other consultative services will become more common during the coming years.

Promotion/Sales

There seem to be many misconceptions regarding the promotion of occupational health programs. Using paid media—in any form—is inadvisable in that they reach too large and broad an audience. Direct mail, likewise, seldom produces tangible results commensurate with the cost of the mailing.

Newsletters, although of some value, tend to consume a disproportionate amount of scarce resources.

The development of personal relationships and one-on-one sales approaches is the key to successful occupational health promotion. The occupational health sales process involves the following basic steps:

1. Identify primary prospects through effective market research.
2. Conduct a sales call that focuses on identifying the employer's specific needs.
3. Develop a written proposal for a company based on its specific needs and the program's capabilities.
4. Conduct a second sales call, with appropriate clinical personnel (that is, "team selling"), in order to discuss and possibly refine the proposal.
5. Follow up and "close" the sales process.
6. Carefully monitor the client's satisfaction with the program's services and be willing to modify the services as necessary.

Brochure Design

Effective brochures and collateral materials do not sell occupational health programs, but poor ones can significantly jeopardize a program. More often than not, occupational health program brochures tend to look the same and are of marginal quality. An effective brochure should possess the following attributes:

- *Simplicity.* We are living in an information-saturated society; people simply don't have time to read. The brochure should convey the intended message in the title and associated graphics.
- *High-quality stock.* Glossy, heavier-weight stock costs a bit more but imparts a far more professional image for the program.
- *Third-party testimonials.* Employers like an established program with a demonstrable track record. Comments from current clients extolling the program permit the employer to hear a testimonial from someone like themselves. For example:

  "Mercy Hospital's WorkWell program has resulted in a 15 percent reduction in lost workdays during the past year."
  —Gerry Gordon, Personnel Director, Garelick Farms

In addition to using testimonial advertising, an established program should take advantage of its track record in marketing. Programs should encourage prospective clients to telephone current clients to discuss their experiences with the program. Programs should also share data summarizing program results (with obvious confidentiality considerations) and invite prospective clients to observe current program activities.

Educational Programs

Educational programs can be a powerful marketing activity. If market research identifies in-service occupational health education as an employer interest, periodic educational programs can be a particularly useful way to introduce personnel managers to a program. Educational meetings or seminars can provide these managers with a better understanding of occupational health issues, and they can serve as yet another avenue for program staff to gain an understanding of industry's perspective.

Educational programs can take the form of periodic presentations (for example, a bimonthly breakfast club), half-day or day-long seminars on major occupational health issues (such as "Getting the Injured Worker Back to Work" or "Drug Testing at the Workplace"), or even a multiweek course such as emergency medical technician training.

Why Programs Fail

Hospital-based occupational health programs fail, or at least fail to prosper, for a great many reasons, many of which are related to inadequate market research and planning. The three most common marketing-oriented reasons for failure seem to be:

- The absence of market research
- Failure to target marketing on a one-on-one basis
- Placing the wrong person in the primary marketing role

The externalization of occupational health services to hospitals provides occupational health professionals with a unique and interesting challenge: to profoundly affect the health of large populations of employees, to assist employers in their goal of attaining a more satisfactory bottom line, and to serve as a vital diversification strategy for their own hospital. Ultimately, a hospital's ability to successfully take up the challenge will be contingent upon its understanding of and response to the specific health care needs of industry. High-quality market research, market planning, and direct sales are essential if hospitals are to meet this goal.

Chapter 14

Sales Strategies*

Richard C. Williams, M.B.A., M.S.
Lynn D. Jones, M.P.S.

The area of hospital sales has emerged with the growing competitiveness of health care. In the late 1970s, the concept of marketing was adopted by a few pioneering hospitals that recognized the importance of matching hospital services with market needs. By the mid-1980s, hundreds of marketing people worked in hospitals. However, their focus was primarily research, planning, development, and marketing communications, not sales.

Although sales is interconnected with marketing and planning, it is the one function of the marketing mix that is highly personal in nature. Sales has become a functional part of the hospital occupational health business because the nature of the business dictates that someone has to contact prospective customers about new hospital programs and services and explain the benefits of the new products. No amount of research or planning can replace the impact of a salesperson's first 10 seconds with a potential customer and the resulting interest that is either generated or lost. For a hospital occupational health service, developing a sales force can mean the difference between success and failure.

Common Misconceptions about Sales

Although hospital management often recognizes the need for a sales force, a hospital's management team may have some serious misconceptions about sales. These misconceptions, or biases, can stymie sales efforts for occupational health services. Managers may view hospital sales as:

*This chapter is adapted from various chapters in *Managing the Hospital Sales Team* by Richard C. Williams (Chicago: American Hospital Publishing, Inc., 1988).

- A "fill the order" function that simply requires the salesperson to "visit" the prospect to get the business
- A natural extension of the fast-talking, slick-dressing stereotype of salespeople
- Part of everyone's job at the hospital
- Something that will have an *immediate* effect on revenue and volume
- A necessary evil in a competitive environment
- A task, not a profession

Many administrators believe that enough customers exist for every service the hospital has to offer. Using this reasoning, administrators assume that by visiting appropriate prospects, salespeople have only to take their orders and leave. On the contrary, sales involves not only finding the best prospects but helping customers to identify a problem that the hospital's services will solve. Few hospital programs or products require only "filling the order." Instead, they require complex selling strategies and skills.

For a personal sales effort to succeed, hospitals must be willing to risk development costs in expectation of long-term results of sales. Often, management expects the new sales program to deliver sales immediately. However, for more expensive services or services that are new to the market (such as an employee assistance program), it may take six to eight months or even a year before a salesperson completes the sale. If salespeople have good products to sell and the appropriate support from the hospital, they can generate significant new business in the occupational health field.

Solution Selling

The most successful salespeople do not sell products or services; they sell solutions. They present their products and services as a solution to a problem. This is one of the most fundamental sales methods in occupational health.

The difference between product selling and solution selling can be illustrated by the following scenario of a salesperson who is trying to sell an industrial medical program to a manufacturing plant with 500 employees. The product approach might yield a conversation such as this one:

Salesperson: Our industrial medical centers are conveniently located.

Prospect: Yes, I have seen them from the interstate.

Salesperson: Our physical examinations are competitively priced, and we guarantee they will take no more than one hour.

Prospect: Yes, we all must deal with a competitive world.

Salesperson: Is this something you would be interested in?

Prospect: I don't know. I need a lot more information, and, frankly, this is not a priority.

The following *solution-selling* approach generates better results:

Salesperson: What issues must your company face if it is to continue to grow as it has over the past five years?

Prospect: Well, our goal is to increase productivity 5 percent per year for the next five years.

Salesperson: What will help you reach that 5 percent?

Prospect: We need to improve our on-the-job performance. In other words, we need to reduce absenteeism.

Salesperson: What is your absenteeism rate?

Prospect: Too high.

Salesperson: So if we could help you reduce that rate, you feel it would represent a big step toward your five-year goal!

Prospect: That's right. If I can reduce absenteeism, I can really get a hold on the problem.

A close examination of these two conversations shows that the product approach was to the point and aimed at selling the product to the prospect. The prospect, however, was agreeable but not interested. Although the salesperson mentioned some benefits, they were not necessarily benefits in which the prospect was interested. The prospect never really got involved in the conversation.

In the solution-selling approach, the prospect determined what the company's priorities were and defined the problem (with the salesperson's assistance). The salesperson asked questions designed to help the prospect identify what was important. Their conversation revealed that the prospect would be receptive to any product that reduced absenteeism. The conversation continued in this way:

Salesperson: Were you aware that one of the principal reasons for excessive absenteeism in certain jobs is hiring a person who is physically incapable of performing a particular job or poorly trained to perform it?

Prospect: I know. Our loading dock people are always hurting themselves. And the production workers are often careless.

Salesperson: So what we need is to find the right people for specific jobs and improve safety.

Prospect: Right.

Salesperson: This preemployment examination can help you. . . .Combined with a safety program, the examination may be a first step in cutting absenteeism. What do you think?

Prospect: I like it. We will have to look at the details, but I like it.

The prospect wanted reduced absenteeism, better-prepared workers, and safety. Hence, the second salesperson sold those benefits to the prospect.

Solution selling involves six simple steps that get the prospective customer involved, generate feedback, and motivate the prospect to buy. A prospect who becomes actively involved by explaining what he or she wants to buy helps the salesperson make the sale.

The six basic steps of solution selling are listed below:

1. *Ask fact-finding questions* to find out as much as possible about the prospect, the organization, and the prospect's needs in order to identify one or more problems.
2. *Develop awareness* to help the prospect visualize the need for the hospital's service by restating the problem from the customer's perspective.
3. *Establish commitment* by helping the prospect to the realization that "I, the customer, want to solve this."
4. *Identify the solution* by helping the prospect to define the problem and identify the solution in the prospect's own terms.
5. *Demonstrate the solution* by referring to testimonials and references to prove that services are effective.
6. *Close* or culminate the solution-selling process by requesting the order.

No salesperson can estimate how much time is needed to follow these steps. However, the typical sale will require more time if these steps are not followed sequentially and the prospect does not get actively involved in the conversation.

Organizational Structure of the Sales Function

Where does the sales function belong? Experience shows that it is easier to create a sales force than to incorporate it within the hospital's organizational structure. Because sales is a new concept, the organizational fit is often difficult. In organizing the sales operation, several options exist, each with advantages and disadvantages that the hospital administration must weigh carefully. Typically, the sales force reports to the general administration, to the occupational health services manager, or to the marketing department.

Placing the Sales Force under the General Administration

Small hospitals or those without a marketing department and hospitals with a chief executive officer who considers sales an important strategy may place the sales function under the general administration (figure 14-1). Reporting to the administrator confers an internal legitimacy on the sales effort that

Figure 14-1. Sales Organizational Chart: The Administration Model

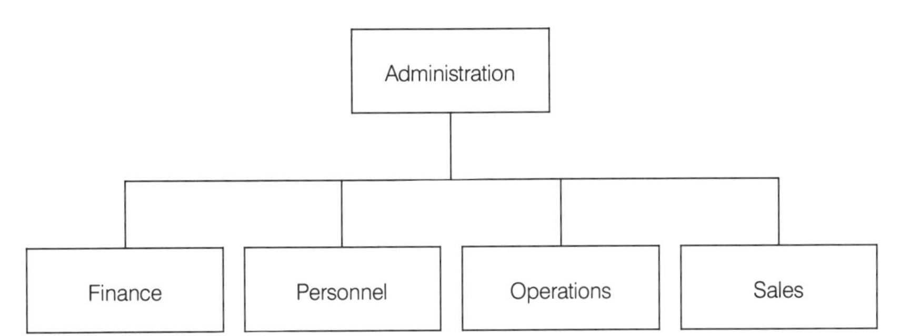

cannot be duplicated through any other type of reporting relationship. This model can be effective if the administrator has sales experience and the time to direct the sales effort. Typically, however, this is not the case, and the administrator ends up delegating the responsibility, leaving the sales force fragmented and without supervision.

Placing the Sales Force under a Product Manager

A common organizational structure adopted by hospitals initiating the occupational health services sales function is to hire a salesperson who directly reports to the occupational health services manager. This organizational structure assumes that the salesperson will be selling only occupational health services (figure 14-2).

The *advantages* of having the sales force report to the occupational health services product manager include the following:

- The occupational health services manager knows the product well.
- If the occupational health services manager has been selling, he or she knows the sales opportunities.
- The occupational health services manager's department is most affected by the results of the sales effort. Hence, the product manager will be the person who is the most interested in the success of that effort.

Some *disadvantages* of having the sales force report to the occupational health services manager are the following:

- The occupational health services manager is usually product oriented rather than customer oriented and is consequently more concerned with product features than with the benefits perceived by the customer.
- The occupational health services manager is often less likely to be open to criticism or suggestions for enhancing the product.

Figure 14-2. Sales Organizational Chart: The Product Manager Model

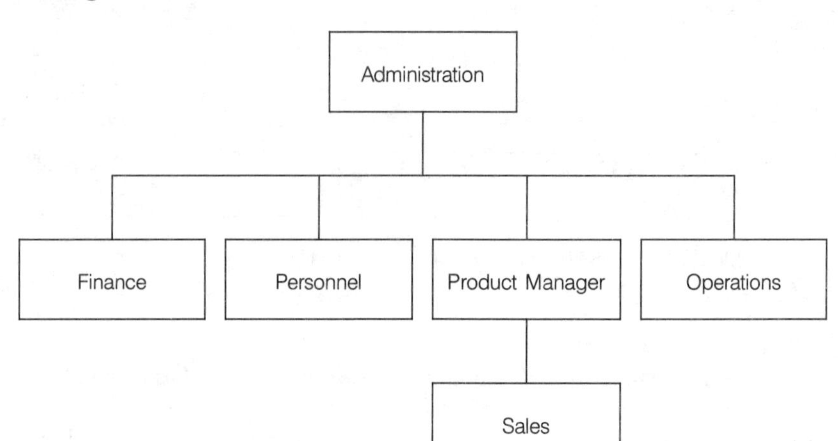

- The hospital sales efforts are focused solely on the services directly provided by the occupational health department and ignore other organizational sales needs (cross-selling opportunities).

As a rule of thumb, unless occupational health services managers have some sales experience, they find it difficult to both manage the product and oversee the sales effort.

Placing the Sales Force under the Marketing Director

The most common hospital option is to incorporate the sales function within the marketing department (or the public relations department in hospitals without a marketing department) (figure 14-3).

The logical arguments for placing sales within the marketing department include the following:

- Selling is the natural conclusion of the marketing process.
- Many sales-support activities emanate from the marketing department.
- In some hospitals, the marketing department is considered the ideal location for new revenue-enhancing products and ideas.
- Locating the sales function in the marketing department can provide broader organizational recognition and greater sales support and resources such as promotional support services.
- The scope of the salesperson's professional responsibilities and job scope is broader and provides more opportunities for growth, thereby decreasing the likelihood of frequent sales staff turnover.

Figure 14-3. Sales Organizational Chart: The Marketing Director Model

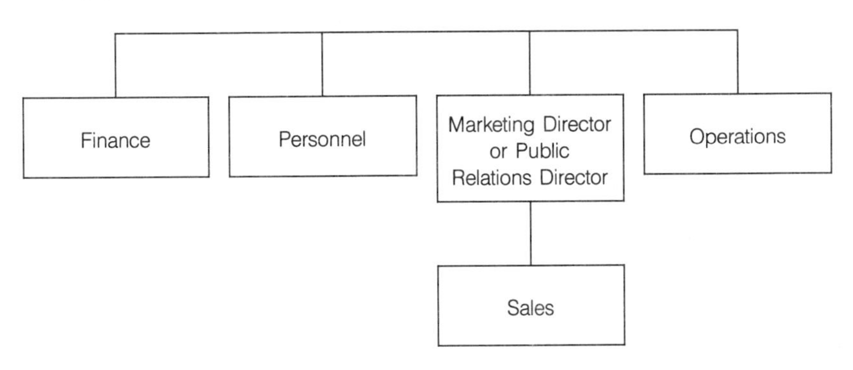

Depending on the hospital, some good reasons may exist for not relegating sales to the marketing department's direction. For example:

- Many marketing people do not have sales experience.
- When the sales function is placed within the marketing department, the salesperson may be required to perform more marketing-related tasks, such as market research and product development, for which he or she is not adequately trained. The salesperson will thus have less time for actual selling.
- Because the salesperson is responsible for a broader array of hospital services, less time may be invested in selling occupational health services.
- The products may be highly specialized and most effectively sold through professional contacts, not salespeople.

Formulating a Team Approach to Sales

One approach to eliminating problems that occur when the sales function is placed within the marketing department is to develop a team approach to the sales function and combine the efforts of both the salesperson and the occupational health services department head or product manager. A successful example of sales staff and department manager collaboration has been implemented at Mills-Peninsula Hospital in northern California.

In 1987, sales representatives at this hospital brought in $1.7 million in new business. Products sold by the hospital include industrial health services, mental health services, employee assistance programs, and chemical dependency, trauma, and fitness programs. The secret to this hospital's success is a coordinated effort of both the hospital sales staff, which consists of a sales director and a two-person sales staff, and the 25 department managers in the hospital.

All 25 departments are linked through Coordinated Health Services, the marketing and sales arm of the organization. Each department manager works with the sales staff to present information about the product or service to prospective customers. The department managers are responsible for all product expertise and for developing the final sales protocol based on the customer's individual needs. The role of the sales staff is to initiate all customer contacts, provide sales information, and negotiate price. A customer service manager handles any complaints or problems.

The sales staff conducts monthly sessions with product managers to review customers' concerns and continually assess customers' service needs. The sales staff also conducts frequent luncheon sessions with department managers to encourage their continued involvement in the sales process. As a result of this organizational structure, a majority of the hospital's sales result from cross-selling different department services to each client. The hospital has extensive tracking and protocol systems in place to make sure that each department staff member knows how to handle patients referred from different customers.

Both occupational health services managers and salespeople can benefit from a sales force that is centrally administered within the organization and encourages a collaborative approach to the sales process. Salespeople who come in daily contact with hospital customers can provide valuable feedback to managers for planning purposes.

At the same time, supportive occupational health services managers can provide leads to help salespeople get off to a successful start. Occupational health services managers can accompany salespeople on calls as "product experts" and can assist in the closing efforts. They can also suggest effective ways for salespeople to present, or position, the product to make the most sales. The more successful the sales effort, the more money salespeople earn.

If occupational health services managers are to support the sales effort actively, they must first understand what sales is and how it can help them. The sales manager should, therefore, plan to have salespeople take managers on sales calls as part of the educational process. Seeing and hearing prospects firsthand is one of the best ways for managers to learn what selling is all about.

The Role of the Administration, the Medical Staff, and the Governing Board in the Sales Process

Administrators, physicians, and trustees all have an important role to play in the hospital's sales success. Whether they monitor or review sales results or assist directly in the sales effort, their input and support can be invaluable.

Administration

The administration's support and monitoring of the sales operation are essential to its overall success. Administrators should ensure that the necessary market research has been done, that sales materials have been produced, that training has been provided, and that products have been developed before salespeople are sent on calls. Administrators also play an important sales liaison role by keeping trustees and physicians informed of products being marketed by the sales force and by reporting periodically on progress.

Medical Staff

The medical staff's involvement and support in selling occupational health services can be crucial to the program's success. At the very least, the medical staff should be kept informed about the development of the hospital's occupational health services. Hospital salespeople should have direct contact with physicians or committees of the medical staff involved in the development and provision of occupational health services. (See chapter 17, "Medical Staff Relations.")

Governing Board

The hospital board also needs to be nurtured. A retreat or special meeting is one of the most effective ways to review the rationale for sales of occupational health services and the hospital's plan of action, as well as to defuse fears about the ethics of sales. Periodic reports and updates about occupational health services should be made thereafter to the board.

Hiring and Training Sales Staff

Several questions face hospital administrators interested in hiring an individual for the hospital sales function. Key questions of concern to most administrators include the following:

- Should internal hospital staff members familiar with the occupational health services product line be hired to staff the sales function, or should external sales specialists be recruited?
- Should sales staff be hired on a full-time or part-time basis?
- How many salespeople will be needed to achieve desired revenue goals?
- What training will be necessary to implement an effective sales effort?

Use of Internal Hospital Staff

A benefit of hiring a current hospital employee to staff the sales force is that the employee knows the hospital resources well and may know the occupational health products well. Some disadvantages are the following:

- The primary focus of current hospital employees is usually their initial area of responsibility, not sales.
- They are usually not trained in sales.
- They tend to be too product oriented rather than oriented toward serving as an advocate of the prospective customer in solving an existing company problem.

The most important factor in considering internal hospital staff members for a sales position is their aptitude for sales. Verbal ability and personality characteristics suited to the sales position are extremely important. A person who can combine product knowledge with selling abilities makes the most effective salesperson. Sales skills can be learned through training if the individual has a strong aptitude and interest in selling. However, adequate ongoing sales training demands a major hospital investment in both time and money.

Use of External Sales Specialists

An alternative to hiring current hospital employees is to hire external sales specialists and teach them about the occupational health services product line. This alternative involves less extensive investment in training programs or direct field supervision of new sales recruits. However, many experienced salespeople may be unfamiliar with the hospital's products and hospital politics. They also may be accustomed to higher commissions or higher-volume sales than a fledgling hospital effort might provide. The result can be rapid staff turnover.

Use of Part-Time Staff

One option for hospitals in need of a sales force is to hire part-time salespeople who are paid on a salary or per-call basis to work in specific markets. The advantages of this option are:

- Low start-up costs, especially when no benefits are paid to the part-time staff
- Potential for specialization and focus on particular markets

Part-time salespeople also present some disadvantages:

- Good part-time salespeople are sometimes hard to find; also, most good salespeople who work part-time prefer to sell on commission rather than on a salary or per-call basis.
- A part-time effort may not yield the results a hospital needs.
- Part-time salespeople often have other jobs or responsibilities that compete for their attention.

- If the hospital pays on a per-call basis, the results are usually quantity, not quality.

Although hiring part-time salespeople sometimes appears to be a good short-term answer, many hospitals find such staff difficult to manage.

Use of a Full-Time Sales Staff

A more frequent choice for hospitals is to hire full-time salespeople, who offer several benefits:

- They devote their full attention to sales.
- They are more likely to regard sales as a career.
- They tend to be experienced in sales.
- Their chances of success are greater. An acceptable hit ratio (number of sales per calls made) may require a larger number of sales calls. Because full-time salespeople make more calls than salespeople who work part-time, they should generate more sales. To hospital managers, full-time salespeople represent an investment; managers may, therefore, be more cooperative.
- Full-time salespeople reduce the length of time required for establishing a hospital sales operation.

The sample job description in figure 14-4 provides criteria and guidelines to consider in recruiting for a sales position.

Size of Sales Staff

How many salespeople to budget for depends on the sales forecast and the resources a hospital can allocate to the sales effort. Largely, however, the number of salespeople depends on market demand and on the product's sales cycle, or how many visits and how much time the sales force needs to make a single sale. Management must determine how many sales calls are required and the total times needed for each sale. With that information in hand, management can determine (1) the number of salespeople required to generate the desired level of business or, if the size of the sales force is fixed, (2) how much business the sales force can realistically develop. A common problem faced by occupational health services salespeople is an unrealistic expectation of sales in the first 6–12 months of the job.

Sales Training

Sales training is a continuous effort to update, upgrade, and improve salespeople's knowledge, technique, and understanding of the product, the buyer, and the sales process. Sales training is essential even if the salespeople

Figure 14-4. Example of a Job Description for a Salesperson

Title:	Corporate Services Representative
Primary functions:	This position involves personal selling to prospective customers, service to existing customers, and generating new business for specific products.
Reports to:	Marketing Director
Responsibilities:	Identifying qualified prospects and selling selected services to the targeted market.
1. Sales planning:	The incumbent salesperson must develop (for approval) an individual sales plan based on specific goals and objectives. This plan must identify market segments, number and type of calls, and projected sales.
2. Account planning:	The incumbent must develop a strategic plan for approaching each prospect.
3. Call planning:	The incumbent must develop a plan for each personal sales call.
4. Personal sales:	The salesperson will make regular scheduled and unscheduled sales visits (cold calls) to qualified prospects.
5. Reporting:	The incumbent is responsible for completing call reports and for performing other related statistical reporting, as determined by management.
6. Follow-up service:	The incumbent is responsible for routine and "emergency" follow-up calls to existing customers to solve problems, to evaluate the level of satisfaction, and to prospect for future business.
Experience/Education:	This position requires either: Two to three years of sales experience, with a proven record of sales success; or Three to five years of health care experience, with demonstrated ability to communicate effectively and to accomplish departmental goals. A college education is helpful but not required, especially if the incumbent has product expertise or considerable experience. Excellent communication skills are essential.

Major accountabilities:

1. Meeting established sales quotas (in unit or dollar amounts) for certain products
2. Meeting sales-call objectives (numbers, type, and results)
3. Assisting management by analyzing prospective new products and their sales potential and customer needs
4. Reporting sales results for analysis by senior management
5. Assessing sales and support materials and making recommendations for improvements, additions, and changes
6. Making recommendations for activities that will promote interest in the hospital's products and services (for example, educational seminars for prospects) and that will lead to sales
7. Providing sales training for others in the hospital who become involved in the sales process
8. Other activities, as assigned

a hospital hires are experienced and have sold for a hospital before. Training orients a sales force to the particular hospital's market, products, and goals. Training sessions are also a time for reviewing and developing sales strategies and even for practicing basic but sometimes forgotten sales techniques. These sessions force salespeople to reflect on past successes and failures, learn more effective ways of approaching problems, and learn from each other.

The value of training is often underestimated, and training is rarely a part of the hospital salesperson's routine. Hospital management should schedule training sessions every 4–6 months to help keep their salespeople sharp, alert, and motivated, as well as to monitor their progress. Department and product line managers as well as administrators and selected physicians should also receive some initial and periodic training. Sales training programs are provided by a number of national sales training organizations, consultants, and health care trade associations.

Motivating and Paying Salespeople

Growth-oriented hospitals with occupational health services need a highly motivated sales force to achieve maximum success. Salespeople who are stimulated by their jobs, by special pay incentives, and by periodic contests tend to consistently meet or exceed quotas and other performance objectives. These salespeople also exhibit good morale and project a winning, positive image to the hospital's customers and new prospects.

Like training, motivating the sales force must be an ongoing activity. Some sales managers believe that a well-designed compensation plan, with many incentives, is motivation enough. Although studies show that money is a powerful sales motivator, successful salespeople also thrive on recognition, competitive challenges, job enrichment and advancement, growth opportunities, and greater authority and freedom on the job.

Sales motivators are both financial and nonfinancial. Nonfinancial motivators include the sales manager's involvement, periodic sales contests, and special honors or recognition. The major financial motivators are the hospital's sales compensation plan and the fringe benefit package it offers.

No one compensation plan is right for all hospitals. Too many variables, such as the competitiveness of the market and the types of products and selling cycles involved, make it virtually impossible to recommend one plan over all others. Instead, hospitals must design their own payment plan. (See figure 14-5 for a model for estimating the annual cost of a salesperson.)

Straight Salary Plans

Hospitals most often use straight salary plans to pay salespeople. Salaries are fixed sums that may occasionally be supplemented by discretionary

Figure 14-5. Annual Cost of an Experienced Hospital Salesperson (1988 prices)

Expense Categories	Low Estimate	High Estimate
Direct selling expenses:		
Total wages (includes incentive)	$32,000	$45,000
Benefits (@ 20%)	6,400	9,000
Travel	2,100	4,200
Administrative expenses:		
Clerical (part-time)	5,000	10,000
Office space (200–400 sq. ft. @ $10 per sq. ft.)	2,000	4,000
Management (assumes no full-time sales manager)	6,400	9,000
General business expenses (such as supplies and telephone)	2,000	3,000
Sales training (10 days)	8,000	10,000
Marketing/advertising expenses	6,000	10,000
Total	$69,900	$104,200

bonuses, prizes, or other short-term incentives. Sales representatives under straight salary plans have a known income and are protected from the wide fluctuations often experienced under commission plans. Hence, straight salary plans create a sense of security. However, incentives are minimal under straight salary plans; the only sizable incentive is the chance to earn a better salary next year. Under a straight sales plan, salespeople have little financial incentive to sell more than the quota.

Straight Commission Plans

Straight commission plans pay salespeople a percentage of the sales volume they generate or, increasingly, a percentage of the gross margin. Commissions can also be based on activities, such as the number of sales calls, rather than strict financial measures. Regardless of the commission's basis, salespeople are paid in direct proportion to the sales they make or the activities they pursue. Salespeople have a direct incentive to work harder and smarter. Hence, salespeople on commission tend to earn more than those on salary. Commission plans often attract salespeople who like risk but who expect the financial rewards associated with success.

Straight commission plans are a good choice when:

- The hospital is using part-time salespeople.
- Most of a salesperson's time can be spent on selling rather than on nonselling activities.
- The hospital's financial position dictates that selling expenses be directly related to sales volume or margins.

Some disadvantages of straight commission plans are the following:

- Salespeople tend to concentrate on easy-to-sell products and ignore the slow-moving products that may generate the best margins for the hospital.
- The hospital will sometimes have difficulty hiring new salespeople if they are only offered a straight commission plan.

Hospitals should be wary of implementing straight commission plans when they have no experience in a particular line of business. If management overestimates sales, commissions will be lower than expected, and salespeople will become dissatisfied and leave. Similarly, underestimating sales can result in some unrealistic and excessive payments to salespeople.

Draws against Commission

To soften the financial impact that commission plans have on new or inexperienced salespeople, the hospital can often add a draw. A draw is essentially front money to meet basic living expenses and level out the peaks and valleys of commission selling. The draw can be a fixed sum advanced at regular intervals, or it can be a pool from which the salesperson draws when necessary. Eventually, what the salesperson makes in commissions should cancel out the draw, much as a loan is repaid over time.

Bonuses

Sales bonuses are paid when the salesperson's activities cannot be directly linked to the short-term sale, when nonselling activities are critical to long-term success, or when identifiable factors can be established as major success criteria. For example, if it takes 20 calls to get one new client, then the salesperson can be paid a periodic bonus for making his or her quota of calls (even though the new prospects called may take months before they actually become customers).

Special Incentive Compensation

Special incentive compensation is awarded for outstanding achievement in meeting a special, often short-term, goal. Special incentive compensation motivates effectively when competition is keen and when the amount and basis for dollar distribution are announced well beforehand. If achieving the goal was a team effort, the bonus is split evenly or according to each salesperson's contribution to the team's success. For example, at Rose Medical Center in Denver, Colorado, bonuses are paid to all employees involved in the sales function, from the product manager to the office secretary responsible for customer phone contacts. In nonteam situations, bonuses are awarded to the top one or two achievers or to all those who exceeded the goal.

Planning and Sales Forecasting

The sales forecast serves as the basis for all planning activities that follow it, namely setting up a sales budget, determining sales quotas, and assigning territories. Simply defined, the sales forecast is a prediction of sales volume for some future period, usually one year. This forecast does not measure the sales effort required to meet it but is simply a projection of sales units or dollars.

Forecasting Sales

In arriving at a sales forecast for occupational health services, hospital managers should evaluate such factors as:

- *The competition.* How many competitors are there? Who are they? How does the product compare with the hospital's own product? What are the competing product's strengths and weaknesses? How does pricing of the product compare with that of the hospital's? Who has been in the market longer—the hospital or its competitors?
- *Market conditions.* What factors affect demand for the hospital's product? What is the current status of those factors?
- *Economic conditions.* What are the general trends? If economic change is predicted, how susceptible is the hospital's product to such a change? What effect does inflation have on product sales?
- *Environmental trends.* What are the current and future employment trends? What are the trends in net income? How do these trends affect demand for the hospital's occupational products?
- *The product's sales cycle.* How long does the sales force typically need to sell a new product? Is it three months or more? If so, management cannot expect to generate any sales in the first quarter after launching the production. Managers often make the mistake of assuming that some quantity of a product will be sold each month without considering the sales cycle. Hence, their forecasts are likely to be too optimistic.

The Budgeting Process

The sales budget, like all budgets, is a financial tool managers use to plan for profits based on expected revenues and expenses. The revenue side of the budget is basically the sales forecast for the coming year. The expense side is far more than direct selling expenses, or what the hospital pays its salespeople (salaries, commissions, bonuses, and benefits) in addition to travel and entertainment expenses. The expense side also includes advertising and marketing expenses in support of sales, such as product brochures, direct mail campaigns, and trade show participation. Administrative expenses such as clerical help, sales training, management time, and the cost of office equipment, supplies, and space must also be factored into the expenses. Marketing and administrative expenses in support of sales can run an additional 30 to 100 percent of wages and benefits. (See figure 14-6 for an example of a hospital sales budget.)

Evaluating the Hospital Sales Function

Salespeople, like other employees, are judged and evaluated according to certain standards, or performance measures. Usually, performance standards are a mix of quantitative and qualitative factors. Quantitative standards set goals for specific sales achievements, such as quota fulfillment, and are totally objective. Qualitative standards reveal personality and job knowledge and attitudes, such as diligence and enthusiasm, and are subjective. The subjective standards are sometimes more important because they form the prospect's first impression of the salesperson, and first impressions are usually lasting.

Periodically, the entire sales organization should be evaluated through a sales audit. An audit analyzes the sales organization in order to identify problems, solutions, and opportunities. Usually done by an impartial third party, the audit shows the administration whether the sales effort is working according to plan and, if not, how it can be improved.

A complete audit includes an analysis of the sales organization, its personnel and policies, and sales results versus the hospital's expectations. In analyzing sales volume, the auditor usually evaluates sale volume by product, territory, and salesperson. This step alone can be highly useful to hospitals wishing to improve sales performance. For example, Hospital X had two salespeople selling a variety of products to general industry. Both succeeded in meeting their quotas. However, inpatient admissions increased in only one salesperson's territory. A sales audit revealed that the other salesperson was selling primarily to companies whose employees lived farther from Hospital X; many of these employees were also enrolled in HMOs and were typically directed to HMO plan hospitals.

At times, hospital sales and marketing personnel are too close to the sales action to see the big picture. They may also be unduly optimistic or

Figure 14-6. Example of a Hospital Occupational Health Sales Budget for One Salesperson and One Product

Revenue	$825,000
Gross sales	
Less contractual allowances (3.5%)	(28,875)
Less bad debt (4%)	(33,000)
Total deductions	(61,875)
Net revenue	$763,125
Direct sales expenses:	
Salary	$40,000
Benefits (@ 20%)	8,000
Telephone	3,300
Rent	4,500
Books/subscriptions	275
Postage	800
Printing	12,500
Travel and entertainment	4,200
Total sales expense	$73,575
Operating (product delivery) expenses:	
Salaries (e.g., staff to deliver the product)	380,000
Benefits (@ 20%)	76,000
Legal fees (for negotiating contracts)	15,000
Consulting services	12,500
Electricity	2,200
Telephone	3,750
Outside purchased services	82,500
Rent	20,000
Office supplies	2,850
Insurance	1,295
Books/subscriptions	500
Travel	700
Depreciation of equipment	8,200
Printing	850
Total operating expenses	$606,345

defensive, or they may exhibit poor judgment. As a result, plans that should be revised are not, and reports of sales progress may be distorted. Although audits can be expensive and time-consuming, they can save hospitals time, money, and effort that would otherwise be misdirected because of poor forecasting or a fast-changing market.

From the results of the sales audits, as well as through performance evaluations and effective supervision, management will be able to continually refine the sales operation. Over time, and after changes and improvements have had a chance to produce results, the sales effort should become a major contributor to the occupational health service's economic success.

Chapter 15

Practical Issues in Operational Design

Philip S. Hanna, M.P.H.

Once research-based decisions have been made about the products to be offered and the clients to be served, there still remain myriad practical decisions about where and how an occupational health program will operate. This chapter reviews some of the basic issues that a program needs to incorporate in its business plan: location, space, staffing, organization, and information management. Although these nuts-and-bolts issues may not be glamorous, they have a major impact on a program's success.

Location

As Frank Leone notes in chapter 13, location is the most important consideration for industry in the selection of an occupational health provider. Here are some key questions programs must answer in determining the optimal location:

- Where are employers concentrated in the service area?
- Where is the greatest concentration of employers that would be likely to use the program's services?
- Is a significant portion of the businesses to be served located in one general area?
- Is the hospital conveniently located to employers that are primary candidates to be served?
- Where are existing occupational health services providers located?
- Are employers expressing concern about general access to acute care or other health care services?
- Are employers expressing concern about 24-hour access to acute care or other health care services?

- How important is it for the service provided to be in immediate proximity to the businesses being served?
- Are the primary businesses to be served heavy manufacturing, light manufacturing, or service industries?
- Are these businesses in which medical surveillance and monitoring will be in demand?
- What are the specific types, nature, and severity of the injuries that will be occurring?
- How far are these employers willing to allow their employees to travel to obtain different services?
- Will ancillary services (radiology, pulmonary function, ECG, among others) from the hospital be used for the program?

The answers to these questions will determine whether the program should be located within the hospital or at a freestanding site. For example, a freestanding satellite location may be desirable if a sufficient client base exists in an area at some distance from the hospital. (See chapter 16 for more discussion of the merits of opting for a freestanding facility.) Projected service needs, however, may necessitate a location within the hospital for cost-effective access to high-technology equipment, assuming that prospective clients have no easier access to such services from a competitor and are willing to allow employees the necessary travel time to the hospital. Projected volume and service needs may also indicate the feasibility of delivering at least some services directly at the worksite.

Space Planning

Once location has been determined, a program must plan for space needs by addressing the issues highlighted in the following section.

Staff Involvement in Space Planning

Both clinical personnel (for example, physicians, nursing personnel, and physical therapists) and administrative personnel should be part of the space planning process. A key member of the administrative staff is the office manager. Because this individual is ultimately responsible for the smooth day-to-day operation of the system components, he or she can provide valuable input into determining business office requirements, storage space needs, and adequate staff work and relaxation areas and can raise such basic questions as "Where will the coats be hung in the winter?"

Patient Access to the Clinic and the Emergency Department

Hospital space that is easily accessible from a nearby dedicated parking facility and that is in close proximity to the emergency department is among the most highly coveted footage in the hospital. However, an occupational health service located in the hospital is less likely to succeed if an injured worker has to drive into a parking structure, go through the main entrance of the hospital, and inquire at the information desk about the exact location of an occupational health clinic located somewhere on another floor.

If one of the program objectives is to offer *convenient* 24-hour access to services at the same location, then program space should be convenient to the emergency department. It is a very effective marketing point to be able to assure a two-shift or three-shift manufacturing operation that its acute injuries will be handled in the same place all of the time and, if an employee's injury is more serious, that the emergency department is "right across the hall."

Program Access to Ancillary Services

A full-service program will have radiographic tests, pulmonary function testing, hearing tests, ECGs, physical therapy, and laboratory services to support the medical services that are offered. It is important to address how effectively outpatients are presently served in the existing hospital departments and to consider which services the occupational health services program should provide for itself. Employers will be critical of an occupational health services program that allows off-work employees to consume excessive waiting time in an inefficient hospital system. Ancillary services that may be provided through the occupational health clinic include the following:

- *Radiographic tests.* If an X-ray room is dedicated to the emergency department already, then that existing resource will work effectively for the occupational health clinic assuming that utilization during the normal clinic hours is not already too high. If all of the X-ray resources in the hospital are committed to scheduled appointments, programs should give serious consideration to adding basic X-ray equipment in the occupational health clinic.
- *Pulmonary function testing (PFT).* Potential volume, especially for occupational health programs committed to providing medical surveillance programs, may dictate that PFT equipment be available in the occupational health clinic.
- *Audiology tests.* If the market analysis identifies a substantial concentration of employers that have work environments exceeding the Occupational Safety and Health Administration (OSHA) noise threshold and therefore require the implementation of a hearing conservation program, then having a hearing booth in the occupational clinic is justified. If an occupational health program objective is to actively promote the availability of hearing conservation programs, a transportable booth should be purchased so that mass annual screening programs can be done at the worksite.

- *ECGs.* Because the demand for ECGs is not great and because they normally are part of a scheduled physical evaluation, it is unlikely that programs will find a need to duplicate existing hospital resources.
- *Physical therapy.* The scope of resources, personnel, equipment, and space required to deliver the various physical therapy services provide compelling motivation to use the hospital outpatient physical therapy program. However, unless there is a unique combination of variables, the most effective and efficient approach is to place office and examination space for a physical therapist in the occupational health clinic.
- *Laboratory services.* This is probably the easiest hospital department to use because the patient does not need to leave the occupational health clinic if the hospital has any type of reasonable internal courier capability.

Space and Design Needs Dictated by Volume and Nature of Patients

Especially if the program serves construction or manufacturing firms, it is best to provide a dedicated waiting area; employees coming to the clinic for urgent care may be covered with dirt or grease. Designers should therefore not use fabric on chairs and should avoid light-colored carpets or carpeting that shows dirt, if carpet is used at all. The resulting utilitarian waiting room, unfortunately, is what many hospitals are currently attempting to avoid. Creature comforts, such as a television, coffee and cold drinks, and a nearby bathroom, should be provided. A sign on the bathroom door should direct people to check with the receptionist before using the bathroom in case they will be required to provide a urine specimen as part of their office visit.

If the program is being planned to serve more than 25 to 30 people each day, then space needs must accommodate the 2 people who will handle telephone calls, scheduling, registration, file maintenance, and chart preparation. Programs should be alert to the problem of inadequate space for medical records and should not use the hospital medical records department.

At program start-up, a physical therapist may be needed only two half-days each week, and space needs may therefore be minimal. However, as the occupational health program grows (to 50 or more people per day), a full-time physical therapist and a physical therapy aide will be needed. Physical therapy may then require space for an extremity tank, ultrasound equipment, and hot/cold packs as well as five treatment areas (beds).

In general, the space needed by clinical staff in occupational health programs is comparable to space required for practices oriented to adult medicine. Physicians should have three to four beds for seeing patients. Depending on the availability of patient intake areas, two or more additional beds could be used to ensure smooth patient flow.

In summary, a busy occupational health clinic should have a dedicated waiting area, a registration area/business office, medical records storage areas, a staff work area (desk space), a supply room, adequate private offices, a clinical workroom (medical intake area), a staff break room with bathroom, and 10–11 treatment areas if the clinic provides both medical and physical therapy services.

Staffing

Like space needs, staffing demands will vary depending on where the program is located and what services are offered. A freestanding facility that services 45 or 50 patients per day and provides a complete range of acute and follow-up care, physical therapy, and physical evaluation services should have the following staff capabilities:

- Radiology
- Pulmonary function testing
- Audiology
- ECG
- Physical therapy
- Phlebotomy

These staffing capabilities would be in addition to the other major staff positions described in the following sections.

Physicians

If the market analysis indicates that the program will see a significant volume of acute care patients, depending on the type and severity of the injuries, it may be appropriate to utilize emergency medicine specialists. A program oriented to physical evaluation may need family practice or internal medicine specialists. A program oriented to disability evaluations would have a greater need for a variety of specialists depending on the nature of the original injury. Orthopedic surgeons and physiatrists have the greatest potential to do disability evaluations, especially if the anticipated types of injuries are those likely to result in a significant period of disability.

Board-certified or board-eligible occupational medicine specialists are difficult to identify and recruit because of their limited numbers and apparent preference for academic and corporate positions. Programs that are able to recruit these physicians can benefit substantially from the physicians' thorough understanding of the interrelationships among workers' compensation, regulatory agencies, employers, and employees.

It is beneficial for physicians without formal occupational medicine training to complete a mini-residency in occupational medicine through one of several available programs. These programs cost from $3,000 to $5,000 and require approximately four weeks of training within one year.

In addition to base salary, a typical compensation package for medical staff will include pension/profit sharing; professional liability insurance; professional development allowance; health, dental, short-term disability, long-term disability, and term life insurance; and paid vacation. When training and experience are included in compensation considerations, it is appropriate to anticipate a range of $75,000 to $140,000 and more for these individuals.

Occupational Health Nurses

As the business and medical communities have grown in their recognition of the complexities of the occupational health needs of the workplace, the demand for professional services is being met by a growing number of nurses with specialized training in occupational health. These nurses are expanding the roles traditionally assigned to nurses employed in industrial settings. (For further information, see chapter 9.)

In the initial program growth phase, the occupational nurse could be utilized in a clinical, a program development, or even a sales capacity. However, as the program grows, a trained occupational health nurse can spend all of his or her time working with client companies in the area of program development.

A nurse may become a Certified Occupational Health Nurse through the American Association of Occupational Health Nurses (AAOHN) after the nurse has five years' experience and has completed 75 hours of continuing education. Thereafter, the nurse must provide documentation that 50 hours of continuing education has been completed every three years. Nursing staff trained in occupational health or certified and active in the AAOHN can lend immediate prestige to an occupational health program. Active participation in the AAOHN can also be an outstanding source of contacts for a developing program.

Nurses expect the same types of benefits/compensation packages that physicians do. Salaries for nursing personnel with occupational health training and experience range from $35,000 to $40,000.

Clinical Support

A variety of clinically oriented personnel can provide substantial support to the occupational health program. Physicians' assistants and nurse specialists can be important supplements to the physicians in a busy program by conducting physical examinations and follow-up visits or by taking care of certain acute injuries. Licensed practical nurses and a variety of nursing aides can perform patient intake procedures, assist nurses and physicians, and perform clerical duties. Their ability to perform both clinical and clerical duties allows for the most efficient utilization of the professional staff.

Clerical Support

It is not uncommon for the clerical support requirements of a program to be overlooked because the individuals actually planning the occupational health program have little practical experience in this area. For this reason, an experienced office manager should be brought into the program early to plan for the clerical staff space needs based on the program objectives. In the early stages of the program, the office manager can provide all of the various clerical support for the clinic. As the program grows, the office manager will be invaluable in identifying personnel and system needs. This capability will be seriously compromised if the approach to clerical support is from the perspective of hiring someone shortly before opening to "schedule appointments and register patients."

Organizational Structure

Decisions about organizational structure and reporting relationships can raise some of the most challenging issues confronting the occupational health program. Organizations usually attempt to structure the environment so that each employee has only one individual with whom he or she has a formal reporting relationship. All pertinent information is conveyed between these two individuals. This traditional pyramid organization is inadequate for occupational health programs.

An occupational program that has multiple physicians involved in clinical practice, 12–15 employees, and over 100 client companies needs an effective matrix reporting structure in place that every employee understands. If responsibilities among personnel are not clearly defined, some of the following problems can occur:

- Staff will begin to question "who is in charge."
- Client companies will quickly perceive that decisions and recommendations from the program are not consistent.
- Some companies will begin to "shop" program staff for the decisions they want.

A lack of clarity regarding reporting responsibilities will also result in individuals on the staff not being aware of new client companies. This is a problem no matter which staff member is uninformed, whether it is the physician who does the wrong preplacement physical or the receptionist who schedules an appointment for the wrong amount of clinical time necessary to complete and document an examination.

There is no one correct way to structure responsibilities within an organization. However, regardless of the particular type of organizational structure, it is important that responsibilities be clearly defined. The best way to accomplish this objective is to have job descriptions written for each position and to review them at least every six months.

Information Management

Information management shifted from a labor-intensive manual process to a computer-supported system with the introduction of "user friendly" computers priced at affordable levels for smaller businesses. This evolution was hastened by the need to downsize companies as a result of the business environment in the early 1980s. However, many businesses found that simply installing computers did not achieve the objective of improved productivity. Unfortunately, this situation largely resulted because the manual system that was being replaced was often ineffective, and the computerized systems did little more than increase the speed at which individuals made errors.

Before a computer system can be effectively implemented, an occupational health clinic must assess the type of information it plans to collect, analyze, and release. The following questions must be addressed:

- Will the clinic do preplacement physicals, acute injury treatment and management, physical therapy, screening tests, and other physical evaluation testing?
- To whom will the information be released?
- How long will it need to be retained in archives?
- If the clinic is going to actively track the process of the employee through the recovery process, how will this be done and under what prearranged system will this information be given to employers?
- If there are multiple facility locations, with different care provision responsibilities, where will the medical record be maintained and how will information from the record be transmitted between the locations?

Information forms are also important. The following forms are essential for a comprehensive occupational health clinic:

- General medical history
- Occupational history
- Pulmonary history
- Registration
- Basic and comprehensive physical examinations
- Report of examination
- Special physical evaluations
  - Surveillance physical

  - Independent medical opinion
  - Disability evaluation
- Occupational medical report
  - Communications report for the employer
- Drug testing
  - Authorization
  - Release of information
  - Specimen verification
  - Chain of evidence

These are just some of the forms that will be used daily to supplement such documentation as the progress notes and test result forms. The clinic will need to coordinate its activities with a wide variety of medical services and specialty testing providers, and the forms that are used must accommodate these multiple uses.

Other vitally important program elements that require well-thought-out management information systems include:

- A system to track sales contacts with employers
- A system to track what services are provided to established clients and identify other sales opportunities for these clients based on standard industrial classification codes (SIC codes identify the employer's primary and secondary businesses by category)
- A system to track when routine contacts should be made with client companies and when follow-up contacts should be initiated with prospective employers
- A system to track when special evaluations (for example, medical surveillance physicals, pulmonary testing, hearing testing) need to be done to help a client comply with various regulatory organizations
- An effective method to transmit routine information between physically separated facilities

Once the program's information needs have been identified, a program can then determine whether computerization of information is appropriate. Chapter 19 provides more discussion of computer applications.

Chapter 16

Service Delivery through a Freestanding Facility

Barbara Robino, R.N.

As stated in chapters 13 and 15, location is the most important factor affecting a company's decision to select a particular provider of occupational health services. If a hospital is located near the industries it serves, a hospital-based program may be sufficient to meet industry needs. If companies are located more than 20 minutes from the hospital, then the hospital should consider having a freestanding center provide occupational health services. A freestanding center can:

- *Strengthen current industry relationships and serve as the basis for new ones.* When occupational health services are available in close proximity to their clients' places of business, the hospital demonstrates its commitment to assisting business and industry in providing high-quality medical care at a reasonable price.
- *Increase the hospital's regional market share.* Generally, 20 minutes of travel time is acceptable for access to occupational health services. Locating an occupational health center within approximately 20 minutes' travel distance from the hospital will significantly increase the infiltration the hospital has in the region. This distance is also attractive to the hospital's medical staff in view of competition for patients.
- *Expand inpatient and outpatient revenue by drawing patients from outside the hospital's normal service area.* These are "new" dollars that the hospital would not have realized without the freestanding occupational health facility.
- *Increase referrals to specialists and subspecialists on the hospital medical staff.* This creates an effective recruiting tool for the hospital and an expanded referral base for the physicians.

- *Improve visibility and community awareness of the institution.* By providing convenient medical care for non–life-threatening injuries, the hospital can position itself as the hospital of choice when an individual requires inpatient services.

Program Planning and Feasibility Studies

Before developing a freestanding occupational health facility, several studies should be conducted: competitive assessment, demographic assessment, market needs assessment, site selection, product line selection, and financial analysis.

Competitive Assessment

Program planners should take a critical look at the competition to identify the type and level of occupational health services that are currently provided in the community. The assessment should include the identification of three different categories of providers with a breakdown of their locations by zip codes on a large map:

- *Hospitals.* Planners should define those programs that are hospital based and those that have freestanding facilities, making detailed listings of each program's service components and collecting any descriptive marketing materials, including printed advertisements.
- *Physicians.* Physicians in private practice, as well as those who operate chains of freestanding clinics, deliver a large portion of the occupational health services in the community. Planners should find out what these physicians' share of the market is, including the range of services they provide.
- *Corporate medical departments.* Planners should find out how many companies in the region have in-house medical departments and what services they provide. These are the hidden competition and, if overlooked, can skew all demographic and market research.

Demographic Assessment

Program planners should find out the total employee population in the region and then use the standard industrial classification (SIC) codes to calculate the number and types of injuries expected to occur in the program's client population. Injury incidence data can be obtained through the state department of labor. Knowing the average number of employees per company will also guide planners in determining product development and sales approach.

Small employers make the decision to purchase health care services differently than large employers do. The local and state chambers of commerce, business and industry coalitions, and unions and trade organizations all have reliable, up-to-date, and inexpensive data. Marketing information is also available commercially, but these publications are often expensive bound copies of the same data duplicated from the organizational sources just listed.

Market Needs Assessment

Chapter 13 reviewed several methods of assessing industry wants and needs. Interviews with focus groups will give a composite of the needs and wants within corporations. To ensure that the program will be broad based, focus groups should include chief executive officers, human resources managers, risk managers, and occupational health nurses. The sizes and types of businesses will determine whether one or more of these decision makers is involved in purchasing occupational health services.

Workers' compensation insurance carriers are regulated by the Workers' Compensation Act and have specific documentation requirements for health care providers. If private insurance companies handle workers' compensation in the program's state, they will be able to inform the program of industry needs. Programs should establish a working relationship with these carriers because they can provide valuable introductions to local business and industry.

Site Selection

Site selection will be based on an analysis of the demographics that have been compiled. Employers should be sorted by SIC code and general categories—for example, construction, manufacturing, transportation, wholesale/retail—and plotted on the map showing competitors' locations. This will identify the zip code or codes that should be targeted for the highest probability of success. Key target areas will have a dense employee population, industries with high injury incidence rates, and minimal competition.

Identifying the right location for the occupational health facility within the zip code can be accomplished by following the criteria for site selection in figure 16-1. A site should score 118 or better to be considered.

Product Line Selection

Program planners should review the needs and wants of the client and insurance carriers and match this information with the location of the freestanding facility. Only those services that the majority of the injured employees will require should be provided at the facility. High-cost, low-volume services should continue to be provided on-campus at the hospital.

Primary care and minor emergency services, including X-ray and basic laboratory services, are usually essential requirements of industry. The

Figure 16-1. Criteria for Site Selection

Location: ____________________

Rank:
Below standard = 1 — Highest above standard score =
Standard = 2 — Highest standard score =
Above standard = 3 — Highest below standard score =

Item	Description	Rank	Standard is	Weight	Rank × Weight = Score
1. Visibility	Easily readable from one main artery, including 2 directions	1 2 3	Description	8	
2. Accessibility	Easy entrance and exit to a main artery	1 2 3	Description	6	
	Able to reach medical center in 20 minutes	1 2 3	20 minutes	3	
		Total		(9)	
3. Signage	Indicates appropriate entrance	1 2 3		2	
	Readable and directional from parking lot area	1 2 3	Description	2	
	Building management and area covenants permit use of medical center signs	1 2 3		3	
		Total		(7)	
4. Parking	Designation of 6 or more parking spaces close to entrance, with adequate lighting	1 2 3	6 spaces	2	
	Access for additional parking (particularly staff)	1 2 3	Description	2	
	Parking is free to employees and patients	1 2 3	Free	2	
		Total		(6)	
5. Competition	No more than 3 facilities offering similar services within a 5-mile radius	1 2 3	3 facilities	3	
	No more than 1 other primary care physician (PCP) in the same building, unless 50% of building is occupied by specialists, and no more than 4 PCPs within a 4-block radius	1 2 3	1 PCP	2	
		Total		(5)	

6. Demographics	Patient population must support 28 patients per day; these encounters must be based on a combination of 2 of the 4 target markets: (1) Industrial employee population and SIC rate is indicative of ______ visits per day (2) Corporate population is indicative of ______ patients per day (3) Residential population is indicative of ______ patients per day for urgent and/or primary care (4) Traffic count is indicative of ______ visits per day Total patients per day =	1 2 3	28 patients/ day	10	
7. Physical plant/building	Square footage for the satellite facility only (excludes other offices, PM&R and time share). The square footage should range from 2,000 to 2,500	1 2 3	2,000–2,500 square feet	4	
	Availability of contiguous space for growth	1 2 3		1	
	Rent should not exceed $15 per square foot in the first 3 years, and be comparable to the area average	1 2 3	$15/square foot	4	
	Easy visibility and accessibility within building	1 2 3	Description	1	
		Total		(10)	
8. Leasehold improvements	Conducive to an effective traffic flow, including wheelchair, ambulance, and ambulance/emergency exit	1 2 3	Description	2	
	Does not affect the start-up cost by 25% or the net income by 20%	1 2 3	Description	3	
	Appropriate plumbing and water taps are available	1 2 3	Description	1	
	Well-regulated HVAC system	1 2 3	Description	1	
	Appropriate electrical and construction for X rays	1 2 3	Description	1	
		Total		(8)	
Grand Total					

Occupational Safety and Health Administration (OSHA) mandates spirometric and audiometric testing for many industries. In addition, treadmill, flexible sigmoidoscopy, and mammography services can be very profitable in the freestanding facility.

Occupational health services should focus on prevention as well as treatment of work-related injuries and illnesses. Preplacement physicals, drug and alcohol testing, and return-to-work evaluations can generate a substantial portion of the facility's revenue. Although programs should consider providing physical and occupational therapy for treatment of acute injuries at the freestanding clinic, specialized therapy and rehabilitation services should continue to be provided at the hospital.

Financial Analysis

Program planners should develop *pro forma* financial statements for the freestanding facility as a final step in the planning process. The *pro forma* statements should include estimated averages for line items that will vary from site to site, such as physician services, minor medical equipment, rent, and equipment and fixtures. The organizational structure of the sponsoring hospital and the number of facilities planned will determine administrative overhead.

Revenue projections should consider that occupational health patients will generate documentable revenue for the hospital's inpatient and outpatient services and the hospital's medical staff. This revenue should be reported as a direct result of the activities of the freestanding occupational health facility. (See tables 16-1 through 16-6 for examples of *pro forma* statements.)

Table 16-1. *Pro Forma* Revenue Projections

	Year 1	Year 2	Year 3
Freestanding center revenue	$ 196,560.00	$ 346,500.00	$ 453,600.00
Hospital outpatient revenue	$ 648,648.00	$1,143,450.00	$1,496,880.00
Hospital inpatient revenue	$ 235,872.00	$ 415,800.00	$ 635,040.00
Physician referral panel revenue	$ 275,184.00	$ 485,100.00	$3,129,840.00
Grand Total	$1,356,264.00	$2,390,850.00	$5,715,360.00

Assume that every dollar generated in the center will generate:

$3.30 for outpatient services

$1.20 for inpatient services

$1.40 for physician referral services

Table 16-2. *Pro Forma* Start-Up Analysis

Total Revenue	$ 196,560.00
Expenses	**Amount**
Human resources	$ 39,374.60
Physician services	$ 71,144.00
Outside medical services	$ 7,862.40
Data processing	$ 6,000.00
Repair and maintenance—equipment	$ 1,000.00
Paging and answering	$ 900.00
Miscellaneous purchased services	$ 1,000.00
Janitorial fees	$ 6,000.00
General medical and surgical supplies	$ 10,862.40
Surgical instruments	$ 1,200.00
Minor medical equipment	$ 2,000.00
Radiology films and solutions	$ 2,500.00
Pharmaceuticals	$ 1,700.00
Printing and forms	$ 5,896.80
Other office supplies	$ 4,948.40
Books and periodicals	$ 1,000.00
Minor nonmedical equipment	$ 2,500.00
Insurance	$ 16,000.00
Personal and professional dues	$ 1,500.00
Postage	$ 600.00
Training/meetings/travel	$ 2,000.00
Utilities	$ 6,000.00
Telephone	$ 6,600.00
Capital investment:	
Equipment	$ 75,480.00
Furniture/fixtures	$ 11,200.00
Leasehold	$ 60,000.00
Rent—buildings	$ 37,500.00
Catering	$ 150.00
Bad debt provisions	$ 8,845.20
Signage	$ 15,000.00
Marketing expenses	$ 33,000.00
Total expenses	$ 439,763.80
Net income	$(243,203.80)

Table 16-3. *Pro Forma* Financial Analysis

	Year 1	Year 2	Year 3
Total Revenue	$196,560.00	$346,500.00	$453,600.00
Expenses	**Year 1**	**Year 2**	**Year 3**
Human resources	$ 39,374.60	$ 43,096.06	$ 47,189.67
Physician services	71,144.00	77,644.00	84,794.00
Outside medical services	7,862.40	14,553.00	19,051.20
Data processing	6,000.00	9,000.00	12,000.00
Repair and maintenance—equipment	1,000.00	1,500.00	1,500.00
Paging and answering	900.00	1,000.00	1,100.00
Miscellaneous purchased services	1,000.00	800.00	500.00
Janitorial fees	6,000.00	7,500.00	9,000.00
General medical and surgical supplies	10,862.40	13,860.00	18,144.00
Surgical instruments	1,200.00	500.00	500.00
Minor medical equipment	2,000.00	500.00	750.00
Radiology films and solutions	2,500.00	2,500.00	3,000.00
Pharmaceuticals	1,700.00	2,900.00	3,600.00
Printing and forms	5,896.80	10,395.00	13,608.00
Other office supplies	4,948.40	5,197.50	6,804.00
Books and periodicals	1,000.00	500.00	500.00
Minor nonmedical equipment	2,500.00	200.00	500.00
Insurance	16,000.00	17,000.00	18,000.00
Personal and professional dues	1,500.00	2,500.00	3,500.00
Postage	600.00	700.00	800.00
Training/meetings/travel	2,000.00	2,000.00	2,000.00
Utilities	6,000.00	6,300.00	6,615.00
Telephone	6,600.00	3,600.00	3,600.00
Depreciation:			
Equipment	1,258.00	1,258.00	1,258.00
Furniture/fixtures	186.00	186.00	186.00
Leasehold	1,000.00	1,000.00	1,000.00
Rent—buildings	37,500.00	37,500.00	37,500.00
Catering	150.00	250.00	250.00
Bad debt provisions	8,845.20	15,592.00	20,412.00
Marketing expenses	18,000.00	18,000.00	18,000.00
Total expenses	$265,527.80	$297,531.56	$335,661.87
Net income	$ (68,967.80)	$ 48,968.44	$117,938.13

Table 16-4. Assumptions for *Pro Forma* Financial Projections: Revenue

The following assumptions and *pro forma* projections were developed to provide a tool for budgeting new sites:

Assume these sites are new practices. Assume marketing efforts equal to or greater than the marketing plan.

Year 1	
First Quarter	
Assume 10 patients/day at $48/visit for 21 days/month	$ 30,240.00
Second Quarter	
Assume 15 patients/day at $48/visit for 21 days/month	$ 45,360.00
Third and Fourth Quarters	
Assume 20 patients/day at $48/visit for 21 days/month	$120,960.00
Total First-Year Revenue	$196,560.00
Year 2	
Assume 25 patients/day at $55/visit for 21 days/month	
Total Second-Year Revenue	$346,500.00
Year 3	
Assume 1 physician a maximum average of 30 patients/day at $60/visit for 21 days/month	
Total Third-Year Revenue	$453,600.00

Table 16-5. Assumptions for *Pro Forma* Financial Projections: Salary Expenses

The following assumptions and *pro forma* projections were developed to provide a tool for budgeting new sites:

Human Resources

Salaries and Benefits

Assume 2 FTEs:	
1 FTE lead medical assistant @ $8.50/hour	$17,680.00
1 FTE medical assistant @ $7.50/hour	$15,600.00
Assume 10 hours of overtime per month @ $12.50/hour	$ 1,500.00
FICA—assume 7% of salaries and benefits	$ 2,434.60
Assume salaries and benefits increase 10% per year for years 2 and 3 ($40,936.06–$45,029.67)	

Contract Labor

Assume 6 weeks' total vacation and sick time per employee. Assume $9.00/hour for temporary help:	
4 weeks (2 weeks/employee vacation)	
+2 weeks (1 week/employee sick time)	
6 weeks × 40 hours/week = 240 hours × $9.00 =	$ 2,160.00
Grand Total Salaries and Benefits:	
Year 1	$ 39,374.60
Year 2	$ 43,096.06
Year 3	$ 47,189.67

Physician Services

Assume the following:	
Physician takes 3 weeks' vacation plus 1 week CME seminars = 4 weeks, plus a temporary physician @ $30.00/hour	$ 4,800.00
Physician earns $65,000/year @ 40 hours/week	$65,000.00
Physician on call 7 nights/month @ $20.00/hour	$ 1,344.00
Physician fees increase 10% per year for years 2 and 3 ($71,500–$78,650)	
Total Physician Services:	
Year 1	$71,144.00
Year 2	$77,644.00
Year 3	$84,794.00

Table 16-6. Assumptions for *Pro Forma* Financial Projections: Other Expenses

The following assumptions and *pro forma* projections were developed to provide a tool for budgeting new sites:

Outside Medical Services

Assume outside medical services are equal to 4% of revenue and include radiology and laboratory services. Assume a 5% inflation factor for years 2 and 3:

Year 1	$ 7,862.40
Year 2	$14,553.00
Year 3	$19,051.20

Data Processing

Assume $500/month for the first year due to low volume, $750 per month for year 2, and $1,000 per month for year 3:

Year 1	$ 6,000.00
Year 2	$ 9,000.00
Year 3	$12,000.00

Repair and Maintenance—Equipment

On the basis of historical data, assume:

Year 1	$ 1,000.00
Year 2	$ 1,500.00
Year 3	$ 1,500.00

Paging and Answering

On the basis of historical data, assume $75/month for the first year:

Year 1	$ 900.00
Year 2	$ 1,000.00
Year 3	$ 1,100.00

Miscellaneous Purchased Services

On the basis of historical data, assume:

Year 1	$ 1,000.00
Year 2	$ 800.00
Year 3	$ 500.00

Janitorial Fees

Assume $500/month based on square footage:

Year 1	$ 6,000.00
Year 2	$ 7,500.00
Year 3	$ 9,000.00

Continued on next page

Table 16-6. Continued

General Medical and Surgical Supplies	
Assume 4% of revenue with additional start-up of $3,000:	
Year 1	$10,862.40
Year 2	$13,860.00
Year 3	$18,144.00
Surgical Instruments	
Assume standard instruments based on historical data:	
Year 1	$ 1,200.00
Year 2	$ 500.00
Year 3	$ 500.00
Minor Medical Equipment	
Assume standard equipment:	
Year 1	$ 2,000.00
Year 2	$ 500.00
Year 3	$ 750.00
Radiology Films and Solutions	
Assume film/solutions and patient volume will increase:	
Year 1	$ 2,500.00
Year 2	$ 2,500.00
Year 3	$ 3,000.00
Pharmaceuticals	
Assume $1,700 in start-up costs:	
Year 1	$ 1,700.00
Year 2	$ 2,900.00
Year 3	$ 3,600.00
Printing and Forms	
Assume 3% of revenue (this does not include marketing materials):	
Year 1	$ 5,896.80
Year 2	$10,395.00
Year 3	$13,608.00
Other Office Supplies	
Assume start-up costs of $2,000 plus 1.5% of revenue:	
Year 1	$ 4,948.40
Year 2	$ 5,197.00
Year 3	$ 6,804.00

Continued on next page

Table 16-6. Continued

Books and Periodicals	
On the basis of historical data, assume start-up costs in year 1:	
Year 1	$ 1,000.00
Year 2	$ 500.00
Year 3	$ 500.00
Minor Nonmedical Equipment	
Assume start-up costs in year 1:	
Year 1	$ 2,500.00
Year 2	$ 200.00
Year 3	$ 500.00
Insurance	
Assume professional liability equals $10,000 per physician, and fire and casualty equals $6,000 (allow for inflation in years 2 and 3):	
Year 1	$16,000.00
Year 2	$17,000.00
Year 3	$18,000.00
Personal and Professional Dues	
On the basis of historical data, assume:	
Year 1	$ 1,500.00
Year 2	$ 2,500.00
Year 3	$ 3,500.00
Postage	
Assume health care center mail only (does not include any marketing activities):	
Year 1	$ 600.00
Year 2	$ 700.00
Year 3	$ 800.00
Training/Meetings/Travel	
Assume 1 out-of-town conference per physician at $1,700 with expenses, and 1 conference per office manager at $300:	
Year 1	$ 2,000.00
Year 2	$ 2,000.00
Year 3	$ 2,000.00
Utilities (excluding telephone)	
Assume $500 per month and an annual inflation factor of 5%:	
Year 1	$ 6,000.00
Year 2	$ 6,300.00
Year 3	$ 6,615.00

Continued on next page

Table 16-6. Continued

Telephone	
Assume a start-up fee of $3,000 and $300 per month:	
Year 1	$ 6,600.00
Year 2	$ 3,600.00
Year 3	$ 3,600.00
Depreciation	
Equipment	
Assume start-up costs for equipment as follows:	
Radiology	$40,000.00
3 examination rooms @ $2,500 each	$ 7,500.00
Microscope	$ 1,200.00
Treatment table	$ 250.00
View box	$ 255.00
Mayo stand	$ 79.00
Utility chart	$ 101.00
Incubator	$ 245.00
Beam scale	$ 225.00
Oxygen set-up	$ 225.00
Spirometer	$ 1,200.00
ECG machine	$ 2,200.00
Signage	$15,000.00
Other	$ 7,000.00
Total	$75,480.00
Depreciated 5-year straight line = $1,258 annual expense	
Furniture and Fixtures	
Waiting Room:	
8 chairs @ $300 each	$ 2,400.00
3 pieces of art @ $150 each	$ 450.00
Children's table, chairs, and toys	$ 500.00
Coat rack	$ 100.00
2 tables @ $250 each	$ 500.00
Front Desk:	
2 secretarial chairs @ $300 each	$ 600.00
1 CRT @ $2,000	$ 2,000.00
1 computer chair	$ 300.00
1 piece of art @ $150	$ 150.00
Examination Rooms:	
3 side chairs @ $200 each	$ 600.00
4 pieces of art @ $150 each	$ 600.00
Blood-drawing chair	$ 300.00
Physician's Office:	
Desk	$ 1,000.00

Continued on next page

Table 16-6. Continued

Credenza	$ 500.00
Executive chair	$ 500.00
2 side chairs @ $200 each	$ 400.00
Bookcases	$ 300.00
Total	$11,200.00
Depreciated 5-year straight line = $186 annual expense	
Leasehold Improvements	
Assume the cost of leasehold improvements at $24 per square foot for 2,000 square feet.	$60,000.00
Depreciated 5-year straight line = $1,000 annual expense	
Rent—Buildings	
Assume 2,500 square feet at $15 per square foot with a 5-year lease equals $37,500:	
Year 1	$37,500.00
Year 2	$37,500.00
Year 3	$37,500.00
Catering	
Assume 1 event at $150	
Year 1	$ 150.00
Year 2	$ 250.00
Year 3	$ 250.00
Bad Debt Provisions	
Assume 4.5% of revenue:	
Year 1	$ 8,845.20
Year 2	$15,592.00
Year 3	$20,412.00
Signage	
Assume cost of appropriate signage at $15,000:	
Start-up	$15,000.00
Year 1	0.00
Year 2	0.00
Year 3	0.00
Marketing Expenses	
Assume marketing plan:	
Start-up	$33,000.00
Year 1	$18,000.00
Year 2	$18,000.00
Year 3	$18,000.00

Product Line Development

Planning for specific products to be delivered at the freestanding facilities can begin in earnest once management is put in place. If possible, the administrative responsibility of the freestanding occupational health facilities should be assigned to a subsidiary of the hospital, either a subsidiary that groups the program with other alternative delivery systems or one that groups occupational health with traditional ambulatory services.

During the 18 to 24 months of program development and implementation, the program director should not have other administrative duties. An additional initial focus for the director will be the development of comprehensive internal and external communications systems.

Injury Treatment Program

The top priority for a freestanding occupational health facility should be the treatment of work-related injuries. Many companies' bottom lines are so eroded by high workers' compensation costs that they have no funds available for prevention programs. The initial objective therefore should be to provide a comprehensive, cost-effective program for the treatment of the company's injured workers. The result will be a client who trusts and values the program and who may later purchase prevention programs when money is available.

Case management by a physician is the key to delivery of a cost-effective program. Occupational health programs should be patterned after other managed medical care programs in that the client's employees should be assigned to a case manager upon entering the system. This case manager should determine appropriate medical care throughout the treatment process until the medical problem is resolved.

A physician referral panel, regulated by well-defined guidelines, should be carefully selected. The specialists and subspecialists that comprise the physician referral panel will be those best suited to deliver the occupational health services the program has defined in its market analysis. The panel also should be composed of competent physicians who have an interest in occupational medicine and who are sensitive to the costs faced by industry.

The program director should provide training for the physicians as well as the physician's office staff. This training should include a review of required procedures and documentation, including an overview of how the state's workers' compensation unit affects the delivery of medical services.

Medical care for the treatment of work-related injuries should be available on a 24-hour basis. This does not necessarily mean that the freestanding facility itself needs to be a 24-hour operation. When an evaluation of the number of employees who work nights in the facility's service area does not justify a 24-hour operation, arrangements can be made with the hospital emergency department to provide after-hours treatment for clients.

Communication and Coordination Systems

Development of the record-keeping system that tracks an injured employee through a program is difficult but necessary. To provide managed medical care, a program must know where in the system the employee is, what services have been provided, and with what results. All health care providers involved with the employee's treatment must have rapid access to this information. All communication and tracking systems currently in use should be evaluated and adapted to comply with the occupational health program's procedures.

External communication involves providing the injured worker, client company, insurance carriers, and often the state workers' compensation department with information about the services provided and the corresponding results of the treatment of work-related injuries.

An effective communication system is a valuable asset in the coordination of occupational health services. In the complex, long-term treatment of certain work-related injuries, the employee must not fall through the cracks of the system. An employee who requires virtually every service available from the emergency department, as well as diagnostic services, medical specialists, inpatient services, and rehabilitation services, will require the coordination efforts of the program director and the physician case manager. Establishment of detailed guidelines in each of these areas and an effective communication system function as the foundation of this coordination effort.

Prevention Programs

Delivery of prevention programs is a common goal of occupational health professionals, and intervention in the workplace to prevent injuries can be rewarding both professionally and economically. The injury incidence rates of client companies will determine the types of prevention programs to be developed. Offering on-site consulting services will provide program planners with the information needed for program development. In addition, occupational health consulting services can generate revenue for departments in the hospital that typically are non–revenue-generating cost centers. For example, the employee health services nurse is an occupational health specialist who can evaluate worksites and design on-site programs for corporations. The hospital's safety engineer and industrial hygienist can also provide valuable services to companies in evaluation of worksite and risk reduction activities.

Program Positioning

Companies are not anxious to change to new health care program providers, particularly if a program is new and has no established track record. One way to successfully position the program and gain credibility is by developing a pilot program. A pilot program can provide the opportunity to fine-tune the system, generate data that prove the program is cost-effective, and deliver quality medical care. The pilot program needs to operate for 6 to 12 months to establish credibility.

State or local government agencies are good candidates for pilot programs. A pilot program does not require a bidding process for a contract. The fact that all statistical information is public knowledge is an advantage in reporting and using the data for marketing the program to employers.

Corporations that are currently "friends" of the institution are also good candidates for a pilot program. They already have an established relationship with the hospital and are usually willing to work with the new program. It is important to get an agreement in the beginning to use data from the pilot program for use in marketing materials. Many corporations will allow only general statistics, rather than actual data, to be publicized.

The pilot program data that will lend the most valuable credibility to the occupational health program include:

- Medical cost per injury
- Quality of communication
- Reduction of lost time from work

Companies are also interested in the acceptability of the program by their employees. Programs can assess such satisfaction with an employee questionnaire (figure 16-2).

Publicity plans to generate interest in the pilot program from the press and from local business publications should be coordinated between the public relations departments of the hospital and the pilot program's client. The program director and the physician case manager should be available for all speaking opportunities in the community. Members of business service and trade organizations are the chief executive officers and managers of prospective client companies. They should know what the program is doing for business in the region. Public speaking engagements represent one of the most effective activities to promote the program, whether presentations include the data from the pilot program or are limited to information on issues employers deal with daily.

The Future for Freestanding Facilities

There are currently numerous roadblocks to establishing a freestanding occupational health facility. The most formidable and complex roadblock is the hospital bureaucracy. Every aspect of an occupational health program is nontraditional. Objections may arise regarding the provision of off-campus services while using the hospital's name. For example, "You have no beds—

Figure 16-2. Rose Network Designated Provider Program Questionnaire

---

Name: ______________________________

Agency: ______________________________

Date: ______________________________

Job Classification	**Please circle correct response.**
1. Manager/supervisor, grade 77 or above	1 2 3 4 5 6 7
2. Manager/supervisor, grade 76 or below	
3. Clerical/technical (includes accounting technicians and computer operators)	
4. Professional (includes JSC and UI reps, admin. officers, accountants, claims adjusters, and auditors)	
5. Trades	
6. Custodial and related services	
7. Other	

---

1. Prior to the Designated Provider Program, did you have one doctor that you called when you had an illness? 1 - Yes 2 - No	1 2
2. What services did you receive from Rose Network Provider? 1 - Office visit 2 - Lab 3 - X ray 4 - Physical therapy 5 - Other	1 2 3 4 5
3. Where did you receive care? 1 - Emergency Room 2 - Outpatient 3 - Inpatient 4 - Other 5 - Specialist physician	1 2 3 4 5

Continued on next page

Figure 16-2. Continued

	Strongly Agree	Somewhat Agree	Undecided	Somewhat Disagree	Strongly Disagree
4. Rose Network facilities have convenient locations.	1	2	3	4	5
5. Scheduled appointment times were convenient for you.	1	2	3	4	5
6. The time spent waiting for a doctor was reasonable.	1	2	3	4	5
7. The doctor explained completely your diagnosis, treatment plan, medicines, tests, and so forth.	1	2	3	4	5
8. The doctor treated you with respect.	1	2	3	4	5
9. The doctor didn't talk down to you.	1	2	3	4	5
10. The doctor gave you a chance to say what's on your mind.	1	2	3	4	5
11. The doctor asked you questions about your job.	1	2	3	4	5
12. The doctor spent enough time with you.	1	2	3	4	5
13. You would use the Rose Network doctor for a non–work-related medical need.	1	2	3	4	5
14. The support staff (other than the physician) at the Rose Network facility treated you in a competent and professional manner.	1	2	3	4	5
15. The support staff (other than the physician) at the Rose facility was polite and respectful.	1	2	3	4	5
16. Overall, your experience with the Rose Network system was positive.	1	2	3	4	5

Comments: ____

____

____

you are not a hospital, so how do you belong? Or more important, why do you have the right to use the hospital's reputation?" It will be necessary to defend the program's identity until the generated revenue quiets the turmoil.

The occupational health program requires that departments work directly with the program as an "outsider" rather than through a committee. As indicated in this chapter, this might lead to non-revenue-generating departments—for example, safety, industrial hygiene, employee health—going outside the hospital to generate revenue via the occupational health program.

The hospital's medical staff will challenge the program as stealing "their" patients and doing nothing for them. "What has gotten into administration?" "Don't they know who delivers patients?" "It's the doctor, not programs!" These will be frequent cries from the medical staff.

In response, occupational health programs must be patient but firm, providing information and support. As the occupational health program becomes successful by delivering both patients and revenue to the institution and the medical staff, supporters will line up. Occupational health services provide an opportunity to generate significant revenue, not only for the freestanding facility but for virtually every division of the institution, including the medical staff. In addition, occupational health services provide an opportunity to build solid and growing relationships with business and industry. The health care provider that can assist businesses in controlling and containing health care costs for work-related injuries will be sought for additional programs to address all of the corporation's health care needs.

Chapter 17

Medical Staff Relations

William L. Newkirk, M.D.
Terry A. Morton, M.A.
Marsha Barnhart Eng, M.S.

Medical staff resistance is a common problem for occupational health programs. These programs often represent a significant change for a hospital and medical staff. Occupational health programs can cause friction between the hospital and medical staff, particularly when the programs manage the care of injured workers or aggressively market or control referral patterns. Thus, working effectively with the medical staff becomes a key factor in the success of an occupational health program.

Understanding Change

To a large degree, when medical staffs resist the development of an occupational health program, they are resisting change. The following pages highlight certain principles that characterize change. Understanding these principles provides insight into the best ways of interacting with the medical staff.

The Evolution of a Change

The process of introducing and implementing a new program can seem chaotic and confusing. However, an examination of the nature of the four development phases through which all new projects pass can help identify the points at which resistance to change can be countered:

- *Phase 1: The Introductory Phase.* This phase is euphoric; it is the one that everyone enjoys initially. The introductory phase is a period of great excitement because new and interesting things are about to happen. Everyone is likely to be swept up with this excitement during this period. During this exciting period, no one ever asks, "If occupational medicine is such a great idea, why did no one do it before?" Such doubts rarely arise because a new crusade is about to begin.

- *Phase 2: The Resistance Phase.* Once the proposed idea sinks in, people begin to see its true impact. The proposed change may disrupt the status quo and create real or imagined hardships. People evaluate this "great idea" in terms of the changes that it will require them to make. This period is the one in which everyone needs to address resistance to change. During the resistance phase, people can easily lose sight of the reasons why they were willing to undertake the change in the first place.
- *Phase 3: The Productive Phase.* Once everyone works through the resistance phase, they enter the productive phase. In this phase, the group actually accomplishes the intended task. If the resistance phase has been handled adequately, people begin to pull together, submerging their reservations. The group begins to see success, and that success is reinforcing.
- *Phase 4: The Termination Phase.* The program is now complete. The time has come to reexamine the total picture. Have all the goals been met? Have any important details been overlooked? Have effective controls been designed to ensure continued success? This phase is also the time to savor the accomplishment of the change.

Resistance to Change

The resistance phase is the most constant and predictable obstacle to successful program implementation, although the degree of resistance will vary from hospital to hospital. Successful program development requires the ability to predict and reduce the severity of the resistance phase. Even though resistance to change may be a natural occurrence, that resistance must be controlled so that the program can move forward.

Normal, healthy people resist change, usually for three major reasons:

- *Fear of losing something of value.* The negative consequences of a proposed change cannot be overlooked. Although change may not have negative consequences for some persons, it may have negative connotations for certain members of the hospital or medical staff. The person in charge of making change happen must take time to understand these negative connotations. During the euphoria of the introductory phase, persons in charge of the change usually assume that they are going to have clear sailing because they do not want to take time to find out all the reasons why they may not succeed.
- *Misunderstanding of the change and its implications.* The persons planning an occupational health program have a fair idea of what

the change involves, and they must accurately communicate this idea. If they do not, others may receive a distorted message. People distort messages because of their existing attitudes. Consequently, when change threatens people who already feel insecure, they may distort the message into something even more threatening.
- *Belief that the change does not make sense.* Staff developing an occupational health program should have a vision of what the program should accomplish. However, they should not expect everyone to accept their viewpoint. Resistance often occurs because people honestly do not believe that the change makes sense.

The sooner that resistance to a project is uncovered, the better. The tendency during the exuberant introductory phase is to ignore potential resistance, and this tendency can become a blind spot. The person in charge should not ignore any comment from a physician that begins with, "That's a good idea, but. . . ." Such comments should not be lightly answered with general statements, such as "Oh, we'll take care of that when the time comes." Now is the time to ask for criticism of the project. Planners who elicit resistance early in a program can plan an approach to it.

Predicted resistance is easier to handle than resistance that comes as a surprise. Resistance that comes as a surprise is both difficult to handle and emotionally stressful. Program planners should ask these questions:

- Who is likely to oppose the occupational health program?
- Why are they likely to oppose it?
- How and when will they express their resistance?

Once the answers to these questions have been determined, the persons in charge can plan an approach to handling resistance. Although all resistance can never be predicted, this approach enables planners to predict much of it.

Planners should adjust the speed of the project to the amount of resistance that you expect. When significant resistance is encountered, planners should slow the program's development so that they can deal with the resistance and form a coalition of the program's supporters. This delay may be impossible if the project has an externally controlled deadline by which the project must be completed. In the absence of such a deadline, however, planners should make sure to consider resistance when a timetable is developed.

Often, new occupational health programs encounter resistance that far exceeds that which would normally be expected. These circumstances usually occur when certain individuals or groups are undergoing significant stress that is often unrelated to the occupational health program itself.

The ability to cope with stress depends on the amount of stress to which the person is exposed. In 1908, Robert M. Yerkes and John D. Dodson of the Harvard Physiologic Laboratory demonstrated that as stress increases, so does performance, but only up to a critical point. Beyond that point, further stress causes a decrease in performance. This relationship is known as the Yerkes-Dodson curve and is illustrated in figure 17-1.

As the curve shows, stress can be a positive force that leads to increased performance. Everyone needs some stress to perform optimally; without it people become bored and unproductive. However, too much stress leads to reduced performance and the downward spiral of burnout. Understanding the impact of stress on performance is important because new occupational health programs being started in the late 1980s are in a period of unprecedented stress and change for hospitals and medical staff.

The Hospital and Medical Staff Environment

Recent changes in health care reimbursement and medical practice have placed tremendous stress on both hospitals and physicians. For the first time, hospitals and physicians are competing for the health care revenue dollar. As a result, the relationship between hospitals and their medical staffs is changing. This change has caused medical staffs to greet some new hospital initiatives, such as occupational health, with resistance. Such resistance is not surprising given the current level of stress and change.

The Physician's View

The traditional medical practice with its high level of independent physician control is dying. It is, of necessity, becoming highly integrated with

Figure 17-1. Yerkes-Dodson Curve—Relationship of Stress to Performance

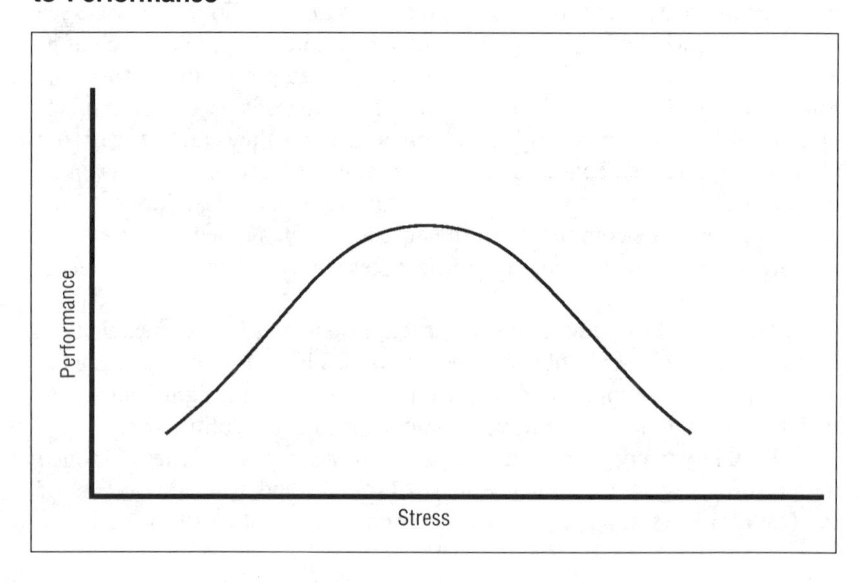

other types of health care delivery sources. No longer is the control of medicine solely in the hands of the physician.

In the 1980s, business and industry are actively involved in the medical care delivery process to an unprecedented degree. Some businesses are even becoming the carriers for their own insurance for health care expenditures. In their search for cost-effective health care, medium- to large-sized buyers of medical services are shopping and actively comparing the prices of services. As government and business gain more control over health care expenditures, physicians see their personal control over the delivery of patient care eroding. Physicians also perceive an erosion of prestige, autonomy, and authority. These changes are threatening and stressful to physicians.

The Hospital's View

Hospitals face similar changes in providing health care. The combined effects of prospective pricing, preadmission testing and certification, quality assurance, preventive health measures, and improvements in medical treatment have significantly reduced the demand for inpatient services. Some hospitals have failed to adapt to this changing environment and have closed. Most hospitals have responded with increased reliance on outpatient services, marketing, and diversification. These changes are transforming the once-sedate hospital industry into a competitive market. It is in this changing environment that hospitals are developing occupational health programs.

Occupational Health Programs and the Environment

Occupational health programs place both the hospital and medical staff in interesting dilemmas. On the one hand, the hospital needs the additional revenues, referrals, and relationships that an occupational health program can provide in order to maintain and generate revenue. On the other hand, the hospital needs to protect and foster existing medical staff relationships.

Physicians, on the one hand, see occupational health programs as further eroding their autonomy and control in the medical marketplace and enhancing their competition with the hospital. On the other hand, they see occupational health programs as providing them with referrals and security in an increasingly competitive marketplace.

Hospital and Medical Staff Expectations

Given the stressful environment and the often-conflicting needs of both parties, generating hospital and medical staff support for an occupational health program requires great care and planning. A key step in the process is identifying what the hospital expects of its medical staff when it calls for medical staff support of an occupational health program, as well as what the medical staff expects to find in an evaluation of the hospital's program.

Hospitals' Expectations of the Relationship

The first step in building effective hospital–medical staff relations is to analyze where the relationship has been in the past, where it is now, and where it is going. Is either group "burned out" by too many recent changes? Who are the key people in each group? How will an occupational health program affect the relationships?

If an occupational health program is to have a chance to succeed, the medical staff should not organize against it. The level of involvement in the occupational health program by the medical staff is influential in their decision to support the program model. The degree to which physicians are involved directly in program planning, implementation, and evaluation varies with each institution, but a willingness to involve physicians in some capacity is critical.

The following are some questions that should be asked about medical staff involvement in the occupational health program:

- Is participation by medical staff in the program valued?
- Is the medical staff allowed to participate in designing the program?
- Is the medical staff allowed to participate in program delivery?
- Is the participation by the medical staff important politically?
- Does the program compete with medical staff? At what level? To what extent?

Although significant medical staff input into the design of the program is important in achieving medical staff support, this approach carries some risk. Most occupational health programs are developed to *correct* current problems in the delivery of health care to workers. Medical staffs have a strong interest in the status quo. As a result, the program design most acceptable to the medical staff is likely to be one that has little impact on identified health care delivery problems.

The hospital and medical staff may have some preconceived ideas and feelings about occupational health programs. The following list identifies some areas about which physician groups may be sensitive:

- Perceived decline of the physician's power base
- Alterations in referral patterns
- Belief that physicians are already delivering the product to industry
- Belief that they already have the relationships with industry and do not need the hospital
- Dislike of marketing and sales
- Perceived loss of primary care business to an occupational health program

- Concern that control of the industrial market alters the entire delivery system
- Concern that the program will be the spearhead of an eventual effort to make the medical staff "employees" of the hospital
- Belief that the hospital will take the primary care physician out of the delivery loop
- Perception that the specialists get the business anyway
- Belief that the hospital will favor certain physicians over others
- General belief that physicians will lose business
- Belief that the hospital will cut the physician out after the program becomes successful
- Concern for the quality of care
- Statement that they "bring the hospital business and create revenue and the hospital turns around and uses the profits to develop programs to compete with physicians"

The physician has the right to expect that the hospital is sincere about the goals and objectives for the occupational health program in relation to the medical staff and is not making only perfunctory gestures aimed at stilling criticism or realistic concerns. Even though hospitals retain the basic right to decide what product lines they want their institutions to be involved in, recognizing the strength of physician interaction is beneficial from the beginning.

Physicians' Expectations of Hospital Programs

The hospital should be sensitive to the criteria physicians use when evaluating the appropriateness of their involvement in an occupational health program. The major concerns of physicians are quality, financial impact, the ethics of sales and marketing in health care delivery, and patient control.

Quality

For many physicians, the basic issue is whether cost cutting and corporate medicine diminish quality of care. Certainly, maintaining the highest quality of medical care in the face of decreasing provider reimbursement is a major challenge. However, because the reputation and success of medical staff members depend on their skill in delivering high-quality medical care, quality is their first criterion in assessing any program. They legitimately fear that competition will create an atmosphere that jeopardizes high-quality care. In addition, some physicians may believe that occupational health programs are not able to deliver a high-quality product.

Financial Impact

Effective targeting of the business market through occupational programs can boost declining utilization patterns for both physicians and hospitals.

The medical staff will ask, and is entitled to know, what impact the services will have on their patient load and referral patterns. They need to understand that the process is designed to channel potential customers through the hospital's system and into the physician's private practice.

Ethics of Sales and Marketing

For physicians, openly seeking business was once considered unethical. Many physicians find it difficult to acknowledge that marketing of health care services is now accepted practice. Most physicians still believe that high-quality work, not advertising, brings in the patients.

However, few businesses today can prosper without some form of marketing, and sales is a key element to success for any occupational health program. Physicians must recognize that marketing helps establish ongoing relationships between the hospital and the businesses.

Patient Control

As hospitals move to expand services and increase revenue, they are increasingly perceived as competitors by physicians. Physicians are concerned that hospitals will try to control and regulate physician practice patterns in order to strengthen the hospital's bottom line.

Developing an adequate patient base is more difficult for physicians, especially new physicians, because of the increasing physician supply. To some physicians who are threatened by occupational health programs, the issue becomes one of who controls the patient flow. Occupational health programs, particularly those that track injured workers and control referrals, can be threatening to those physicians with inadequate or marginal patient bases.

Strategies for Gaining Medical Staff Support

Many methods can be used to work through resistance with the medical staff when an occupational health program is being introduced. In deciding to venture into occupational health, each hospital must work within its particular circumstances to respond to the criticisms of physicians. In chapter 23, Dr. C. Kirby Griffin reviews some successful approaches used in developing a comprehensive occupational health program. In general, hospitals use four tools in handling medical staff resistance.

Education and Communication

Because a misunderstanding of change and its implications is a major cause of resistance, one method of countering resistance is through education and communication. Listening skills are helpful here. The hospital must understand the exact problem and misunderstandings that people have concerning the program.

Example: Hold educational sessions for the medical staff. Bring in expert speakers from successful outside programs. Discuss how a similar program could be developed in your hospital.

Participation and Involvement

Whenever possible, the hospital should present only the general outline of a proposed change. The medical staff should be allowed to fill in the details. Participation and involvement are critical. People support ideas more when the ideas are their own. The medical staff should be allowed the opportunity to propose changes whenever possible.

Example: Establish a professional advisory committee with broad representation from the various clinical departments. During regular meetings, the group should be encouraged to critique and modify the plans. The hospital should get the group's "stamp of approval" on all programs being developed for implementation. If a colleague later challenges the program content, the committee can run interference on the program's behalf. In addition, seek out the most credible member of the medical staff and make that person the medical advisor for the program.

Facilitation and Support

Every change causes stress and anxiety. Support during this period is helpful to everyone. Representatives from the hospital should be visible and available. The person in charge of the change should not propose a change and then hide in his or her office to work on it. Instead, he or she should spend time with the people who will be affected.

Example: Hold informal personal meetings with key medical staff members on a regular basis. Brief private meetings over coffee or lunch can uncover resistance and help allay fears. Leave the door open, walk the hallways, and do not take vacation during key resistance periods, such as when the program is being introduced.

Negotiation and Agreement

One cause of resistance is a desire not to lose something of value. If a proposed change will mean that certain physicians will lose out, the hospital should try to negotiate acceptable settlements.

Example: In effective occupational health programs, some traditional physician services lose out. When physicians who will be affected are identified in this way, the hospital should try to provide alternative business to those physicians. For instance, a physician may be offered the opportunity of working some shifts in the occupational medicine clinic.

Chapter 18

Hospital-Physician Joint Ventures

R. Kevin Smith, D.O.
Timothy R. Patten, M.B.A.

Joint ventures in occupational health are a new and uncommon phenomenon. The American Hospital Association surveyed 6,264 member hospitals in June 1984 concerning their involvement in health promotion and occupational health programs. Of the 3,565 hospitals that responded to the survey, 226 reported that they have occupational health programs. None of the 226 hospitals reported participating in joint ventures, and only 21 percent reported using a separate corporation from the hospital for their program.[1]

Advantages and Disadvantages of Joint Ventures

The decision to joint venture an occupational health program is complex and requires careful analysis. Anyone considering the development of such a venture should undertake this critical appraisal in consultation with legal counsel. Studying the advantages and disadvantages of such an approach for both the hospital and the physicians is essential to ultimately choosing the best structure among several options.

For both the hospital and the physicians, the most commonly cited advantage to involvement in a joint venture is the reduction in capital outlay and the risks for both parties. Most important, the hospital and the physicians work as partners for common goals rather than as potential competitors. The venture maximizes the expertise of each party. The hospital brings its business acumen to the venture, and the physicians provide their clinical expertise.

Advantages to the Hospital

By joint venturing with physicians, a hospital will avoid the loss of revenue from a physician's clinic for X rays, physical therapy, laboratory medicine, pulmonary medicine, and other services. Most important, a hospital will have a major say about other important aspects of the program, such as admissions, outpatient surgery, and special procedures and tests, such as nerve conduction studies, CT scans, and magnetic resonance imaging (MRI). A physician-owned-and-managed occupational health program could choose among several providers for these services.

A hospital has more to gain from an occupational health program than the physicians because it can benefit from both the primary profit of the program as well as secondary revenue that the program can generate for the hospital. Secondary revenue includes that from inpatient admissions, outpatient surgery, or special procedures and tests for injured workers, as well as revenue from "nonoccupational" utilization of the hospital by employees and their families and friends who have been introduced to the hospital through the occupational health program. It is estimated that 3–4 percent of all occupational health clinic visits result in hospital admissions.[2] A hospital might also experience an increase in secondary revenue from potential health maintenance organization or preferred provider organization customers referred through business leaders. Therefore, giving part ownership to physicians might be a wise move because the hospital can benefit significantly from the secondary revenue generated by an effective program.

Physicians' expertise in occupational medicine is the most important factor to the hospital. However, only 16.8 percent of all hospital occupational health programs report that a physician is director of the program, according to a 1984 American Hospital Association survey.[3] It is difficult for a hospital to manage services such as health screening, clinical diagnosis and treatment, rehabilitation, industrial hygiene services, consultative services, hearing conservation, and health promotion programs without the expertise of an occupational health physician. Strong physician presence in an occupational health program adds to the credibility of a program. Businesses are particularly impressed with physician involvement.

Another key reason for a hospital to joint venture is to use the physician as a buffer between the hospital and the medical staff. Medical staff resistance can be significant and can cause many problems for a hospital occupational health program. Physicians involved with the program can help reduce resistance among other medical staff.

Physicians can operate as employees, independent contractors, or equity partners with the hospital in an occupational health program. In a joint venture arrangement, a hospital would expect more involvement and commitment from the physicians who are equity partners because the success and failure of the program would directly affect them. Physician turnover and contract disputes should be less of a problem with joint ventures than with employee or independent contractor relationships. The biggest problem is finding a qualified occupational health physician in a competitive market, whether it be as an independent contractor, as an employee, or as a joint venture partner.

The formation of a separate corporate entity in an occupational health program reduces hospital bureaucracy. The program can respond more quickly to the needs of the business community instead of being restricted by laborious hospital policies and procedures and restrained by complex budgetary processes. This separate entity can be accomplished without joint venturing, but a corporation that is clearly distinct from the hospital, with physician involvement, can operate more effectively. The separate corporation can negotiate with departments and use its clout in making changes while avoiding the often-complicated hospital bureaucracy.

Advantages to Venture Physicians

The primary goal of physicians is to gain stability from the hospital while avoiding competition with it. A joint venture can accomplish both objectives. With hospital support, an occupational health program is less expensive and risky for the physicians and gives them easier access to cash.

In a hospital-based occupational health program, physicians do not have to develop and fund services such as the laboratory, X rays, or physical therapy, but at the same time they gain the benefit of the revenue. Physicians can offer more services to companies through the hospital than they could alone. They are able to utilize the hospital's expertise in areas such as marketing, billing, collections, and accounting and can supplement the hospital in medical service areas such as health promotion, physical therapy, and rehabilitation. It could cost physicians as much as a million dollars to develop a comprehensive occupational health program, but venturing with the hospital could reduce the amount by 60–80 percent. Most important, the hospital will not be competing with the physician for investment dollars.

A joint venture program in occupational health may include the hospital as one of the clients. This could be a significant account that the physician probably would not have an opportunity to service outside a joint venture.

Physicians have more control in a joint venture program than they would have as an employee or an independent contractor with the hospital. Most employees and independent contractors lack stability, because they usually have contracts with 60–90-day termination clauses. These physicians often have limited say on such vital matters as the budget, marketing, staffing, and growth and expansion. As an owner and a partner in a joint venture, the physician not only knows and reviews all aspects of the program but has an obligation to develop and support them. Similarly, specialist referral is usually determined by a hospital in an employee or independent contractor relationship, whereas the joint venturing physicians have an important voice in this matter. This may be an important factor to the stability of the joint venturing physicians.

Disadvantages of Joint Ventures

There is loss of flexibility to both parties in a joint venture. The joint venture will usually have a management team for day-to-day operations, but major issues need the consensus of all parties. A separate hospital or physician program answers only to itself and is not restricted by contractual issues.

Friction may develop between the joint venture staff and hospital departments in a hospital-based joint venture. The joint venture staff, although in many ways similar to hospital employees, will be distinct in other ways. Joint venture staff may not have to work weekends and holidays, and they will work only day shifts. The benefits package provided to joint venture staff may be different from that available to hospital employees. Most important, the joint venture will be viewed as a different entity from the hospital, and negative attitudes toward helping a separate program may arise. The joint venture will likely form separate agreements with various hospital departments in the form of discounts or preferential treatment for injured workers. The department personnel will perceive this as additional work without any benefit to the hospital. The joint venture will want to respond quickly to the needs of business and may be frustrated by the lack of concern and responsiveness from the hospital departments. The hospital should be aware of these potential conflicts and communicate to the departments the importance of the occupational health program.

The joint venture will probably have more implementation costs for the hospital than a separate hospital service. A joint venture will need to develop separate services apart from the hospital, whereas a separate hospital program can use existing staff and services. A joint venture, for example, may need a full-time occupational nurse at its inception, whereas a hospital-only program could utilize staff from existing areas until the program could support full-time staffing. If the joint venture program were treating acute injuries, it would need the staff and equipment to operate on its own, but the hospital program might utilize the emergency department in innovative ways to provide services at a lower cost owing to existing staffing, equipment, and supplies. The same is true for ECGs, pulmonary function tests, and audiograms. The pharmacy, in particular, needs careful separation from a joint venture. Many hospital pharmacies are not set up to supply medication to a separate corporation.

The same principles apply for administrative services, such as medical records, printing of various patient forms, and marketing. Billing and collection within a joint venture require separate equipment and personnel, whereas a hospital service could incorporate these services into existing ones.

Issues of conflict are sure to arise and may cause considerable problems within a joint venture. In an employee or independent contractor relationship, these issues are confined within the structure of the contract, and ultimately conflicts can be resolved with the termination of the contract. Conflict resolution among owners in a joint venture is more complicated. Conflicts may arise over capital expenditure, program development, share of the work load, profit or losses, and expansion. However, because both parties share common goals and have equal access to corporate knowledge and books, there is less of a chance for conflict.

Legal Structures of Joint Ventures

Once the decision has been made to joint venture, the involved parties must decide on the appropriate legal structure. Several alternatives exist:

- Corporation
  - For-profit
  - Not-for-profit
- Partnership
  - General
  - Limited

It is beyond the scope of this chapter to discuss these options in detail. Most legal experts recommend the corporate structure to limit the liability or risk to both parties. A for-profit status is presumed by a hospital involved with physicians.

Contractual Issues of Joint Ventures

The initial agreement for a joint venture should include provisions dealing with impasse disagreements and deadlock between the parties. It is much easier to consider options such as arbitration, mediation, or buyout provisions prior to incorporation than it is after problems arise.

Ownership

During the process of negotiating and finalizing the joint venture, the partners must decide how the ownership is to be divided. A hospital's general liability and malpractice insurance carrier may dictate that the hospital have a majority interest in order for it to participate in the joint venture. In such a situation, the hospital may have to give special provisions to the venturing physicians to equalize the contract. Such provisions might include requiring more than a simple hospital majority agreement for passage on major program issues such as election of officers, expansion, and the budget.

Noncompetition Provisions

Noncompetition provisions should address competition within both the hospital service area and the physicians' practices as well as future program expansion where the "intelligence" developed from the original program may be used. This could range from not allowing any separate expansion by either party, which may be illegal, to not addressing the expansion issue, which is careless. Placing limitations and a price tag on such expansion is necessary from the outset.

Transfer of Shares

Another important consideration is the transfer or sale of shares within the corporate structure of the venture. Neither party would want the other to sell its shares to a hostile third party. A way to manage this provision is to allow first right of refusal to the other shareholder with equitable terms for the transfer.

Business Issues for Joint Ventures

Once the contract issues have been formalized and the entity has been incorporated, a number of start-up issues demand immediate priority.

Capital Contribution

The most important business issue is the capital contribution or the start-up capital required from all parties for the venture. The venture may borrow the capital or require proportionate contributions from all parties. It is necessary to have capital to cover 3–6 months' operating expenses as well as enough money to cover initial expenses for legal matters, marketing, equipment, and supplies. Collection for workers' compensation cases takes from 60 to 90 days, with some accounts requiring months to close. It may take the program one to four years to become self-supporting, so realistic cash flow projections are necessary.

Budget

A realistic first-year budget is needed. Revenue projections should be conservative and based on market research data. There will be fixed and variable expenses. Fixed expenses will include base salaries for clerical, administrative, marketing/sales, billing, and secretarial support staff. In addition, there will be fixed expenses for equipment, office supplies, rent, accounting, legal matters, education, business development, and marketing. Variable expenses will depend on the setting and structure of the venture. They include expenses that will vary with volume and revenue, such as medical supplies. Variable expenses may also include certain salaries and radiology, laboratory, and physical therapy expenses.

Accounting and Banking

Accounting and banking relationships are needed at the outset for payroll, expenses, and cash flow. Resources within the hospital can offer sound business advice at a reasonable price until relationships with outside accounting or financial management firms are feasible.

Billing

Billing is a particularly crucial issue. It is possible that the venture could subcontract with the hospital for these services, but more commonly, the hospital billing system will not accommodate the unique needs of the smaller occupational health program. The venture will often have to do the billing or contract with an outside billing firm at significant expense. If the venture manages its own billing, then a part-time biller/collector will be needed with a provision to expand into computerized billing as the need dictates.

Operational Structure

A day-to-day operating structure must be developed early. The corporation's board of directors cannot deal with day-to-day operating issues. An effective management team should be formed. It is best to include both hospital and physician representatives in the management team. The team will be involved in employee supervision, clinic management, accounting, bookkeeping, billing, and relationships within the hospital.

Staffing

The venture must make arrangements for the hiring and management of its employees. It should consider purchasing employee benefits from the hospital, which would likely be cheaper and more comprehensive than trying to find benefits as a small corporation. Gradually bringing on staff and using existing staff whenever possible is most important. For primarily clinical programs, an occupational nurse will be the minimum staffing requirement.

The same issues of staffing apply to the physicians as well. Ideally, the joint venturing physicians will be active participants, but contractual agreements with other physicians may be necessary.

Purchasing

The venture must make arrangements for purchasing supplies and office and medical equipment, among other things. It will probably have to go outside the hospital for these purchasing services, particularly for pharmaceutical supplies. A number of group purchasing arrangements are available from state hospital associations and other organizations.

Insurance

General liability and malpractice insurance must be obtained for the venture. Physicians must secure their own malpractice coverage for clinical services. In certain circumstances, general liability can be included under the hospital's existing policy, although this might be extremely complicated. If this is not feasible, alternative sources should be explored with local insurance brokers.

Service Relationships

The venture must establish relationships for services within hospital departments. This might include preferential treatment or discounted service agreements. The venture should make a special effort to inform the hospital departments and medical staff of how the venture affects them. It is particularly important that those physicians who will be working closely with the program, such as the radiologist and orthopedic and physical medicine specialists, be well informed. Agreement on policies and procedures and even contracts may be needed to establish these relationships.

Joint Venture Example

The following is a brief example outlining major aspects of a joint venture in occupational health between a hospital and physicians. It utilizes actual experience from the authors' joint venture in conjunction with other practical matters that will likely arise. The hospital is a not-for-profit institution that has a separate for-profit investment company (figure 18-1), which arranged the joint venture with two physicians.

Figure 18-1. Example of a Legal Structure for a Joint Venture

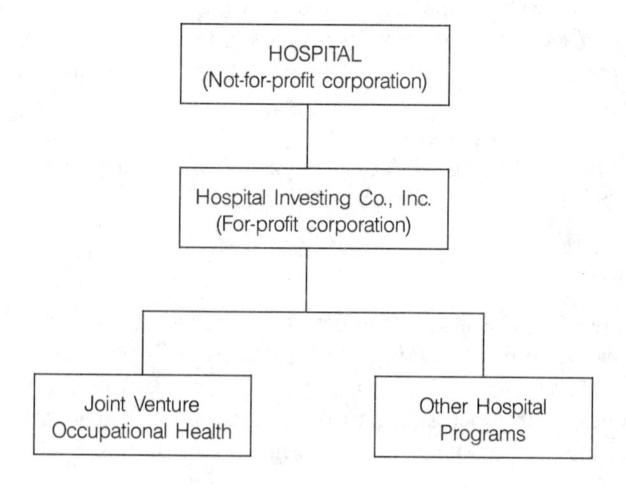

Environmental Assessment

After definite interest is expressed in a joint venture by all parties, an environmental assessment is performed. Marketing research is conducted by a combination of the hospital marketing department, the two physicians, and an outside marketing firm that obtains the pertinent business data. The marketing research takes four months, at a cost of $15,000 for the outside marketing firm.

Location

An on-campus location is selected based on the funding available and on information provided from the environmental assessment and marketing research.

Advantages and Disadvantages

All parties weigh the advantages and disadvantages of the available options. After careful consideration, they believe that the best arrangement is a joint venture.

Legal Structure

The joint venture chooses a for-profit corporation as the best organizational structure. The board of directors of the corporation consists of five members: three individuals from the hospital and the two physicians.

Contract Terms

The following four items are included in the contract:

1. *Ownership.* The hospital must have majority ownership for liability coverage, so equity is divided as follows:

Hospital	*Physicians*	
	A	B
51 percent	24.5 percent	24.5 percent

The physicians wanted an equal split in ownership, with the hospital having 50 percent. A compromise was agreed upon wherein a 60 percent majority is required for major issues—budget, expansion, major purchases, and so forth.

2. *Noncompetition.* No competition is allowed in the immediate service area (defined by zip codes) for the occupational health services provided by the venture. Further expansion is allowed by any party outside the service area for a fee of $10,000 to the joint venture. This amount is subject to amendment annually.

3. *Impasse.* Any impasse or disagreement will be sent to a mutually acceptable third party for mediation. The joint venture also has buy-out provisions during an impasse.
4. *Transfer of shares.* If a shareholder wishes to dispose of any or all of his or her shares, the first right of refusal must be given to the remaining shareholders.

Business Issues

The following business issues are agreed upon:

1. *Services.* The physicians are experienced and trained in emergency medicine and occupational medicine so that acute care and follow-up care are promoted. A location next to the emergency department is selected. Minor occupational injuries are referred to the occupational medicine clinic during its hours of operation, 9:00 a.m. to 5:00 p.m., Monday through Friday. The total services include:
   a. Acute injury and illness care
   b. Follow-up and referral care
   c. Case management
   d. Physical therapy
   e. Medical screening
   f. Worksite walk-through assessment
   g. Wellness program
2. *Budget.* The joint venture projects a realistic first-year budget based on conservative estimates (table 18-1).
3. *Capital contributions.* The venture requires all parties to make an initial capital investment equal to 50 percent of the first-year budget in amounts proportional to their equity interest.
4. *Operational structure.* Figure 18-2 outlines the operational structure of the venture, which combines hospital and physician representation.
5. *Accounting.* The joint venture utilizes the hospital accounting department for assistance with corporate books, banking, payroll, and taxes.
6. *Billing.* A part-time biller/collector is hired. In the first five months of operation, the billing is performed manually, and thereafter a computer program is used.
7. *Staffing.*
   a. Nursing: The joint venture hires a full-time nurse, who is a major focal point among the program, the hospital, and the business community.
   b. Medical assistant: A medical assistant is required on a part-time basis (four hours per day) at the ninth month of operation.
   c. Physician: One of the joint-venturing physicians is the medical director of the program and also provides the majority of physicians' clinical services. The physician is hired as an independent

Table 18-1. Example of a First-Year Budget for a Joint Venture

I. Fixed Expenses	
A. Staff[1]	
1. Nurse (1 FTE)	$ 27,000
2. Marketing/sales rep (1 FTE)	32,000
3. Physician administrator	25,000
4. Biller (0.3 FTE)	6,000
5. Secretarial staff (0.25 FTE)	3,000
6. Medical assistant (0.25 FTE)	4,000
B. Equipment[2]	12,000
C. Office supplies	4,000
D. Marketing[3]	14,000
E. Accounting	4,000
F. Legal[4]	13,000
G. Education/business development	5,000
H. Rent	10,000
I. Market research	15,000
Subtotal	$174,000
II. Volume-Driven Expenses[5]	$100,000
Total Expenses	$274,000
III. Revenue	$200,000
IV. Net Loss	$ (74,000)

1. Staff salaries include benefits.
2. Equipment—computer, desks, chairs, ECG, audiometer, typewriter, storage, and so forth.
3. Marketing—includes sales material, development, and expenses.
4. Legal—includes incorporation expenses.
5. Volume-driven expenses based on 50% of estimated total billing of $200,000 in the first year—includes expenses for radiology, radiologist, laboratory, pulmonary medicine, physical therapy, medical supplies, and clinical physician services.

Figure 18-2. Example of an Operational Structure for a Joint Venture

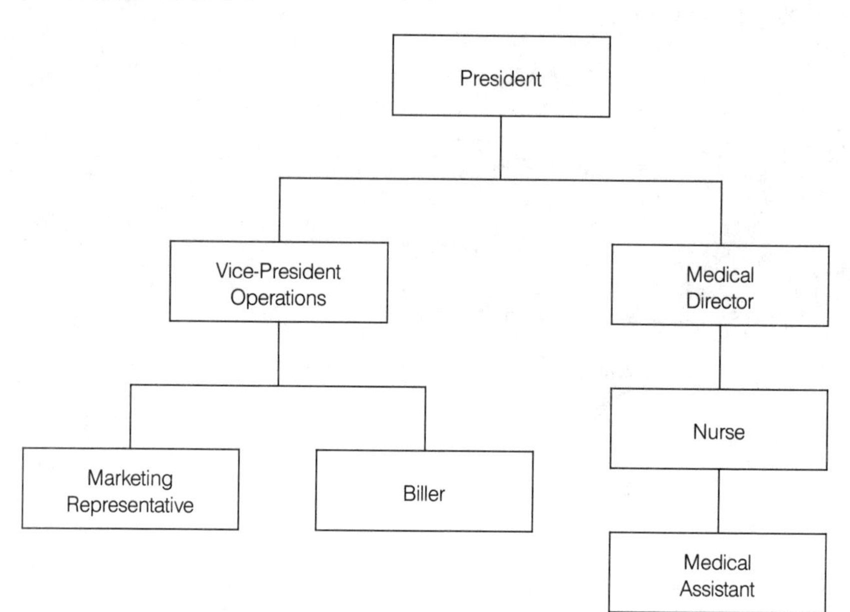

contractor and receives a stipend for administrative duties and a fee-for-service arrangement for clinical services. The venture saves a significant amount of money by paying the physician only for the clinical services performed instead of paying an expensive hourly wage for a physician who sees few patients in the initial months of operation.

d. Marketing representative: A full-time marketing sales representative establishes a marketing plan and personally calls on businesses in the service area.
e. Secretary: A part-time secretary is utilized from existing resources within the hospital on an as-needed basis.
f. Benefits: The venture purchases a comprehensive benefits package for its full-time employees (nurse, marketing representative) from the hospital, at a cost of 20 percent of their salary. The hospital system is utilized for payroll as well.

8. *Insurance.* The hospital's general liability and malpractice insurance covers the venture itself. The physician must purchase his or her own malpractice insurance.
9. *Service relationship.* The venture contracts with the hospital for radiology, laboratory, physical therapy, and health promotion services. Discounted and preferential treatment is given to the venture by these departments, which allows the program to be competitive in the

marketplace. In addition, the joint venture establishes formal relationships with key medical specialists for prompt treatment and timely reporting in return for additional patient referrals.

Summary and Recommendations

In the authors' experience, the following should serve as useful guidelines for those considering the formation of a joint venture in occupational health services.

1. A joint venture is not for everyone. In fact, it will work only in a minority of situations.
2. The joint venture should be given consideration if most of the following factors are present:
   a. The hospital and the physicians are compatible.
   b. A program would not be as well developed if it were a solo entity.
   c. Time constraints are a major factor; that is, a program could be developed without a joint venture, but it would take much more time.
   d. Capital is a major issue.
   e. The hospital's medical staff would be a major hindrance to a hospital-only program.
3. Hospitals have much to gain from an occupational health program, including the primary revenue of the program; the secondary revenue from admissions, outpatient surgery, and major procedures; and the added benefit of influencing business to utilize the hospital and develop preferred provider arrangements.
4. Physicians gain not only the revenue from the program but also stability and cooperation from the hospital in a very competitive medical environment.
5. A thorough environmental assessment and marketing research are essential.
6. A hospital should select physicians experienced in occupational health. These physicians should understand local business needs and be willing to become a major focus of the program in meetings with business leaders.
7. A for-profit corporation is the most likely legal structure for a joint venture.
8. The contract must be fair to all parties and address key issues of ownership, competition, expansion, impasse, and the transfer of shares.
9. When setting up the venture, it is best to utilize existing resources within the hospital as much as possible, including staff, equipment, accounting, billing, liability insurance, and compensation packages.

If possible, the emergency department should play a key role in the program, as it is often the business community's link to the hospital.

References

1. American Hospital Association. *Profile of Hospital Occupational Health Services.* Chicago: AHA, 1986, p. 20.
2. Droste, T. Occupational health: profits and problems. *Hospitals* 61(12):92, June 20, 1987.
3. American Hospital Association, pp. 12, 14.

Chapter 19

Computer Systems

William L. Newkirk, M.D.

Modern medicine relies on technology. Developing a successful occupational health program requires an understanding of when it is appropriate to apply new technologies to occupational health problems. This chapter provides a framework for assessing how and when to use computers in occupational health programs.

Computer Applications in Occupational Health Programs

Computer systems are helpful in solving a variety of occupational health program problems, such as injured worker tracking, preplacement screening, biological monitoring, communications, and clinic administration.

Injured Worker Tracking

The greatest contribution of computer systems to occupational health program development and worker health care has been in the area of injured worker tracking. Chapter 4 discusses how injured worker tracking can form the backbone of an occupational health program. In its simplest form, injured worker tracking is a commitment by the hospital to the injured worker, the employer, and the employer's insurance carrier that the injured worker will be carefully followed during the course of his or her injury rehabilitation. Worker tracking reduces the time a worker is off the job by speeding referrals, improving communication, and preventing the worker from "falling through the cracks" of the workers' compensation system.

Obviously, an occupational health program can track workers without a computer system. However, the greater the program volume, the more difficult it is for the program to track workers manually. As programs grow, they often begin to rely on computers.

Computerized worker tracking systems also offer the ability to develop statistics of injury incidences, evaluate injury trends, assess the efficacy of the occupational health program, and compare the performance of different health care providers. The worker tracking reports are often effective communication and marketing tools.

Preplacement Screening

Computers can assist the preplacement screening process in several ways: specific job assessment, job matching, probability projections, and large population screening.

Specific Job Assessment

For preplacement screening to be valid, a specific worker must be assessed against the Bona Fide Occupational Qualifications (BFOQ), or the identified risks of a specific job. Computerized job assessment systems provide a way of assessing and storing records of job demands so that they are available for the examining physician.

Job Matching

Computerized systems can match workers to jobs for which they are qualified. The computer's capacity to compare a handicapped worker's skills to the risks of a large number of jobs to find an acceptable position helps an employer provide reasonable accommodations or alternative duty placement (see chapter 6 for legal obligations of employers of disabled individuals).

Probability Projections

In some states, an employer can reject an otherwise qualified employee if the employer has a factual basis to believe, with a reasonable probability, that the worker will suffer a significant deterioration in his or her health. The courts have not clearly defined what level of probability is "reasonable." Nonetheless, occupational health programs have the responsibility to determine the probability of a specific worker suffering a deterioration in health in a specific job. Computers can help in this task. Computer models, using Bayesian or logistical regression equations, can provide estimates of risk that are useful in arriving at clinical assessments of probability.

Large Population Screening

Legally, preplacement screening can be used to reject only a small percentage of potential workers. Rejected workers are those who cannot fulfill the

BFOQ of the job and, in some states, those who have a reasonable probability of suffering a significant deterioration in their health because of the job. As a result, if the sole purpose of a company's preplacement screening program is to identify workers who should be rejected, then applying the traditional physician preplacement screening to all workers is not the most cost-efficient approach for most companies. A multistep screening process that utilizes computerized screening as the first step is more cost-efficient.

Suppose the occupational health program is doing preplacement screening for a worker for a secretarial job that has an insignificant injury incidence rate. The worker is in good health, has worked without difficulty in secretarial jobs before, and has no significant injury history. Given this circumstance, it is extremely unlikely that the company could reject this worker for health-related reasons. A computerized system can screen such workers and pass them without utilizing limited and expensive physician time. This reserves the physician for a more in-depth evaluation of workers where rejection is a possibility.

Biological Monitoring

The Occupational Safety and Health Administration (OSHA) requires medical surveillance for the biological effects of a very limited group of workplace exposures. The National Institute of Occupational Safety and Health (NIOSH) makes recommendations for medical surveillance for a much larger group of exposures. Frequently, hospital occupational health programs participate in this mandated or recommended medical screening, called "biological monitoring." (See chapter 5 for more information about OSHA, NIOSH, and medical surveillance services.)

Computers can assist this task in several ways: automating the testing process, analyzing trend data, and identifying whom and when to test.

Automated Testing and Analysis

Computers can automate the testing process, diminishing the need for highly qualified and expensive personnel to perform routine, repetitive tasks. This automation occurs at three levels: data gathering, data interpretation, and data storage.

Intelligent testing equipment can assist in data collection. A good example of this is automated audiometric (hearing testing) equipment. These devices can perform a hearing test and, in some cases, analyze and store the data.

Computers can aid in data interpretation. Intelligent computer programs contain the logic physicians use to interpret such tests as audiograms or pulmonary function tests. Use of these computer programs to perform routine data analysis is faster, more consistent, and significantly less expensive.

Finally, automated testing can provide electronic data storage, which facilitates comparison test results and saves time in filing and sorting analyses.

Trend Analysis

From a clinical perspective, the greatest advantage of computers in biological monitoring is the computer's ability to analyze trends and manipulate data. For the most part, biological monitoring looks for long-term adverse effects of toxic exposures. As a result, observing the trend of a worker's biological performance is extremely important. Computers aid this process in several ways:

- They can display data in useful pictorial formats so that trends become more visible.
- They can select workers who meet predetermined trend criteria who might otherwise be missed in large population bases.
- They can group workers so that negative group trends become obvious, often indicating the failure of protective measures.
- They can manipulate data to assess the effects of age, sex, amount of exposure, and protective devices.

Testing Requirements

Computers are also helpful from an administrative perspective in determining which workers require which tests at specific times. Computers can electronically link the workers to their jobs, the jobs to chemical exposures, and the exposures to OSHA and NIOSH recommendations. In this way, each worker can have a profile of recommended initial, periodic, and emergency screenings. Trying to manually perform this task for a large population base can be extremely time-consuming.

Communications

Hospital occupational health programs are just beginning to recognize the power of computer systems as communication devices. The number of computer-to-computer communication applications is certain to grow in the future. At present, the two major computer communication applications for occupational health programs are retrieving information from scientific data bases and sending information to employers and insurance companies.

Retrieving Scientific Information

Hospital occupational health programs retrieve scientific information from a broad range of disciplines, including medical advances, industrial toxicology, and legal changes. An effective way to rapidly access this information is to use the occupational health program computer to connect to large computerized data bases. These data bases usually contain more recent information than is available in textbooks. They can search the medical literature to find articles that address specific medical problems. In many hospitals, computerized literature searches have become a standard way of reviewing medical information. (For information, check with National Library of Medicine Specialized Information Services, Bethesda, Maryland 20894, 301/496-6531.)

Transmitting Medical Information

The prospect of immediate transfer of medical information from the occupational health clinic to the industry and to the insurance company holds great promise. Hospitals are notorious for their inability to provide timely information to industry about the status of injured workers. This leads to increased workers' compensation costs because injured workers miss more work than is necessary. In addition, if companies do not understand the nature of the worker's injury and physical limitations, companies can place the worker in inappropriate jobs, risking further injury.

The capacity exists to directly transmit medical information about a worker while at the same time protecting the injured worker's rights to medical confidentiality. This can improve the worker's care at the worksite. Another advantage is that direct transmission can tie the industry closely to the health care provider, providing a significant marketing advantage. Similar advantages exist for transmitting information to the insurance company.

Clinic Administration

Computer systems offer advantages in the administration of medical clinics. These advantages fall into two categories: clinic management and financial management.

Clinic Management

Computer systems can help clinics to have smooth operations. Systems can manage scheduling, first reports of injury, OSHA logs, clinic logs, and medical records. They can track client company statistics and medical staff referrals. The number of applications are limited only by the ingenuity of the clinic and its programmers.

Financial Management

Computer systems can assist a clinic with billing and financial management. Systems with report-writing capability allow clinic administrators to customize their financial management reports. In a hospital setting, clinic computers can interface with the hospital's mainframe computer to ensure an integrated billing system.

Development or Selection of Computer Systems

The balance of this chapter examines the considerations that should guide occupational health programs in their decisions to develop customized systems or to purchase existing hardware and software.

Basic Rules

Hospitals can avoid some of the problems that frequently occur when applying computer systems to their occupational health problems by following these five rules:

1. *Avoid computer jargon whenever possible.* Effective communication is essential to occupational health program development. Computer jargon short-circuits communication. Although jargon can save time when one computer person is talking to another, it intimidates noncomputer people. If you are a noncomputer person, particularly if you are in a managerial or clinical role, you must ensure that you understand what your computer people are telling you. Don't be afraid to ask a dumb question. Often, computer jargon covers up sloppy thinking.
2. *Don't computerize any task that doesn't need to be computerized.* Computers are seductive. Without experience with computer systems, it is easy to expect computers to solve every problem. In fact, computers rarely solve problems; they just substitute one set of problems for another. Ask, "Can the task be performed adequately without computers?" If it can, don't computerize it. Ignore the claims of computer people who say they can improve your performance on that task.
3. *If an important task is computerized, make sure there is a back-up system.* Computers break down. If the essential tasks of an occupational health program are computerized and the computer fails, then the program fails. If a computer is used to perform essential program functions, back-up capability must be available to perform those tasks when the computer fails.
4. *Software is more important than hardware.* Software (computer programs) is more important than hardware (the machines themselves). Good occupational health software is scarce; the machines to run the software are plentiful. Software should be selected before the hardware. Computer decisions should never be based on hardware alone!
5. *Don't computerize meaningless or redundant information.* There should be a good reason for saving any data in a data base. Data entry and maintenance cost money. Computer people have a saying: "Garbage in, garbage out." Only meaningful data should be

entered into the computer, and the information should be analyzed in a useful way. If the computer buries data in irrelevant information, it will become more a hindrance than a help.

Promise versus Reality

Computer systems can significantly assist in the development of hospital occupational health programs. However, many times computer systems do not work out. Even when systems do work well, they often do not reach their full potential. There are several reasons for this:

- *Hospitals frequently underestimate the cost and time involved in developing a comprehensive occupational health computer system.* Developing comprehensive occupational health computer software is expensive; hospitals often substantially underestimate development costs. Professional-level, comprehensive, mainframe systems rarely cost less than $1,000,000 to develop. Comprehensive microcomputer systems often cost $250,000 or more to develop. In addition, systems usually take considerably longer to develop than initially estimated.
- *Hospitals underestimate the importance of computer training and support for the clinic staff.* For many occupational health program staff members, computers are threatening and confusing machines. Computers rarely solve problems; instead, they substitute one set of problems for another. For example, computers can make it possible to track hundreds of workers simultaneously. However, to accomplish this task, a clinic staff member must enter data, endure "bugs," make back-up copies of information, and perform other computer-related functions. Hospitals often underestimate the amount of computer training and support necessary for staff members to accomplish these tasks.
- *Hospitals fail to recognize the long-term effects of committing to an occupational health computer system.* Certain occupational health functions, such as biological monitoring, require data maintenance for long periods of time. This period is likely to extend beyond the life span of the computer, the computer language, and the operating systems. When hospitals decide to computerize such data, they must understand how they will deal with the changing technologies. Who will rewrite their programs when they are obsolete? Who will modify their data?

Hospitals successful in developing occupational health computer systems recognize that the systems take time and money to develop, require significant commitments to staff training, and need long-term technical support and development.

Hospitals can develop their own computer systems or lease or purchase systems from other hospitals, hospital groups, or developers. Systems vary greatly in design and cost. To determine which system is right for a particular program, the hospital should assess its expectation and duration of use.

Expectations from Use

Imagine that you are selling word processors. A man buys a word processor from you and states, "I'm going to write a best-seller!" He returns two years later and says that your word processor wasn't any good. You ask about bugs, features, spelling checking, and other possible problems. He states that the word processor performed well in all those areas. "So what's the problem?" you ask. He looks you in the eye and says, "The book wasn't a best-seller."

In this example, the word processor performed a specific *task*—the manipulation of words. The user was looking for a specific outcome—the production of the best-seller. What is a similar occurrence in occupational health? Suppose that a hospital purchases a computer system to help with hearing conservation programs. The hospital can expect that the system will effectively perform a task (for example, read audiograms and determine threshold shifts promptly and accurately) or that it will produce a specific outcome (that is, effective hearing conservation programs). Obviously, producing an effective hearing conservation program is much more complex than merely reading audiograms. It requires more than just computer software. It requires training, policies, surveillance, and record keeping. As a result, computer systems designed to produce specific outcomes are more comprehensive, more training-oriented, and usually more expensive than task-oriented systems.

Controlling Human Behavior

Computer systems designed to produce outcomes deal as much with managing human behavior as they do with managing data. A common mistake in preplacement screening programs, for example, is for the occupational health program to perform a preplacement screening on a worker without having assessed the worker's job. This violates legal principles of preplacement screening, such as worker-specific job screening and limitation of preplacement inquiry to job-specific tasks. Computer systems designed to produce a successful preplacement screening program can prevent occupational health clinic staff members from performing a preplacement screening without first having assessed the job.

Physicians resist efforts to change their practice behavior. Often, a physician's practice pattern may have a strong negative effect on the success of a hospital occupational health program. Directly addressing the problem with the physician can sometimes solve the problem. Often, however, the physician resists. An intelligently designed computer system can often redirect the physician's behavior in a subtle way.

Suppose, for example, that the physician fails to closely follow his or her patients—letting them fall through the cracks of the workers' compensation system. If direct efforts to convince the physician to change his or her habits are unsuccessful, providing the physician with a computer system that assists with many office functions and, in addition, makes sure that workers do not get lost can solve the problem.

A second area where computer systems are helpful in controlling behavior is in multifacility occupational health networks. In these networks, it is often important that hospitals provide similar services to industry. A large employer, for example, may want to have similar preplacement screenings performed at several hospitals. If each of the hospitals uses the same kind of computerized preplacement screening, the screenings are likely to be more uniform than if the hospitals provide their own brand of screening.

Finding commercially developed software for the purposes just outlined may prove difficult. Computer systems designed to control human behavior in occupational health clinics are much more difficult to develop than other computer systems because they require a specific knowledge of how occupational health clinics function.

Software Selection

For most hospitals, it is impossible to develop comprehensive software for their occupational health program. There are several reasons for this:

- Software development is expensive.
- Hospitals often lack the appropriate computer expertise.
- Hospitals often lack the necessary occupational medicine expertise.
- Hospitals need to bring their occupational health services to market and do not have the time to spend on software development.

For these reasons, and others, hospitals seek to lease or purchase software systems from third parties. Hospitals that seek to do this must be aware of two major problems:

- *There are no accepted standards for occupational health software.* As of early 1989, no accepted testing criteria or certifying agency for occupational health software exists. For example, there is no system or agency to verify that software designed to read audiograms correctly performs that task. In addition, there is no requirement that software developers have a background or training in occupational health or that they have any medical training or expertise whatsoever.
- *Most occupational health software companies fail.* Although exact figures for the failure rates of occupational health software products and companies are not known, experts in the field estimate the failure rate at 60–90 percent. This is significant for hospitals because it means

that the company from which the hospital obtains its software may not be available to support that product for the long term.

There are three major reasons for the failure of occupational health software companies:

1. *The occupational health software market is very small and as a result does not command the attention of the large software providers.* In addition, large software providers often lack the specific occupational health expertise necessary for a comprehensive occupational health product.
2. *Occupational health software companies are poorly capitalized.* Often, they are a sideline or hobby of a person who works in occupational health. Rarely do these operations have adequate survival strategies or a commitment to meeting hospitals' long-term development and maintenance needs.
3. *Occupational health software is often underpriced.* One major flaw of small software developers is that they fear rejection more than they want success. As a result, they price their software so low that the long-term survival of their service is unlikely unless they achieve unrealistic market penetration.

For hospitals who are making a decision about software use, evaluating the viability of the software provider is as important as evaluating the quality of the software.

Summary

Occupational health computer systems offer benefits and pose risks for hospital occupational health programs. Hospitals can increase a computer system's chances for success by:

1. Understanding how computers are beneficial in occupational health and clearly defining how the hospital expects to use the computer to perform those functions
2. Making a significant investment in personnel training and technical support
3. Using realistic cost and time estimates for completing a project if the hospital chooses to develop its own software
4. Selecting software from an outside source by investigating how well other hospitals have fared with the outside provider and determining the capitalization and financial viability of the provider

Chapter 20

High-Technology Equipment

Thomas F. McCoy, D.O.

Hospital occupational health programs are increasingly relying on high-technology equipment to help them diagnose, rehabilitate, and evaluate injured workers. This equipment is expensive: A fully equipped laboratory can cost several hundred thousand dollars. Programs are willing to pay that amount in the belief that high-technology equipment will allow them to use more accurate, reproducible, and legally defensible measures of a prospective or injured employee's capacity for work. In the process, the programs hope to expand existing markets or develop new markets for their services. Some hospitals have reasonable assumptions about high-technology equipment. Others see the equipment as a panacea for their program's problems. This chapter evaluates the process of selecting equipment and the reasonable and unreasonable expectations programs have about the equipment.

Needs Assessment

In order to establish the need for high-technology equipment, the hospital occupational health program must answer two basic questions. The first is, "Why does the program need the equipment?" If the equipment is needed to increase referrals in response to a waning market share, it is best to question whether equipment is the answer. The program should review why referrals are dropping off and why the services are no longer competitive; it is unlikely that equipment will solve such problems. Three common market goals usually affect the perception of equipment needs:

- *Expanding an existing market.* If a hospital is driven by an already successful market to expand services, new equipment will serve a specific and useful purpose. Certain equipment needs will be obvious from daily practice. Existing services should provide reimbursement for equipment use. Usually, the personnel needed to run the equipment are already on hand.

- *Adding new markets.* Adding a different but proven market also makes it easier to identify equipment needs. Proven markets have consultants who can address the type and value of the equipment, as well as the reimbursement protocols and staffing needs such an endeavor will require.
- *Creating a new service.* Creating an entirely new service, especially one directed at a new market, is the most speculative situation for properly selecting high-technology equipment. Often, the opportunity that the new service and equipment address is poorly understood. In addition, third-party payers may not reimburse the new services if they perceive them as unproven or experimental. In this situation, a well-planned market study should precede the decision to purchase expensive equipment.

The second basic question the program needs to answer is, "How will the equipment be used?" There are four basic equipment functions:

- *Diagnosis.* This is the prerogative of the physician. The physician should have training and familiarity with the particular type of equipment under consideration. Certain government regulations control the sale and use of diagnostic equipment. The need for equipment can be estimated by reviewing incidence data on medical disorders within the target population.
- *Treatment.* Treatment applications most often involve the physical therapist or occupational therapist in rehabilitation services. By far, treatment of the musculoskeletal system is the greatest application for high-technology evaluation equipment today. Systems for evaluating and treating back and extremity disorders represent the most competitive equipment markets. This competition among product firms makes them more willing to help the consumer evaluate and develop the market in which such equipment will be used.
- *Special measurements.* These are usually limited-application services related to permanent impairment evaluations, work fitness studies, and musculoskeletal retraining programs. In general, these systems depend on equipment that tests a specific function, such as lift capability. This equipment market is growing as recognition is given to the role of cost containment in work-related injuries.
- *Screening.* These applications are usually a part of occupational medicine services. These, too, are special measurement systems but dedicated to earlier identification of health disorders arising in industry. Equipment in the category of physiological evaluation is most appropriate to screening services.

Equipment Selection

There are four general categories of high-technology equipment that occupational health programs buy or lease:

- *Diagnostic.* High-technology diagnostic equipment, as opposed to more common diagnostic instruments, is frequently hazardous to use. Because the use of such equipment often involves invasive and painful procedures and may increase health risks to the patient, the equipment is rigidly controlled in terms of product testing and availability. Although diagnostic equipment has some proven value and relevance to particular medical specialists, it is important to ensure that the physician operating the system has adequate qualifications and training before the equipment is used.
- *Regional.* Regional equipment measures performance of a body part, most often the extremities or the spine. This category is often associated with treatment programs administered by physical therapists, kinesiotherapists, and occupational therapists. Orthopedic applications predominate. Recent developments in spine measurement systems now provide four different back machines, from different companies, to study and condition back and abdominal musculature. In addition, new software programs have permitted computer assistance to some leg machines that were previously purely mechanical, making older regional equipment more useful. Common names associated with these service products are Cybex, Isotechnology, Lido, and Kincom.
- *Functional.* Functional evaluation systems measure performance of a goal-directed activity. The use of tools can be evaluated with a work simulator (BTE), lifting capacity can be studied with lift-task devices (ISTU, Lift-task), and gait can be evaluated with ambulatory monitoring systems. These devices are especially useful as part of work fitness evaluations, impairment measures, and activity-related rehabilitation programs. Names associated with functional tool systems are Baltimore Therapeutic Equipment, Ergometrics, and Biodex.
- *Physiological.* Physiological systems study the activity of the cardiovascular system (Pulse-Tach, Performance 2000 ergometry), muscle activity (Bioscan, surface EMG systems), blood flow (photo-pulse plethysmography, Doppler flow systems), autonomic activity (surface thermistors, thermography, galvanic skin resistance), sensory acuity (vibration threshold testing), and nerve conduction systems. Names commonly associated with physiological systems are Davicon, Biotech, Sensortek, Neuromed, Everest & Jennings, and Flexitherm.

Expectations, Reasonable and Unreasonable

Occupational health programs face a variety of complex social, legal, and medical challenges. High-technology equipment is often perceived and frequently marketed as a method of resolving some of those challenges. Equipment capabilities often are misunderstood, and their true use as scientific instruments is likewise overlooked. As a result, programs' expectations for equipment are sometimes unrealistic. The following pages review a series of unreasonable and reasonable expectations, that is, what we want to believe about high-technology equipment versus what we should believe.

The following are the five most common *unreasonable* expectations about high-technology equipment:

- *It prevents legal difficulties.* It is often argued that high-technology equipment prevents the legal difficulties that arise from preplacement screening and return-to-work assessments. Consequently, programs often have mistaken impressions about high-technology equipment. Programs may believe that the courts have generally held that assessments performed with a particular brand of high-technology equipment are acceptable and supportable, whereas other more traditional evaluations are not. For the most part, such claims represent misunderstandings or unsubstantiated marketing. Legal success is more likely to rest on understanding job risks and requirements and having medical opinions from competent physicians who have performed appropriate evaluations.
- *It determines injury cause.* A critical issue in litigation surrounding many workers' compensation cases is whether work caused or contributed to the development of a health problem. High-technology equipment cannot provide this answer. Determinations of causation rest, for the most part, on historical information.
- *It proves malingering.* A difficult problem for occupational health programs is the injured worker who malingers and does not return to work. High-technology equipment cannot prove malingering, despite claims to the contrary. Proving that an individual is a malingerer is often difficult and requires medical, social, and psychological data.
- *It prevents injury.* The use of high-technology equipment in preplacement or return-to-work assessments cannot, by itself, prevent injury or reinjury. Injury prevention requires a combination of factors: ergonomic changes, work selection, and safety rules, among others.
- *It accelerates recovery.* High-technology equipment cannot, by itself, accelerate recovery. Numerous effective worker injury rehabilitation programs exist that do not use high-technology equipment. Exercise performed on high-technology equipment can, in most cases, be reproduced without such expensive equipment.

The following are four principal *reasonable* expectations for high-technology equipment:

- *It controls test administration.* High-technology equipment controls the way tests are administered. As a result, the data resulting from such tests are likely to be more consistent and reliable than data derived from tests that are not as well controlled.
- *It provides precise measurement.* High-technology equipment provides more precise measures of performance. Such equipment often quantifies data that are difficult to quantify and permits complex measurements. With quantified data, performances can be compared, allowing the precise measure of recovery.
- *It documents consistency of performance.* High-technology equipment can determine whether the person being measured is performing consistently. Inconsistent performance can be a tip-off to symptom exaggeration and malingering.
- *It provides instant feedback.* High-technology equipment can perform certain roles of a therapist by providing rapid, accurate feedback to the injured worker using the equipment. As a result, the worker can modify performance to meet accurately defined targets.

From these lists, it becomes clear that sophisticated testing equipment does not replace professional judgment. Normative data bases and computer-assisted evaluation systems may make machine interpretations more believable, but in order to be useful such interpretations must be endorsed by the professional.

Caution is warranted regarding statements about equipment providing better safety, accelerated recovery, or improved validity. Safety may be improved by reducing the variables that lead to injury, but no system guarantees safety with injudicious use. Similarly, although no high-technology training system alters the body's recovery process, some are more efficient in eliminating unnecessary delays to recovery that an inexact training program would create. Finally, the statement "this is a valid measure" often relates more to the accuracy of a particular measurement technique rather than proof that it is the only or even the best measurement available.

Characteristics of Good Equipment

Good equipment advances our ability to measure, study, and interpret performance data. Here are fourteen characteristics of good-quality high-technology equipment:

- It is well designed.
- It provides accurate/precise measurement.
- It can be calibrated when needed.
- It is sturdy.
- It is easy to use.
- It has normed data.

- It has testing protocols.
- It is efficient and compact.
- It can be easily upgraded.
- It is supported by good research.
- It has adequate data storage capacity.
- It employs standard computer languages.
- It has component parts that are readily replaced.
- It permits measurement in the most natural manner.

Equipment that allows performance to be evaluated in its most natural configuration, at normal speeds and full motion, most closely approximates human use and physical demands. Therefore, if one can gain the same or at least acceptable precision from such a fluid device that one would get from a more rigidly constrained system, choosing the former is preferable. It permits more useful inferences about every function and increases the relevance of the measurement technique.

If the program plans to use the equipment for high-volume and rapid services, attention to efficiency and compactness becomes more important. An efficient piece of equipment is easily calibrated, requires little time to start, provides minimal time for patient set-up or protocol changes, has few delays during testing, prints hard copy quickly, allows contiguous testing while data are being stored or dumped, and gives usable report formats that decrease or eliminate dictating time. Compact machines take up little space, are easily moved, and require no additional hardware purchases to operate. Several compact machines can operate in a small space, increasing the number of people who can be evaluated at one time.

Cost of Equipment Decisions

When evaluating equipment, monetary costs, space limitations, and professional concerns must be assessed:

- *Monetary costs.* Monetary costs extend beyond the initial outlay of capital. The cost of future upgrades, auxiliary computers and printers, paper supplies, computer desk space, and maintenance agreements are also important factors. Downtime is likely to occur and can significantly reduce revenue. For this reason, one should ask vendors about the average turnaround time for repairs and the availability of a replacement when equipment is down for repairs.
- *Space limitations.* Space limitations may also have a monetary impact. The size of the equipment may require redesign of some work space or special handling to get it into the clinic. Also, once the equipment is installed, it may be difficult to move without the additional effort and expense of breaking down the system and recalibrating it in the

new location by company technicians. Size may limit equipment placement and alter the flow of foot traffic through the facility. If space is fixed, new equipment may force services to be relocated.
- *Professional concerns.* Professional concerns may arise about learning computer languages or about eyestrain from constantly being exposed to a video display terminal. The novelty of the equipment may be attractive, but its presence may also be anxiety-producing for clinical staff. Introducing evaluation techniques may make services more accountable but can raise concerns about what determines effective treatment. Also, changing professional habits may take time and create a drop in productivity while training is under way. Finally, competence in the use and interpretation of the equipment and reports may become an issue, especially if training programs are inadequate or impractical.

If the equipment selected does not fulfill its intended function, is unreliable, or becomes obsolete compared to other systems, the future cost of the unit may include decreased program referrals and increased overhead.

Future Trends in Equipment Design

In assessing high-technology equipment for use today, it is important to be aware of the future trends for equipment development. Equipment with configurations approximating future design considerations should not become obsolete as fast as less-developed tools. In the future, equipment will be smaller, lighter, less energy demanding, and more portable. Following the lead of microcomputers, equipment will be more memory-rich, more automated, and more easily upgraded. The decrease in size and portability of equipment will allow measurement to take place in more natural settings (for example, the workplace). Workers will be evaluated while they perform their jobs. Biofeedback is likely to be used to help direct the worker to safer, more effective work practices.

Summary

High-technology equipment is an effective, though expensive, method of ensuring standardization of test administration, quantification of difficult-to-measure data, measurement of consistency of performance, and provision of rapid and meaningful performance feedback. These factors, and others, make high-technology equipment an attractive adjunct to an occupational health program.

Although it can be helpful in improving the assessment of prospective or injured employees, high-technology equipment does not solve a program's legal problems relating to screening and return to work. It does not prove injury causation or determine malingering. And it does not esure improved rehabilitation of workers.

Although high-technology equipment can be helpful in expanding existing markets or allowing an established program to add new markets, hospitals should carefully determine whether the equipment costs can effectively be borne by an entirely new service. In addition, if a hospital occupational health program is losing its market share, high-technology equipment is rarely a good solution to the problem.

Chapter 21

Ethical Issues

Peter Orris, M.D., M.P.H.
William L. Newkirk, M.D.

Hospital occupational health programs frequently face ethical conflicts. Some of these ethical conflicts have concerned physicians since antiquity. Historically, occupational health conflicts have occurred most commonly between the health care provider and the employer. The recent trend of hospitals using occupational health programs as a marketing tool and limiting referrals to members of the hospital's medical staff raises further concerns. These ethical dilemmas often defy simple solution. This chapter discusses how the core precept of occupational medicine—ensuring the health and safety of employees—conflicts with the economic needs of employers, employees, and health care providers. In the process, the chapter demonstrates how the American College of Occupational Medicine (ACOM) Code of Ethical Conduct provides guidelines for dealing with these conflicts.

Core Precept of Occupational Medicine

The primary responsibility of the occupational health physician and the hospital-based occupational health program is to promote the health and safety of the employee. This responsibility embraces the highest aspiration of medicine, described well by Dr. Patrick Derr.

> The fundamental value in medicine is life and health. The physician is expected to use his knowledge and technique to secure life and health for his patients. The corollary of health is that a physician must have a commitment to the truth and logical deductive reasoning to apply this technique. These are not only desired, but required for a physician to practice medicine as a professional.[1]

The American College of Occupational Medicine Code of Ethical Conduct (the appendix to this chapter) states that physicians should "accord highest priority to the health and safety of the individual in the workplace." In occupational medicine, ethical conflicts arise primarily when this core precept collides with the economic interests of the involved parties.

Employers' Perspectives

The occupational physician's ethical conflicts with the employer have been recognized for centuries. In the seventeenth century, the Italian physician Ramazzini, author of the first text in occupational medicine, while writing about working people, observed that:

> Whatever metal they mine, they invite dreadful diseases which too often mock at every remedy, even supporting that some suitable remedy is duly prescribed; though it would seem to be a question whether it can be considered a pious duty to administer medical aid to men of that class and thus "prolong their lives to the bitter end."... Moreover, the use of metals is essential for nearly all arts and crafts. We ought to study carefully the diseases of these workers with a view to their safety and suggest precautions and remedies as was the custom in antiquity and is today also.[2]

Employers' concern for the health and safety of employees has increased since Ramazzini's time. The recent dramatic escalation in employer costs for injured employees (for example, workers' compensation premiums) and liability for employee exposure (for example, asbestos lawsuits) have increased many employers' awareness of the priority for employee health and safety programs. The Occupational Safety and Health Administration (OSHA) provides further emphasis in this area through its regulations.

In many circumstances, the employers' financial interests are consistent with these health and safety needs. In general, a corporation does better financially if its employees are healthy and productive, its injury rate is low, and injured workers are rehabilitated promptly and effectively. However, inevitable conflicts arise between employee health and the bottom line. The costs of reengineering a production facility for safety are always weighed against the medical and production costs of allowing injuries to occur.

At some level in the corporation it is essential to balance employee health against corporate finances. At a 1978 NIOSH/New York Academy of Medicine conference, a corporate medical director summarized this position by stating "... not only may our patient be an actual flesh and blood person but also that legal fiction of a person, the body corporate."[3] In a 1987 article on medical ethics, an author noted that the task of the corporate physician is "to seek the greatest good for all legitimately interested parties (stockholders, customers, public, and managing and nonmanaging employees), yet preserve and enhance the health of the individual employee."[4] These views argue that it is the occupational physician's responsibility to balance employee health and safety needs against corporate finance.

There is a danger in accepting this view. To effectively fulfill his or her function to "accord highest priority to the health and safety of the individual in the workplace," as indicated in the ACOM code of ethics, the physician must, of necessity, be an employee advocate. If the physician relinquishes this role, in the misguided notion that he or she is responsible for ensuring corporate financial viability, then the debate on employee health and safety issues becomes unbalanced. Financial issues become unopposed in the corporate decision-making process. In addition, if physicians and employers have learned nothing else from the asbestos lawsuits, they have learned that neglecting to deal with employee health and safety issues appropriately can have a catastrophic long-term financial impact on the corporation.

Some companies will demand that the physician place the needs of the company over those of the employee. The demands may be so unreasonable as to force the occupational health program to sever the relationship with the employer in order to ensure the continued ethical practice on the part of the health care institution. One method to reduce the likelihood of such problems is to resolve ethical issues with the company before establishing a relationship with them. Dr. Barry Hainer, in his monograph for family physicians providing occupational health services, suggests that agreements be established between client companies and the hospital before entering into a relationship. These agreements should address:

- Physician access to the workplace and workers
- An understanding that the physician will inform workers evaluated by the program of any abnormalities detected and, if they relate to the worker's job, the physician's opinion as to the occupational relationship
- An understanding that the physician will inform management of the existence of hazards requiring correction, and in the absence of corrective action, the physician's obligation to communicate directly with employees or responsible governmental agencies
- A procedure to maintain confidentiality of medical records[5]

The more specific the procedures agreed to before the establishment of the contracted relationship, the fewer problems that will subsequently arise.

Employees' Perspectives

Ethical conflicts also arise with employees because "according highest priority to the health and safety of the individual in the workplace" often conflicts with employee economic and job-related interests. Physicians often mistakenly believe that because they are advocates for employee health and safety they become advocates for all employee needs. This is not the case. Just as the physician should not be the corporate financial officer, neither should he or she be the shop steward.

The occupational health physician's conflict with the employee's economic needs takes many forms. Dr. Alice Hamilton, the pioneer of American occupational medicine, wrote in 1937 that an employee threatened with loss of a job if occupational disease is detected may refuse "to submit to an examination, he prefers to keep his skilled job and die at an earlier age, rather than join the unskilled or the unemployed and lower his or her family's social standing and standard of living. And his objections cannot be really met until we assure him that what we advocate for him as a protective measure does not carry with it such a menace."[6]

The threatened loss of job is a powerful reason why workplace hazards are not reduced. For example, although OSHA ostensibly guarantees protection for employees reporting hazards, many employees believe the protection worthless—particularly in nonunionized companies. As a result, work hazards continue to exist. An employee will frequently caution an occupational health physician not to raise concerns about a safety violation for fear that the report will be traced back to the employee. Although the physician has a clear responsibility to employee confidentiality, he or she also has a conflicting responsibility for public health and safety. In this regard, the ACOM code of ethics states that the physician should "treat as confidential whatever is learned about individuals served, releasing information only when required by law or by over-riding public health considerations. . . ."

Another conflict with employees arises because safe work often involves unwelcome modifications of the way the job is performed or the way employees conduct their lives. Wearing hearing protection or steel-toed shoes, using guards on machinery, working at a slower pace, and many other factors affect employee safety. Physicians often shy away from vigorous advocacy of these safety measures out of a misguided notion that they do not want to interfere with the way employees want to perform their jobs or live their lives. This is incorrect. The physician is the advocate for employee health and safety. When the physician fails to fulfill that role, debate about safety measures becomes unbalanced.

In cases of employee injury, the physician must often act counter to the injured employee's expressed wishes and financial interest. It has long been known that the best outcome in rehabilitation occurs when the injured employee is returned to work promptly. Occasionally, the employee does not want this. One reason is that if the employee has disability insurance on his or her mortgage and car loan, the employee may be financially advantaged when disabled. In addition, returning to work may jeopardize an employee's chances for a large cash settlement for the injury. The employee may not want to work in a modified work situation. In these cases, the physician must recognize that being an employee health and safety advocate will not solve all of the employee's social problems at work.

The physician can also be in conflict with employees' financial needs in preplacement screening. In order to effectively perform the role of ensuring employee health and safety, the physician must on occasion find certain prospective employees unsuitable for particular jobs. Under law in most states, the employer can reject a prospective employee if that employee cannot do the job or has a reasonable probability of suffering significant injury on the job. (Handicap discrimination legislation is discussed in depth in chapter 6.) The vague aspect of this standard becomes apparent when one considers an employee who is at higher risk than average, yet is capable of doing the work. Clearly, an employee with uncontrolled grand mal seizures should not be driving the company shuttle bus, yet occasionally a personnel department may request eliminating all hypercholesterolemic applicants from jobs requiring manual labor. In this context, the physician's advice must balance the need to protect the workers and others from harm with the positive benefits that a job provides for the worker and his or her family.

Hospital and Medical Staff Perspectives

Hospitals also pose ethical dilemmas for occupational health programs. In fact, some argue that the physician's objectives for the workers he or she treats are more consistent with employers' objectives than with the hospital's. Hospitals' economic benefits are often directly opposite those of industry. Hospitals benefit from high industry injury rates through increased utilization of hospital facilities for injury treatment and rehabilitation. The more serious the injury, the more the hospital benefits. As a rule, the more invasive the therapy, the more the hospital benefits. Back surgery, for example, often earns hospitals more than does conservative back treatment. Occupational health programs that feature injury treatment and rehabilitation do better economically than those featuring prevention and wellness.[7,8]

Given this economic reality, do hospitals really want programs that prevent injury? Programs that prevent injury should reduce hospital utilization and revenue. This runs directly counter to one of the fundamental reasons hospitals have surged into the occupational health market since 1981. Would hospitals embrace occupational health programs as warmly if the programs reduced hospital utilization as opposed to increasing it? Probably not. Therein is the ethical dilemma.

A hospital's decision whether to support programs that will, if successful, reduce hospital utilization is rarely explicitly discussed in that context. Prevention programs are poorly funded because "it is not the hospital's role" or "it is not a high priority." Never does one hear that the prevention programs are not being adequately funded because "we are not adequately utilizing our new rehabilitation facility," even though that consideration may be a major one in making the decision.

Prevention plays a major role in ensuring the health and safety of the individual in the workplace. Occupational medicine is, after all, organized under the Board of Preventive Medicine. Medical directors must continually fight to have prevention programs be a featured part of their occupational health programs. Effective occupational health programs must be able to gradually reduce the need for injury treatment and rehabilitation by reducing the rate of injury. An occupational health physician should work hard to eliminate the need for the injury treatment component of his or her program. Because the injury treatment component of the occupational health program is likely to provide the bulk of the occupational health program's revenues and the physician's salary, then, in a sense, the occupational health physician's actions are designed to put him or her out of a job. Is it likely that the physician will vigorously pursue this goal?

A second ethical dilemma involves the marketing of hospital occupational health programs. Until relatively recently, marketing by hospitals or physicians was considered unethical. The great interest in occupational health programs over the past few years has corresponded, not coincidentally, with the rise in hospital marketing. Done well, the marketing of hospital services can be a benefit to both the hospital and the consumer. Unfortunately, the marketing of hospital occupational health services is often designed by a person who has little knowledge of health care and even less knowledge of occupational health. As a result, problems can occur.

Imagine the outcry if a hospital marketed its cancer chemotherapy program by making unsubstantiated claims that patients treated in its program lived longer than those treated in a competitive hospital's program. Such behavior would be scorned, and rightly so. However, it is not uncommon for a hospital marketing department to advertise that the hospital's occupational health program will "make more productive employees" or "reduce lost time" with very little empirical evidence that these claims are true. Such misleading claims can even relate to whether the hospital has an "occupational health" program at all. A large number of hospital marketing departments have created hospital occupational health programs seemingly "out of air" by combining existing hospital services. These programs bear little resemblance to the American College of Occupational Medicine (ACOM) standards for occupational health programs (see chapter 1).

The ACOM's Code of Ethical Conduct (appendix) states that physicians should "avoid solicitation of the use of their services by making claims, offering testimonials, or implying results which may not be achieved, but they may appropriately advise colleagues and others of services available."

The occupational health program director must resist the hospital's efforts to misrepresent the program or its capabilities. The same standards of scientific investigation must apply to claims made for an occupational health program as they do to claims made for cancer chemotherapy programs.

The third area for ethical conflict involves the referral of patients from an occupational health program. One reason that a hospital develops an occupational health program is so that it can refer patients from that program to members of the medical staff and to hospital-owned or hospital-supported services. This referral system can create problems such as the following:

- Does the occupational health physician refer a patient to a physician on call when he or she knows that another physician on a competitor hospital's staff is more competent to deal with the problem?
- Does the occupational physician utilize hospital-based ancillary services (X rays, laboratory services, and so forth) when he or she knows of other services that are of equal quality and lower cost?
- Does the occupational health physician refrain from referring to physicians of low competence even though the hospital medical staff says the physician must refer to all the physicians on the staff?

The ACOM Code of Ethical Conduct states that physicians should "avoid allowing their medical judgment to be influenced by any conflict of interest." Physicians must not allow hospital economic or political influences to affect their decisions. If the hospital wishes to receive the referrals from the occupational health program, it must provide as good or better services than its competitor in the referral areas. The mere fact that the occupational health program is hospital-based or hospital-owned does not mean that the hospital is entitled to referrals when the hospital's referral services are substandard.

Conclusion

Occupational health physicians should accord highest priority to the health and safety of individuals in the workplace. This will, however, bring the physician into conflict with the economic needs of the employer, the employee, the hospital, and in some cases, the physician's own beliefs. In these conflicts, the physician must at all times remember that he or she is a health and safety advocate—not a corporate financial officer, shop steward, lawyer, or hospital sales agent. The workplace is a complex place in which the physician has a specific role to play. When the physician abandons his or her role or adopts that of another, the workplace debate becomes unbalanced and the health of the employee may suffer.

References

1. Derr, P. G. Ethical considerations in fitness and risk evaluations. *Occupational Medicine State of the Art Reviews* 3(2):194, Apr.-June 1988.
2. Ramazzini, B. *Diseases of Workers.* Chicago: University of Chicago Press, 1983, p. 19.

3. Dinman, B. D. The loyalty of the occupational physician. *Bulletin of the New York Academy of Medicine* 54(8):730, Sept. 1978.
4. Deubner, D. Ethics. *Seminars in Occupational Medicine* 2(3):177, Sept. 1987.
5. Hainer, B. L. *The Role of the Family Physician in Occupational Health Care.* Chicago: American Medical Association, 1984, pp. 10–11.
6. Sicherman, B. *Alice Hamilton—A Life in Letters.* Cambridge, MA: Harvard University Press, 1984, p. 359.
7. Sabatino, F. G. The diversification success story continues: survey. *Hospitals* 63(1):26–32, Jan. 5, 1989.
8. Health Care Advisory Board. *Marketing to Employers.* Vol. 2, *Occupational Health Programs.* Washington, DC: HCAB, July 1988, p. 17.

*Appendix. ACOM Code of Ethical Conduct for Physicians Providing Occupational Medical Services**

These principles are intended to aid physicians in maintaining ethical conduct in providing occupational medical service. They are standards to guide physicians in their relationships with the individuals they serve, with employers and workers' representatives, with colleagues in the health professions, and with the public.

Physicians should:

1. Accord highest priority to the health and safety of the individual in the workplace
2. Practice on a scientific basis with objectivity and integrity
3. Make or endorse only statements which reflect their observations or honest opinion
4. Actively oppose and strive to correct unethical conduct in relation to occupational health service
5. Avoid allowing their medical judgment to be influenced by any conflict of interest
6. Strive conscientiously to become familiar with the medical fitness requirements, the environment and the hazards of the work done by those they serve, and with the health and safety aspects of the products and operations involved
7. Treat as confidential whatever is learned about individuals served, releasing information only when required by law or by over-riding

*The code is reprinted with permission of the American College of Occupational Medicine (ACOM). As of October 27, 1988, the American Occupational Medical Association and the American Academy of Occupational Medicine officially merged into the American College of Occupational Medicine. At the first board meeting of the new College, the Board voted to adopt the "Code of Ethical Conduct" as the code for the American College of Occupational Medicine and reaffirm these principles. The original code was adopted in July 1976 and has had minor revisions since that time.

public health considerations, or to other physicians at the request of the individual according to traditional medical ethical practice; and should recognize that employers are entitled to counsel about the medical fitness of individuals in relation to work, but are not entitled to diagnoses or details of a specific nature

8. Strive continually to improve medical knowledge, and should communicate information about health hazards in timely and effective fashion to individuals or groups potentially affected, and make appropriate reports to the scientific community
9. Communicate understandably to those they serve any significant observations about their health, recommending further study, counsel or treatment when indicated
10. Seek consultation concerning the individual or the workplace whenever indicated
11. Cooperate with governmental health personnel and agencies, and foster and maintain sound ethical relationships with other members of the health professions
12. Avoid solicitation of the use of their services by making claims, offering testimonials, or implying results which may not be achieved, but they may appropriately advise colleagues and others of services available

Chapter 22

Occupational Health Services: A Labor Perspective

James L. Weeks, Sc.D.

Workers need occupational health services that are technically competent, prevention oriented, and socially conscious. Workers do not need "company doctors," that is, physicians who place the employer's economic welfare above workers' health.

The Company Doctor

The company doctor originated in its purest form in coal company towns[1] with the full complement of company stores, company currency, company housing, company schools, and company preachers. Other historical examples can be found in the lead producing and consuming industries[2] and in the cotton textile industry.[3,4] Contemporary examples occur in the production and use of asbestos[5] and in the chemical industry.[6]

According to the stereotype, the company doctor is ill-informed, attributes workers' illnesses to anything but occupational exposure, blames workers' own actions for illnesses or injury, accuses workers of malingering, places the employer's economic welfare above workers' health, suppresses knowledge that is harmful to the employer, and provides confidential information about workers' health to the employer.

The stereotype is the product of history and of the current organization of corporate occupational medicine. This social structure produces an inevitable dilemma for the physician. A physician who works for a large international labor union describes the situation as follows:

> While the process of policy development [within a business organization] is strengthened by the involvement of those who identify strongly with their organizations and are confidants to those at their highest

levels, the clinical process requires physicians who can be unfettered advocates for the health of individual workers. It is difficult, probably impossible, to wear both hats at the same time.[7]

Elements of Programs Responsive to Employee Needs

Hospital occupational health programs can escape the stereotype of the company doctor by doing four things. First, the program must have the appropriate technical expertise. Second, providers should know the workplace. Third, they should be committed to prevention. Fourth, they should be conscious of the social structure and potential for social conflict in the workplace and should establish working relationships with workers and employers as early as possible. Each of these four elements is discussed in the following pages.

Technical Expertise

The essential foundation of any health practice is technical competence. As discussed in chapter 1, occupational health is a broad field that includes many disciplines. Proficiency in occupational medicine requires knowledge of toxicology, epidemiology, industrial hygiene, biostatistics, ergonomics, and related topics. One of the most vexing situations in occupational medicine is that most health professionals lack this expertise.[8,9]

Some hospitals have compounded this deficiency by marketing "occupational health programs" that are little more than collections of existing hospital services repackaged for industry. These programs often have little or no technical expertise in occupational health. The consequences of the lack of expertise are that occupational diseases can go unrecognized and uncounted,[10] as well as uncontrolled and uncompensated.[11] Sentinel health events,[12] which are preventable conditions whose occurrence signals the failure of prevention efforts, are often missed. As a result, workers unnecessarily suffer from diseases that arise from occupational exposure.

Knowledge of Workers and the Workplace

In order to recognize occupational diseases, clinical prowess alone is insufficient. A successful occupational health program must combine clinical competence with knowledge of workers' exposure. If this knowledge is missing, diagnosis of occupational contributions to disease is difficult if not impossible, just as it is difficult to diagnose other diseases without information about the environment from which a patient comes. One can obtain information about exposure from the employer, from the workers, or from other sources. Most employers must make available information about potential exposure as required by the Occupational Safety and Health Administration

(OSHA).[13] A common form used for this information is the Material Safety Data Sheet.

If industrial hygiene measurements of exposure have been made, an occupational health program should obtain this information and make arrangements to receive it routinely for future use. The employer, a consultant, an insurance carrier, a government agency, or an academic researcher might have made measurements in the past. If measurements of exposure have not been made, the worksite should be assessed to determine whether they should be made. The occupational health service can retain an industrial hygienist to provide such a service.

To obtain more insight into working conditions, an occupational health service should visit the workplace itself on a regular basis. During worksite tours, health professionals should talk to workers on the job and not limit their information to what the employer shows them. For every private discussion with the employer, there should be a similar private discussion with workers or workers' representatives.

The complementary side of assessing hazards on the job is evaluating workers' health, usually in the form of medical examinations. Medical assessment of workers, which is treated in detail elsewhere in this book, should be designed to monitor the effects of specific workers' exposures. By itself, this is sound practice; it is also required by NIOSH criteria documents and by the American Conference of Governmental Industrial Hygienists.[14,15]

Information gathered in periodic examinations *combined* with information about exposure is the principal means of identifying work-related health or safety hazards. By using some elementary epidemiologic methods such as comparing the incidence or prevalence of certain conditions among groups of workers classified by exposure, one can identify health hazards and better focus prevention efforts.[16]

Medical examinations are excellent opportunities for educating workers and health professionals. During these examinations, workers can learn about hazards and hazard controls on their jobs and physicians can learn about jobs of individual workers. Well-informed workers and physicians can together better prevent disease.

It is important, however, to avoid abuse of medical examinations. Historically, the purpose of medical examinations in industry has been limited to evaluating whether a worker was physically able to work. Little attention was given to diagnosing occupational disease or disability.[17] Given this limited purpose, information about individual workers that in any other form of medical practice would be considered confidential was freely given to employers. As examinations have become more sophisticated, employers often receive information for which they have no need and no right to know. Such breaches of confidentiality can undermine the credibility and effectiveness of an entire program. As a general rule, no medical information should be shared with the employer unless the individual worker has provided informed written consent. There must be a clear relationship between the information provided and the specific job requirements.

Another form of abuse is conducting tests or research (for example, pregnancy or drug tests) without workers' knowledge or consent. The results of the tests can affect employment. Although universities and other institutions that receive government funds for research must submit their research protocols to human experimentation review committees, employers who use their own funds are under no such formal obligation. Yet ethical concerns that require review for government funds also apply to any other medical research.

Some medical tests are presumed to have predictive value for persons at increased risk of disease or disability, despite evidence to the contrary. Such tests include low back X rays (to predict back injury), genetic testing for alpha-1-antitrypsin heterozygotes (to predict increased risk of chronic lung disease), G-6-PD testing (to predict persons at increased risk of hemolytic anemia if exposed to certain toxic substances), and others. The predictive value of these tests is weak, the effect can be discriminatory, and the tests tend to be substituted for control of hazards on the job.[18]

And, finally, medical testing is sometimes used as the primary means of monitoring workers' exposures. Testing, by itself, is not harmful, but it can lead to harmful results if it is used instead of workplace monitoring or if it leads to worker placement rather than hazard control as the means of preventing disease and injury.

Commitment to Prevention

Occupational diseases and injuries are man-made; therefore, they are preventable. Occupational medicine is, appropriately, a subspecialty of preventive medicine.

The need for prevention arises from two important factors. First, many occupational diseases, especially those that arise from chronic exposure (for example, pneumoconioses, malignancies, noise-induced hearing loss), are irreversible, untreatable, disabling, and often fatal. Prevention is the principal means of disease control for these ailments. Second, workers' compensation for occupational diseases is often difficult to obtain because precise causes cannot be easily identified in the individual.[19] The compensation system is inherently more responsive to injuries than to illnesses, especially chronic illnesses.

There are some significant obstacles to a practice of prevention by hospitals. Hospitals are organized to treat the sick rather than to prevent illness in the healthy. Hospital hierarchies often favor procedure-oriented physicians over prevention-oriented physicians. Hospitals are better compensated for treatment than they are for prevention. In addition, hospitals are more likely to be compensated for treating injuries than they are for treating occupational diseases. Thus hospitals' basic orientation and financial rewards discourage prevention.

In the workplace, primary prevention is basically an engineering rather than a medical problem in much the same way that primary prevention of cholera is a problem for plumbers and sanitary engineers. The engineering subspecialty devoted to primary prevention is industrial hygiene, a field with which most health care professionals are not familiar.

Industrial hygiene is the practice of anticipating, identifying, evaluating, and controlling occupational health hazards.[20] Occupational medicine can and should play an important role in anticipating and recognizing hazards and being an active participant in intervention. In general, the hygienist uses a hierarchy of controls, from the most effective to the least. The best form of hazard control is positive engineering. Inevitably unique to each job, this approach implies that hazard control is built into each job, by using less toxic, less noisy, and less dangerous materials and methods. A second method is environmental control, by using ventilation, shielding, muffling, and the like. In situations where other controls are clearly not feasible or during the time they are being installed, the least effective means of control is the use of personal protective equipment such as dust masks or special clothing.[21] Occupational medical care providers should be familiar with this bare outline of standard industrial hygiene practice because it is the principal means of achieving primary prevention, by altering the workplace rather than the worker.

Social Consciousness

What occupational diseases have in common is not so much any common biology as a common social etiology—the workplace. To be effective in disease control, therefore, requires that practitioners know the social structure of workplaces. Just as those who combat malaria have had to learn a lot about mosquitoes, one needs to know the workplace to combat occupational disease.

Virtually everyone at work has a material interest in activities at work—to make a return on investment, to produce a product or service, to keep one's job, and so on. These interests directly affect viewpoints, actions, and policies. In order for an outsider (for example, a hospital-based health professional) to obtain a reasonably accurate picture of events on the job, he or she must be aware that what workers on the job do and think about what they do depends on their interests.

The workplace is, as one writer concisely put it, contested terrain where people take sides.[22] The minimal step for health professionals is not necessarily to choose sides between the employer and workers—although this is necessary occasionally—but rather to recognize that sides exist.

Typical employer-provided medical programs inevitably function between conflicting interests and competing loyalties. On the one hand, medical ethics require primary loyalty to patients and patients' welfare. On the other hand, medical care providers hired by an employer are almost always accountable to the employer in terms of their financial status and their status in the organizational hierarchy. Moreover, by education, income, and social class, most health professionals are more inclined to employers than to workers. This can result in health care providers not recognizing conflicts of interest and embracing an employer's viewpoint by default or consciously choosing the employer's viewpoint to maintain the provider's employment. As a result, patient care suffers.

Partly because of the historical recognition that the industrial health professions could not by themselves achieve the ends of hazard and disease control, governmental regulatory agencies were created. The principal federal government agencies are the Occupational Safety and Health Administration (OSHA), the Mine Safety and Health Administration (MSHA), and the National Institute for Occupational Safety and Health (NIOSH). They are an important part of the arsenal of occupational disease control. (See chapter 5.)

With the nearly 20 years' experience with these regulatory agencies, it is evident that they can be effective at reducing risk of disease and injury.[23-25] Moreover, they do a more thorough job at worksites where the workers are organized to represent themselves as a union.[26]

Another factor affecting occupational health issues between employers and workers is the labor–management contract. Labor–management contracts existed before the creation of the aforementioned government agencies and exist alongside them in many workplaces today. Most of them contain some language pertaining to occupational health and safety. These contracts are working documents for workplace self-government that arose as a need to accommodate conflicting interests of employers and workers. Providers of occupational health and safety services should also become familiar with provisions in local labor–management contracts.

Workers who are not covered by contracts also have certain legal rights that pertain to occupational health and safety matters. These too should be understood. (See chapters 5–8.)

Because any workplace environment is laden with potential for conflict over occupational health issues, successful hospital-based occupational health programs must have ways to obtain the views, the information, and the advice of the workers themselves as participants in the program rather than as patients only. In workplaces where workers are organized into a union, this can be accomplished by formal liaison with local (or higher level) union officials. An advisory board, consisting of employer and union representatives, would be a useful formal mechanism for program planning, implementation, and evaluation. Information about workplace hazards could be shared with this group. At workplaces where workers are not organized to represent themselves, obtaining the views and advice of workers is much more difficult, although here, too, an advisory board could be helpful.

Third parties (such as hospitals) are largely outside the legal environment framed by OSHA, MSHA, NIOSH, and labor laws within which employers and employees function. For example, third parties do not have the legal right to request OSHA inspections or to call for health hazard evaluations by NIOSH. As a practical matter, however, if a third party knows of a workplace hazard and has credible documentation, it would be possible to contact a local OSHA office and persuade them to inspect a workplace.

However, a note of caution is in order. If a third party obtains information about hazards on a job from an individual worker, requesting an inspection, a health hazard evaluation, or even bringing the information to the attention of the employer may put that worker at risk of some form of adverse personnel action. Although workers are, in principle, protected from discrimination under the Occupational Safety and Health Act of 1970 and the Mine Safety and Health Acts, this right is not well defended. Therefore, as a general rule, such actions should *never* be undertaken without an individual worker's informed consent.

Some of the concerns discussed in this chapter can be illustrated by describing the limitations of certain kinds of "common sense" advice—such as an admonition to wear a dust mask, a suggestion not to use certain chemicals, or a hint to seek another line of work. Individual workers may resist such advice, passively or actively, not because of ignorance or stubbornness but from a common sense born of a different life. Dust masks are uncomfortable, interfere with communication, and often leak. It is partly for these reasons that they are low on the priority of industrial hygiene methods of hazard control. Moreover, well-managed programs for respirators[27,28] are the exception rather than the rule, which leads to widespread skepticism about respirator usage. In addition, the choice of substances to use on a job is most often not within a worker's control.

Changing jobs is an option only if another job is available. If a worker quits "voluntarily," he or she is not eligible for unemployment insurance and loses whatever seniority, pension, and other benefits that have accrued. It is, in principle, possible to quit a job and receive unemployment benefits if the job can be shown to be dangerous, but this requires documentation, which often does not exist. Further, the employer can and often will contest such a claim, which results in a lengthy delay and an uncertain outcome. An occupational medical service at a hospital may be recruited by an employer into an effort to discredit an individual worker's claim. Therefore, a health professional should consider carefully what kinds of advice to give individual workers with occupational health problems.

Conclusion

Workers don't need company doctors. Hospitals that provide occupational health services must avoid the trap of becoming a company doctor by developing programs that are technically expert, knowledgeable of the workers and worksite, prevention oriented, and socially conscious. This is nothing less than the best that modern health care and industrial hygiene can provide, living up to these professions' own best principles.

References

1. Boone, J. T. *A Medical Survey of the Bituminous-Coal Industry. Report of the Coal Mines Administration, U.S. Department of the Interior.* Washington, DC: U.S. Government Printing Office, 1947, p. 91f.

2. Sicherman, B. *Alice Hamilton—A Life in Letters.* Cambridge, MA: Harvard University Press, 1984, pp. 170–72.

3. Levenstein, C. *Byssinosis: The Recognition of an Occupational Disease. A Report to the National Institute for Occupational Safety and Health, 1984.* Ithaca, NY: Cornell University Press, 1984.

4. Rosner, D. and Markowitz, G., editors. *Dying for Work: Workers' Safety and Health in Twentieth Century America.* Bloomington, IN: Indiana University Press, 1987.

5. Brodeur, P. *Expendable Americans.* New York City: Viking Press, 1974.

6. Randall, W., and Solomon, S. D. *Building 6: The Tragedy at Bridesburg.* Boston: Little, Brown & Co., 1977.

7. Silverstein, M. Presentation to the American Occupational Medicine Association, May 2, 1983.

8. Rothstein, M. *Medical Screening of Workers.* Washington, DC: Bureau of National Affairs, 1984.

9. Committee on the Role of the Physician in Occupational and Environmental Medicine, Institute of Medicine, National Academy of Sciences. *Role of the Primary Care Physician in Occupational and Environmental Medicine.* Washington, DC: National Academy Press, 1988.

10. U.S. Congress, House of Representatives, Committee on Government Operations. *Occupational Illness Data Collection: Fragmented, Unreliable, and Seventy Years Behind Communicable Disease Surveillance.* Washington, DC: U.S. Government Printing Office, 1984.

11. Selikoff, I. J. *Disability Compensation for Asbestos-Associated Disease in the United States. Environmental Sciences Laboratory, Mt. Sinai School of Medicine. Report to the U.S. Department of Labor.* Springfield, VA: National Technical Information Service, 1981.

12. Rutstein, D. D., Mullan, R. J., Frazier, T. M., Halperin, W. E., Melius, J. M., and Sestito, J. P. Sentinel health events (occupational): a basis for physician recognition and public health surveillance. *American Journal of Public Health* 73(9):1054–62, 1983.

13. 29 C.F.R 1910.1200.

14. Rothstein, cited in reference 8.

15. American Conference of Governmental Industrial Hygienists. *TLVs: Threshold Limit Values and Biological Exposure Indices for 1988–1989.* Cincinnati: ACGIH, 1988.

16. Weeks, J. L., Peters, J. M., and Monson, R. R. Screening for occupational health hazards in the rubber industry. *American Journal of Industrial Medicine* 2:125–41, 1981.

17. Nugent, A. Fit for work: the introduction of physical exams in industry. *Bulletin of the History of Medicine* 57:578–83, 1983.
18. U.S. Congress, Office of Technology Assessment. *The Role of Genetic Testing in the Prevention of Occupational Disease.* Washington, DC: U.S. Government Printing Office, 1983.
19. Weeks, J. L., and Wagner, G. R. Compensation for occupational disease with multiple causes: the case of coal miners' respiratory diseases. *American Journal of Public Health* 76(1):58–61, 1986.
20. Plog, B. A., editor. *Fundamentals of Industrial Hygiene.* 3d ed. Chicago: National Safety Council, 1988.
21. First, M. W. Engineering control of occupational health hazards. *American Industrial Hygiene Association Journal* 44(9):621–26, 1983.
22. Edwards, R. *Contested Terrain—The Transformation of the Workplace in the Twentieth Century.* New York City: Basic Books, 1979.
23. Boden, L. I. Government regulation of occupational safety: underground coal mine accidents, 1973–75. *American Journal of Public Health* 75:497–501, 1985.
24. Mendeloff, J. *Regulating Safety: An Economic and Political Analysis of Occupational Safety and Health Policy.* Cambridge, MA: MIT Press, 1979.
25. Braithwaite, J. *To Punish or Persuade—Enforcement of Coal Mine Safety.* Albany, NY: State University of New York Press, 1985.
26. Weil, D. Government and labor at the workplace: the role of labor unions in the implementation of federal health and safety policy. Doctoral thesis, Harvard University, Cambridge, MA, 1987.
27. 29 C.F.R 1910.134.
28. American National Standards Institute. *Practices for Respiratory Protection, ANSI Z88.2-1969.* New York City: ANSI, 1969.

Part 3

Summary and Conclusions

Chapter 23

A Comprehensive Occupational Health Program—A Case Example

C. Kirby Griffin, M.D.

In chapter 1, the introduction to this book, we reviewed several factors that led to the growth of occupational health services during the 1980s. The shrinking hospital inpatient market, competition between hospitals and physicians, and the shift in power from providers to payers have all led to hospital diversification strategies that have targeted corporations as clients. This chapter describes how one hospital and medical center developed a wide-ranging occupational health services program to meet the needs of companies in its service area.

At the St. Vincent Center for Occupational Health (Portland, Oregon), program planners recognized that wellness and health promotion services were only a partial answer to the needs of business and industry. The planners at St. Vincent Hospital and Medical Center proposed that the hospital and its medical staff forge a *comprehensive* occupational health program. Such a program would directly address the needs of the business community and emphasize those services that were not currently available and that could not be provided solely by an individual physician or office. Saint Vincent's planners also recognized the need for a much more complex and well-integrated structure and organization if it was to accomplish the program's objectives.

This chapter begins with an examination of the principles on which the St. Vincent Center for Occupational Health was founded. It then shows how St. Vincent's applied these principles to its program and how it has evaluated its success.

Principles of Program Design

If there is one important caveat for a health care facility interested in offering occupational health services, it is this: Before jumping in, the facility must spend sufficient time to research the field and must base its decisions on the recommendations of knowledgeable people in the field.

The seven principles that guide and serve as the foundation for St. Vincent's program are:

- The program must be comprehensive.
- Service excellence is a byword for all personnel.
- The program staff must adhere to impeccable ethical practices.
- The program must be flexible enough to adjust to the needs of various clients.
- Data collection and data management systems must be superb.
- There must be tight central control of program operations and activities.
- The program and personnel must be in place before the program is offered to industry.

Comprehensive Program

To assess business and industry needs, St. Vincent's conducted a series of focus groups composed of health benefits managers and health/safety managers of large private and public employers. When the focus groups were asked what occupational health services they needed, their response was "everything." The more comprehensive the program, the better for all concerned.

A sizable parent institution is necessary in order to provide the support for a comprehensive program. It is neither necessary nor desirable for the occupational health program itself to be involved in the ownership or management of all the services utilized in the program. That is to say, it would not be desirable or necessary for the occupational health program per se to own or manage such supporting services as, for example, a work hardening program, a physical therapy department, a respiratory challenge booth, an employee assistance program, or an industrial dermatology clinic. What *is* necessary is for the program to develop good working relationships with the providers whose services will round out the comprehensive program.

The key to a comprehensive program is having a mechanism for centralized coordination of all services, including those of the physicians. This means that at least one individual's primary function must be program coordination. It also means that there must be the computer capability to accomplish the tracking and data management involved. Although the more specialized services will be available on a statewide or regionwide basis, the concept of centralized coordination requires that any client company be accommodated by calling a single telephone number.

Excellence of Service

There must be no compromise in quality of service. Clients will select excellence of service even if the cost is greater. Both the medical care and the quality of the client's experience in dealing with the program must be superb. There should be little tolerance for delays, confusion, poor communication, or faulty reporting.

It is a great asset to have a parent institution of proven excellence and reputation for high quality. Saint Vincent's has been able to build much of its program because of the excellent reputation of the parent institution and the medical staff. However, the focus groups for St. Vincent's indicated that the quality of the individual providers is much more important than the perceived quality of the sponsoring organization. An excellent program requires trained, knowledgeable physicians. A comprehensive program will need the services of many specialists and generalists who are well informed about occupational health and workers' compensation laws. They must have a commitment to doing those things that will make the program work, such as communication, quality reporting, and preferred referral.

The central direction of a comprehensive occupational health program must reside in the hands of a full-time occupational health physician. The occupational health physician must be well informed in regard to the occupational health literature, regulations, legislation, and specific occupational rules and must have a clear understanding of what goes on at the workplace.

The health care professionals selected as consultants must be highly skilled. Just as primary physicians have a moral and ethical obligation to obtain the best surgical care, orthopedic care, and other appropriate care for their patients, so too must the comprehensive occupational health program be very selective in finding the best consultants for the program. It is not advisable to offer every specialist on your medical staff an equal opportunity to participate. To follow a random call list or in some other way avoid being highly selective would lead to a wide range in the standard of care and ultimately to the decline of the occupational health program.

Impeccable Ethical Practices

All occupational health programs should adhere strictly to the *Code of Ethical Conduct for Physicians Providing Occupational Medical Services* adopted by the board of directors of the American College of Occupational Medicine on October 27, 1988 (reprinted as the appendix to chapter 21).

Occupational health professionals who remain objective and act in an ethical manner will be respected and will maintain their integrity even when conflicts arise. The occupational health physician must avoid becoming "the company doc," or "the insurance doc," or "the lawyer's doc." There are times when it may be difficult to remain objective. In such cases, physicians should ethically disqualify themselves and turn the situation over to another party.

Flexibility

Comprehensive occupational health programs must have the flexibility to adjust to the needs of the various parties. They must take into account the employer's need to maintain productivity and control costs, as well as consider the employees' travel time, comfort, and so forth. There must be flexibility in hours of operation, location of service, and range and price of services. The program must be capable of providing services in the office, at the worksite, at central locations, and at remote sites. The final decision as to who, where, what, and how needs to be reached through dialogue with the various participants. Often, it will be the health care provider that will have to make the adjustment in order to achieve the best balance for all parties.

Flexibility also means being able to quickly expand staff and equipment as demands dictate. A comprehensive program must have sufficient resources to accommodate a sudden demand for large-scale evaluations or increased demands for care.

Superb Data Collection and Data Management

The data collection and data management system is the glue that holds comprehensive occupational health programs together. Meaningful workers' compensation case tracking depends on an automated system of high quality. The communication requirements and integration requirements of a comprehensive program cannot be accomplished without the use of computers.

Having a superb data collection and data management system allows for significant utilization of all clinical data in research. In addition, the sophisticated use of the data system is the most powerful marketing tool.

Tight Central Control

Control is an important but troublesome issue. The larger, more complex, and more comprehensive the program, the greater the importance of systems that guarantee quality, uniformity, and communication. Responsibility, accountability, and authority must all reside together. The medical director of the comprehensive occupational health program does not necessarily need to be directly involved in the details or decisions relevant to occupational health planning or occupational health services, but absolutely everything involving occupational health in the institution must go by the occupational medical director's desk.

Validation of Program Capabilities

In competitive occupational health markets, there is a strong urge for providers to promise the services an industry requests even if they have never delivered those services before. Don't make such promises. Although it may take longer, thoughtful and thorough planning, coupled with careful implementation of a service, will be much more effective.

One of the key concepts for St. Vincent's program has been to recognize that St. Vincent's employee health program could be an ideal model for what could be accomplished in business and industry at large. With 2,200 full-time equivalents, St. Vincent Hospital is one of the largest employers in its service area. The goal has been to make the employee health service at St. Vincent's the model company occupational health program to which all of its clients and potential clients should aspire. Saint Vincent's strives to perfect any new service within its own employee health program as a first step to offering that service to other clients.

Development of the Center for Occupational Health at St. Vincent's

By 1985, St. Vincent's had developed a sound, carefully drafted comprehensive plan based on the seven principles for a successful comprehensive occupational health program just described. The first task was to secure top-management support. A series of presentations was made to the hospital administrative council and to the medical staff executive committee. These presentations gained the program the high-level support it needed, and the planners were given the "go-ahead" to develop the business plan. The business plan proposed a start-up phase consisting of core, hospital-based occupational health services including clinical facilities, a coordinating center, a data collection and data management center, and a workers' compensation case tracking center.

Securing overall high-level support is only the first step in implementing an occupational health program. In addition, the critical issues of control and technical competence must be addressed. These issues require agreement between top management and program directors if the programs are to have enduring success.

Control issues involve giving *authority* along with responsibility and accountability to the occupational health directors and occupational health providers. Although there is a willingness to accord program staff responsibility and accountability, the authority necessary to ensure program flexibility, quality, and central control can only come through top-management support.

Competence issues involve ensuring that only knowledgeable and committed people are active in the program. This is not to say that individuals without previous knowledge or experience in occupational health would be excluded. However, before such individuals could participate they would need the requisite training and orientation.

In a comprehensive occupational health program, the occupational health team must not only be competent but also have high visibility and high involvement. Key members of the team should be very active in the appropriate professional societies. They should have a presence at local, regional, and national meetings and at all business and industry meetings and societies where occupational health matters might be relevant.

Finally, to maintain top-management support, the occupational health program must ensure that its accomplishments are routinely brought to the attention of top management through regularly scheduled meetings between the program medical director and top management.

Medical Staff Support

Medical staff support is a vital element of program development. At St. Vincent's, the approach to creating medical staff support consisted of three elements: (1) involvement, (2) education and communication, and (3) referral policies.

By using these three steps, St. Vincent's has developed a positive, supportive relationship with its medical staff. The direct and indirect advantages accruing to them as a result of the program have proved to be of significant value while fears of competition have proved nearly nonexistent. As the program has become established, the reporting and communication that flows from the data management system and the workers' compensation case tracking program maintain a positive link between the Center for Occupational Health and St. Vincent's medical staff.

Involvement

Two medical staff surveys were completed at St. Vincent's in order to ascertain the medical staff physicians' current involvement in occupational health activities and to assess their interest in becoming involved in the occupational health program. It was a surprise to find that of 95 primary care physicians, only 15 expressed significant interest in occupational health matters.

Saint Vincent's then conducted focus groups with the medical staff physicians who were practicing occupational medicine to some degree. These physicians demonstrated that they were already acutely aware of the need to improve the system for occupational health services and enhance their own capabilities in occupational health. They concluded that it was necessary for the hospital to develop a comprehensive occupational health program.

To ensure ongoing medical staff involvement, a medical staff occupational health committee was established. This committee has been a major source of strength at St. Vincent's. It has assisted in defining the program and acquiring medical staff support. The recommendations of the occupational health committee communicated to the medical staff executive committee and to hospital administration are the instruments by which official policy has developed.

Education and Communication

Saint Vincent's uses four educational and informational techniques to increase medical staff awareness of occupational health matters.

- Noted occupational medicine specialists present at grand rounds.
- Key members of the medical staff visit successful occupational health programs and meet with noted occupational medicine specialists.
- Publications are distributed and articles are printed in medical staff newsletters.
- Seminars on workers' compensation law and workers' compensation billing are held for physicians and their office staffs.

These four activities have kept the medical staff informed about the progress of the program referrals and have kept lines of communication open.

Referral Policies

Beginning in 1986, St. Vincent's started a series of meetings with some physicians through their individual departments, those of orthopedics, neurosurgery, and cardiology. Individual departments were encouraged to recommend referral policies and methods for selecting department physicians as consultants. The departmental recommendations were then sent to the medical staff executive committee.

The major policy governing referral of ill and injured workers was established by the medical staff executive committee based on the recommendations of the occupational health committee and the individual medical departments (appendix A).

You will note that the second priority for referrals stated in the policy is to the physician or group designated by the company. As St. Vincent's has established relationships with companies, many have designated its Center for Occupational Health as the "preferred provider" for their employees. Updated lists of those companies naming St. Vincent's as their provider are kept in the emergency department and the family medical care unit. Personnel in those departments are then obliged to contact the Center for Occupational Health in regard to referral, follow-up, or both.

Saint Vincent's has emphasized to its medical staff that those who will benefit the most from the occupational health program are the specialists in orthopedics, neurosurgery, neurology, gastroenterology, cardiology, and some surgical subspecialties. Those who will not be affected are pediatricians and, for the most part, specialists in obstetrics and gynecology. The primary care practitioners are the group that can either benefit or be unaffected by the program depending on their own level of commitment.

Program Description

The process of defining and establishing St. Vincent's occupational health program began with a definition of the tasks that would need to be accomplished at four phases: immediate tasks, tasks preliminary to opening the occupational health clinic, tasks during clinic start-up, and tasks during the development of additional services. The tasks in each of these phases are listed in appendix B, "Key Steps in Establishing the Center for Occupational Health."

In the first two phases of program development, the scope of services was defined (appendix C). This was done to ensure that the program's services were comprehensive and that St. Vincent's had the expertise to provide them.

Saint Vincent's approach to workers' compensation case treatment and management reflects its understanding of business and industry's needs. Throughout the treatment process, St. Vincent's has tried to address the following needs expressed by the business community:

- High-quality medical care
- Convenience
- Optimal communication
- Availability
- Clear, precise medical directives from the physicians
- Compensation cost reduction

The initial care needs to be prompt and provided by physicians experienced in the management of work-related illness and injury. Those physicians must also be oriented to good occupational health practices, and they must be knowledgeable of the workers' compensation law. The physicians who work best in the initial care setting are family practitioners or emergency medicine physicians. At St. Vincent's, it is believed that 80 percent of the reason for program success is related to the quality of the physicians.

As in many states, compensation law preserves the right of the individual to select his or her physician. However, that right is exercised by less than 5 percent of acutely ill or injured workers. Ninety-five percent of acutely ill or injured workers go to the most convenient source for quality medical care or to where they are directed. In recognition of this need to provide convenience, initial care in St. Vincent's program is available at four locations: emergency department (with a 24-hour capability), family medical care unit, occupational health clinic, and some private physicians' offices. Fifth and sixth locations will be added as satellites for the convenience of employers in areas remote from the hospital.

As described in chapter 2, workers' compensation case tracking is vital to program success. At St. Vincent's, the following goals for the tracking program were set:

- To provide excellent and optimal health care to the ill or injured worker
- To improve the efficiency and quality of information for the employee, the employer, the insurance carrier, and the physician
- To coordinate the employee's treatment and rehabilitation program, facilitating optimal recovery and return to work

- To achieve cost savings for the employer and the insurance carrier by decreasing claims, decreasing time loss, and maintaining productivity
- To promote referrals to the St. Vincent Hospital medical staff
- To build knowledge and familiarity of St. Vincent Hospital and medical staff among the work force in the business community as a means of promoting utilization of St. Vincent Hospital and medical staff for occupational and nonoccupational health care needs

The tracking system begins with initial treatment. The employer is notified by telephone either at the time of service or on the next working day. All pertinent information is communicated to the insurance carrier and the treating physician. Throughout the case, tracking is the glue that binds the illness and injury management system together. It is the primary means of achieving optimal care, communication, and workers' compensation cost reduction. This link instantly solves the problems of late reports, lost reports, no reports, slow referral, slow rehabilitation, and no communication. (See chapter 4, "Injured Worker Tracking.")

The roles of those involved in tracking are defined as follows:

- *The initial treating physician.* The initial treating physician gives high-quality medical care and formulates a *plan* for the patient's optimal recovery and rehabilitation.
- *The workers' compensation specialist.* The workers' compensation specialist sees that the plan is followed. As the plan is subsequently altered by further physician input, the workers' compensation specialist sees that the new plan is followed accordingly.
- *The occupational health committee.* The basic role of the occupational health committee together with the occupational health medical director is to see that the plan is a good plan.

In order for the system to work, the treating physicians must understand the fundamental differences between the management of work-related problems and the management of non–work-related problems. For a non–work-related problem, the cost of care is not significantly affected by delays, as long as the delay is not deleterious to the particular illness or injury. For a work-related problem, the added costs of time loss are stacked on top of any medical costs. Delays in diagnosis and treatment of work-related problems quickly increase their overall cost.

From 1986 through 1988, the Research and Statistics section of the Oregon Workers' Compensation Department tracked the average cost of care for injured workers in cooperation with the Bureau of Labor Statistics of the U.S. Department of Labor. It found that in Oregon, the three-year average cost for care was as follows: Forty percent of the workers' compensation dollar went to medical costs, about 40 percent went to compensation for lost time, and the remaining 20 percent was divided among vocational counseling, rehabilitation, and disability prevention.

If the treating physician isn't well oriented to the differences between occupational and nonoccupational treatment, he or she might say, "If your condition does not improve in four or five days, then call (the follow-up physician)." This may be a reasonable approach for the non–work-related illness or injury, but for the work-related problem, leaving the decision about scheduling follow-up care with the employee/patient almost invariably leads to increased costs. The employee/patient usually tries to get a follow-up appointment only after the recommended number of days. At that point, whatever follow-up appointment is available usually requires several more days or weeks of waiting. During that wait, the time-loss meter continues to tick. It is a much better practice, and far less costly, for the treating physician to make specific arrangements for both treatment and follow-up.

The employee/patient should have all that is needed in terms of medical care and time in order to recover and return to work. Tracking does not reduce actual time for recovery, but it can reduce unnecessary delays. Cost savings do result from control of time loss and disability prevention. Early and accurate diagnosis with optimal treatment and early intervention for complicated cases reduce the injured worker's risk of developing long-term disability.

Program Results

The most important goal for St. Vincent's comprehensive occupational health program has been met: The program has developed a higher standard of occupational health activity that affects employees, employers, insurance carriers, and physicians in a positive way. Sooner or later, however, the secondary goals must be addressed, namely, "What are the fiscal results of the program?" To answer that question, several different parameters must be considered because the fiscal intent of a comprehensive occupational health program is to raise the entire base of occupational health activity in the institution and among medical staff.

The first parameter is a measure of how the occupational health program has increased the entire base of workers' compensation case activity throughout the institution. The measurement of the base activity includes the activity in the emergency room, the family medical care unit, the ambulatory surgery department, the occupational health clinic, as well as the activity of hospital inpatients and all ancillary services such as radiology and laboratory. The second parameter measures the revenue generated from the occupational health clinic alone. The third parameter measures what we call "spin-off" activity. This is activity generated in any of the hospital departments or in offices of the medical staff that comes to them by virtue of the client's previous contact with St. Vincent's through its occupational health service.

The data presented in figures 23-1 through 23-3 reflect St. Vincent's experience from the opening of the Center for Occupational Health in

Figure 23-1. Census of Workers' Compensation Patients at St. Vincent Hospital, January 1987 to February 1988

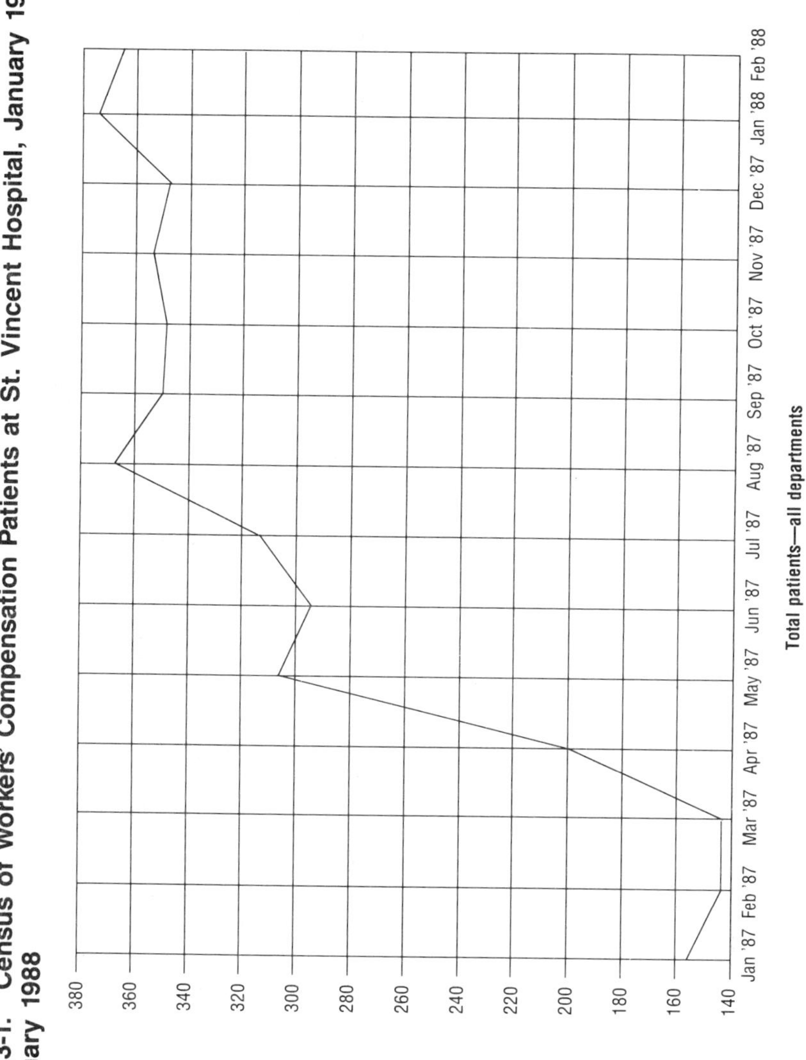

Figure 23-2. Number of Patients by Cost Center from Workers' Compensation Patients at St. Vincent Hospital, January 1987 to February 1988

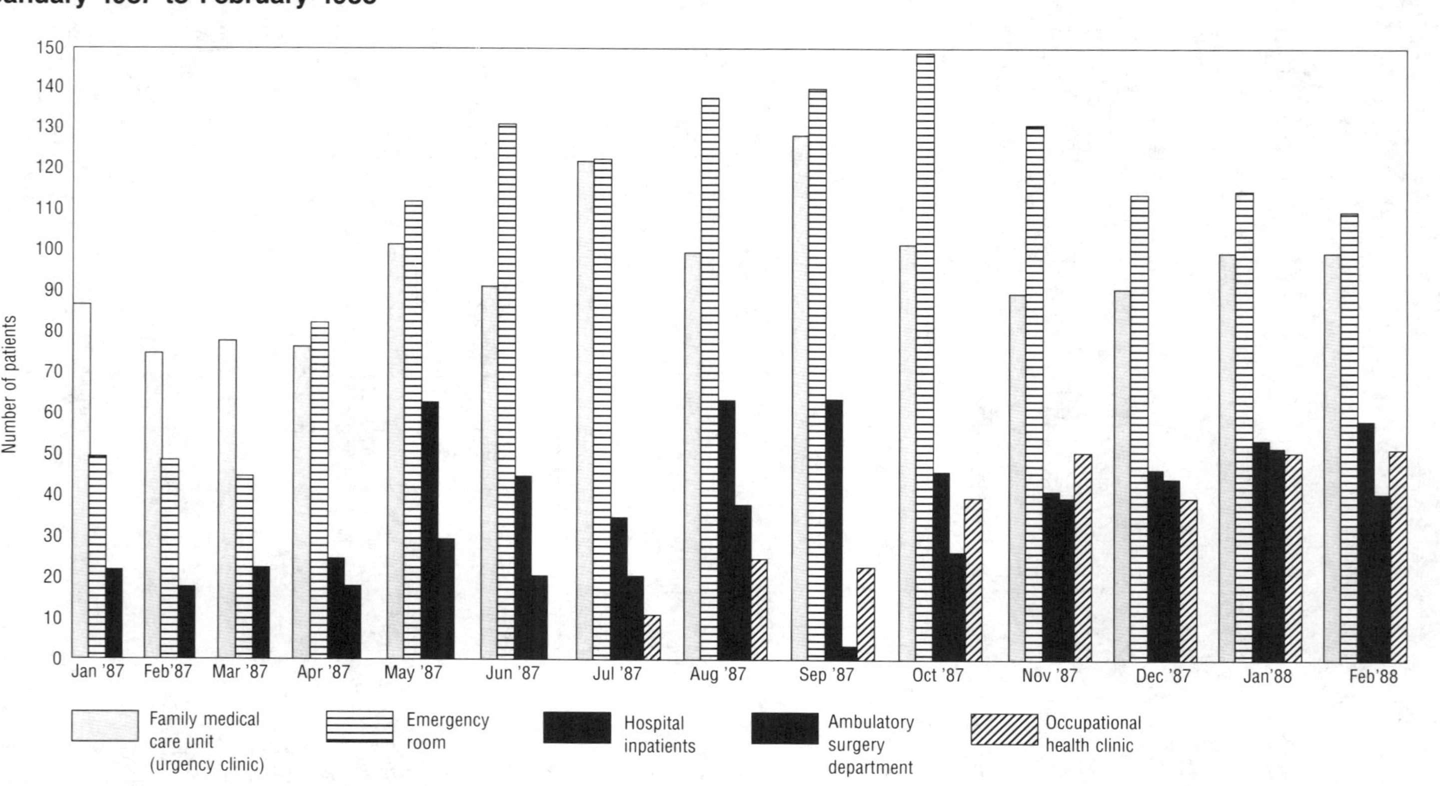

Figure 23-3. Total Workers' Compensation Revenue at St. Vincent Hospital, January 1987 to February 1988

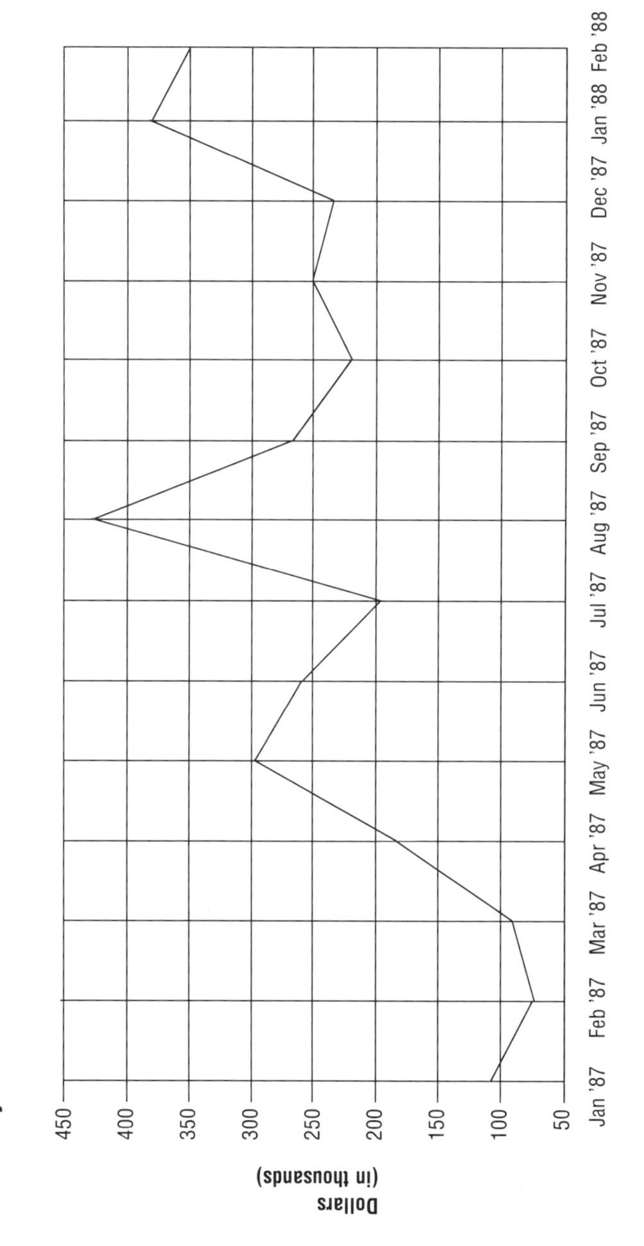

May 1987 to March 1, 1988. In that time period, the Center for Occupational Health has been designated as the preferred provider for some 30 companies. The center has tracked 2,357 injuries involving 1,100 different companies. As a result of the tracking program, referrals have been made to 110 different physicians on St. Vincent's medical staff.

The best estimates are that for each 100 work-related illnesses or injuries treated, 5 or 6 admissions are generated. These numbers are somewhat higher than those of other programs because of the secondary and tertiary nature of St. Vincent Hospital.

Using St. Vincent's own employee health department as a model, a reduction in workers' compensation costs has been demonstrated. One example is the back program. Through this program, a reduction in back injury claims that equates with a $120,000 savings in the hospital's workers' compensation costs has been achieved.

It has not been possible to accurately measure the "ripple" effect for this program (the number of visits for nonoccupational health care resulting from the familiarity that patients gain with the institution and medical staff through an earlier occupational-related visit).

The best measure of success is the measure of the increasing total workers' compensation revenue, the increasing workers' compensation visits, and the changing ratios of occupational health-related activity. Figure 23-1 shows the census of workers' compensation patients by month from January 1987 until February 1988. Figure 23-2 shows the total revenue broken down by cost center. Figure 23-3 shows the total workers' compensation revenue per month from January 1987 until February 1988. The graphs speak for themselves. The increased workers' compensation revenue generated represents a 61 percent increase over St. Vincent's previous base revenue from workers' compensation!

For St. Vincent's, this is the best of all possible worlds. The comprehensive occupational health program allows St. Vincent's to offer meaningful service, stand on solid ethical grounds, and pursue scientific and medical goals while producing positive financial results for the hospital and medical staff.

Appendix A. Center for Occupational Health Executive Committee Referral Policy

1. That the following policy statements and documents be approved as policy of the St. Vincent workers' compensation case management program:
   a. First, the stated wish of the patient to see a personal physician
   b. Second, the physician or group named by the company as the company medical director or preferred doctor
   c. Third, a physician of appropriate specialty on the workers' compensation case referral list, or
   d. The St. Vincent Center for Occupational Health.

2. There shall be a separate physician referral list developed for use by the St. Vincent emergency and clinic staff for referrals of patients who have work-related problems. This list is to be developed in cooperation with each clinical committee after opportunity in clinical committee meetings for learning the special needs and expectations of the workers' compensation case management program. This list will be provided by the medical staff office, just as the existing list for all referrals has been and will continue to be.

Appendix B. Key Steps in Establishing the Center for Occupational Health

I. Immediate Tasks
   A. Define occupational health team
   B. Order equipment
   C. Name the program
   D. Order library materials
   E. Acquire computer hardware and software
   F. Plan clinical and office suites
II. Tasks Preliminary to Opening of Occupational Health Clinic
   A. Begin search for personnel: workers' compensation specialist, occupational health nurse
   B. Hire clinic secretary
      1. Begin secretary's training on word processing and other software applications
      2. Design and acquire paper goods: stationery, business cards, brochures, and pamphlets
   C. Install computer hardware and software
   D. Begin training on software: medical director, occupational health nurse, secretary, workers' compensation specialist
   E. Complete program design: daily operations, policies, policy and procedure manual, clinical training manual
   F. Develop quality assurance program
   G. Orient and instruct occupational health staff
      1. Workers' compensation seminars for staff physicians and their office staffs
   H. Develop program guide for medical staff physicians
   I. Complete details of registration and preregistration
      1. Admitting department
      2. Data processing
      3. Information services
   J. Complete details of billing system
      1. Provide for single bill—make specific arrangements with hospital departments that charge a physician's fee, such as the radiology department

2. Establish charges
3. Complete charge ticket
4. Establish billing procedure for workers' compensation, including forms and reports

K. Complete details of record storage system
1. Information services
2. X rays
3. Laboratory results
4. Permanent charts to be maintained in Occupational Health Clinic

L. Complete encounter form for workers' compensation case management program
M. Develop and complete forms, contracts, agreements
N. Complete program brochures and maps

III. Clinic Start-Up Phase
A. Hire workers' compensation specialist
B. Hire clinic nurse
C. Conduct orientation and instruction seminars for emergency department and family medical care unit
D. Conduct orientation and instruction seminars for referral physicians
E. Complete details of phase I physical therapy and rehabilitation program
F. Conduct team-building sessions with carriers and medical management groups
G. Establish protocols for interfacing with hospital services

IV. Additional Services Development Phase
A. Begin marketing program
B. Develop complicated case panels
C. Prepare medical staff presentations
D. Develop resource network
1. Subspecialists' and specialists' network including respiratory challenge booth, dermatology clinic, and so forth

E. Develop relationships with other occupational health providers, such as industrial hygiene and safety personnel
F. Begin phase II testing and rehabilitation program including disability prevention program and work hardening
G. Establish areawide contacts through meetings, seminars, journal club, professional organizations

Appendix C. Scope of Services of Center for Occupational Health

I. Treatment of Work-Related Illness and Injury
A. Initial care

- B. Follow-up care
- C. Workers' compensation case tracking
- D. Ancillary services
- E. Job reentry/work modification/light duty

II. Medical Surveillance
- A. Initial appraisal
- B. Required or regulated evaluation
- C. Evaluation after accidents
- D. Evaluation of complaints
- E. Periodic evaluations
- F. Executive evaluations
- G. Biologic surveillance
- H. Drug screening

III. Complicated Cases
- A. Disability evaluations
- B. Complicated case panels
- C. Independent medical evaluations
- D. Closing evaluations
- E. Specialist consultations

IV. Consultations
- A. Company physician or advisor
- B. Consultation in regard to specific problems
- C. Developing company health programs
- D. Developing medical standards
- E. Plant surveillance

V. Education
- A. Seminars for office staff
- B. Workers' compensation case management seminars
- C. Physician education
- D. Regional and national educational programs
- E. Research

VI. Health Promotion Services

VII. Political and Legal Involvements

VIII. Community and Environmental Relations

Chapter 24

Challenges and Future Trends

William L. Newkirk, M.D.

For many hospitals, occupational health programs play a key role in the hospital's plans for the 1990s and beyond. Several recent surveys have identified occupational health as one of the key areas targeted for diversification. In a 1988 American Hospital Association survey of Ambulatory Care Professionals, occupational health was the most requested topic for continuing education programs.

As this book has demonstrated, developing occupational health programs is a complex task. The programs require a broad range of medical, legal, managerial, and marketing skills. The previous twenty-three chapters have provided a view of the topics that programs must address. As programs look to the twenty-first century, new issues will arise. This chapter briefly highlights the key trends to watch for in the next decade. These trends include the following:

- Competition for the occupational health services market will increase between hospitals, between hospitals and freestanding centers, and between physicians and hospitals.
- Medical reimbursement will be controlled.
- The occupational health nurse at the worksite will be a key player in generating program referrals.
- Physicians will recommend less surgery and more exercise for occupational injuries.
- The Occupational Safety and Health Administration (OSHA) will become more active in establishing and enforcing medical standards.
- Occupational health delivery systems will become larger, more controlling, and more sophisticated.
- More emergency medicine physicians will move into occupational medicine.

- Legal issues such as drug testing and preplacement screening will be further clarified.

Competition

In the next decade, competition for the corporate market will undoubtedly heat up. Hospitals are reactionary institutions. As hospital-sponsored occupational health programs appear in the marketplace, more hospitals will undoubtedly follow suit. Providing occupational health services will probably not become the sine qua non of hospital success; certain hospitals will shun the market and do well because of excellence in other areas. Nonetheless, it will be very difficult for hospitals to ignore the industrial market if their competitors have targeted the worksite as a key audience.

A second area of competition for the occupational health market will be between hospitals and entrepreneurial freestanding centers. The promise of freestanding emergency centers has diminished since they first entered the marketplace. With waning profitability, many of these centers are diversifying into occupational health. Because their overhead is less than that of hospitals, they can often very effectively compete on price. In some markets, these centers will do extremely well. In most, however, diversification into occupational health will be a last-ditch strategy to save what is, in many cases, a nonviable business operation.

The third area of competition will be between physicians and hospitals. As noted in chapters 1 and 17, this competition is a fact of life in many areas. It is likely to become worse as physicians are caught in the squeeze between stable revenues and increasing overhead. Expect physicians to increasingly diversify into higher-profit areas such as physical therapy, work hardening, and rehabilitation. This approach will make physicians less reliant on the hospital while at the same time reducing hospital referrals and revenue.

These competitive forces are likely to lead to a shakeout in the hospital occupational health program market in the 1990s. Hospitals that entered the market with poorly conceived or supported programs are likely to drop their services. The number of hospitals offering such services will level off after several years of rapid growth.

Reimbursement

The introductory chapter of this book described the rapid escalation of workers' compensation costs in the 1980s. Corporate America is not going to accept this continuing escalation without a fight. In 1987, for example, a well-financed and coordinated corporate effort in Maine succeeded in limiting several workers' compensation benefits in an effort to control the rapid escalation of costs.

Some states have control of medical reimbursement in workers' compensation cases; some do not. Uncontrolled reimbursement is unlikely to survive the 1990s. From a political perspective, it is difficult to imagine that any group with sufficient clout will maintain high rates of reimbursement for medical services. Corporations, faced with an increasingly competitive world market, will seek cost reductions. Labor, with its declining power, will adamantly fight to maintain or improve workers' compensation for disability. It is unlikely to fight to maintain physicians' and hospitals' fees.

Physicians and hospitals will fight alterations in reimbursement, but other issues (Medicare reimbursement and malpractice, among others) are likely to be more pressing ones. As controlled reimbursement schemes (fee schedules, prospective payment, capitation) become the norm for other reforms of health care, reimbursement for workers' compensation is likely to be reined in. Because one of the reasons hospitals are becoming involved in occupational health is the high rate of reimbursement, the capping of workers' compensation reimbursement rates will force some hospitals to reevaluate their commitment to occupational health and will lead to a shakeout in the hospital occupational health market.

The Occupational Health Nurse at the Worksite

The trend for employers to disband their own occupational health departments and rely on outside resources for staffing is likely to continue. In many markets, the worksite itself will be the marketing battleground of the 1990s. One of the major reasons hospitals are pursuing occupational health is to increase or protect the hospital referrals in a competitive market. In many cases, the on-site occupational health nurse makes the referral. As a result, providing the occupational health nurse to the company on a contract basis will become an increasingly important marketing strategy. The strategy is: If you control the nurse, you control the referrals.

The nurse will play an increasingly larger role as industry recognizes that surgery and invasive medical treatments are poor and expensive substitutes for prevention and ergonomic job modification. Office and hospital treatment, with its high cost and employee downtime, will increasingly be replaced by worksite treatment and intervention. In the 1990s occupational health market, the occupational health nurse will be the key player.

Treatment

As a rule, hospitals are more impressed by surgeons than are employers. Certain forms of surgery, such as back surgery, are widely criticized in the business community. In the 1990s, surgery rates for occupational health problems are likely to decline. Back surgery will, in many cases, be replaced by aggressive strengthening and rehabilitation programs featuring swimming, aerobics, and strength training. Arm and carpal tunnel surgery will be replaced by early intervention and ergonomic job modification. The common practice today of the physician operating on a patient and then returning the patient to work without rehabilitation or job modification will be increasingly viewed as substandard care.

In the 1990s, physical therapists, exercise physiologists, and athletic trainers will become more important and in greater demand in the occupational health market. Passive treatment modalities (ultrasound, electrostimulation, massage, and the like) will be replaced with active strengthening and conditioning programs. Swimming programs are likely to become much more common. With the advent of computerized tracking systems, rehabilitation will start earlier, helping to ensure better results.

The Occupational Safety and Health Administration

Public concern about exposure to toxic and potentially toxic substances will increase in the 1990s. The Occupational Safety and Health Administration (OSHA) will reemerge as an important player in the workplace. Two factors combined to significantly weaken OSHA's effectiveness in the 1980s. First, the standards-setting process has become so cumbersome that developing new standards for toxic substances has slowed to a snail's pace. In the 1990s, OSHA will probably succeed in developing generic standards that provide the framework for regulating classes of toxins in a more efficient and responsive manner. Second, the political climate in the 1980s opposed federal regulation, and OSHA became a target. For a period in the 1980s, OSHA was largely reduced to a clerical organization—replacing worksite inspections with paperwork inspections. This trend has reversed in the late 1980s. The 1990s are likely to see OSHA as a more potent force in the workplace.

The significance of the reemergence of OSHA in the 1990s for hospital occupational health programs is that the market for medical surveillance is likely to grow as OSHA becomes more active in establishing and enforcing medical standards. In addition, having trained occupational health physicians and nurses to implement the new standards is likely to become more important.

Systems

In the 1980s, a hospital that could offer an occupational health product line that featured emergency department care, freestanding clinics, and in-hospital rehabilitation programs and on-site nursing was considered advanced. In the 1990s, occupational health delivery systems will become more comprehensive and more controlling.

Three factors will encourage this system growth. First, hospitals will join together in networks capable of delivering standardized products to larger employers. Second, information transfer networks will link hospitals, insurance companies, and employers. No longer will it be acceptable for cases to be held up because of delays in the medical records department. Information will be electronically transmitted either by FAX machines or linked microcomputers. Third, hospitals will integrate occupational health with their managed care products. Employers are likely to have the option to purchase prepackaged occupational health programs in a manner similar to the way they will purchase other managed health care products.

In the 1990s, employees are likely to demand more accountability from the health care system. This will force more hospitals to join more sophisticated occupational health delivery systems.

Physicians

The number of board-certified or board-eligible occupational health physicians is grossly inadequate to meet current needs. Moreover, the closing of the practice-eligible option, which allowed practicing physicians to become board-certified, is likely to help keep this shortage in place. As a result, other physician groups will move in to fill the void. The most likely source for new physicians in occupational health is the emergency department. Many emergency medicine physicians are reaching an age where the excitement of emergency medicine is colliding with the realities of middle age. As a result, they are seeking to shift careers. Often, they are moving into occupational medicine. This development, which began in the 1980s, directly coincides with hospital needs. The first step in developing an occupational health program is often to start in the emergency department. As the program grows, it frequently leaves the emergency department and takes one of the physicians with it.

Legal Issues

The 1990s should bring some clarification of the murky legal issues affecting occupational health. Two areas will be highlighted: drug testing and preplacement screening. As cases move through the court system and the state legislatures deal with the issues, drug testing controversies should be, to some extent, resolved. Occupational health programs should have clearer guidelines for who can be tested and under what circumstances and how the information can be used. Specific issues such as specimen collection should be resolved: Do you watch the employee urinate and risk "unreasonable search," or not watch the employee urinate and break the chain of evidence?

In the preplacement area, predictive screening should have further court decisions regarding the meaning of "reasonable probability" of illness and injury. In most states, an employer can reject an otherwise qualified employee if the employer has factual information that the employee has a reasonable probability of suffering a deterioration in health. The current problem for occupational health programs is that the courts have been reluctant to define what they mean by "reasonable probability." Cases in the 1990s should help clarify the issues.

Occupational health programs will need greater legal sophistication in the 1990s, particularly in the area of employee screening. Instead of marketing a "physical examination" to employers, programs in the 1990s will need to provide a spectrum of examinations for preplacement, medical surveillance, and return to work, among others—each examination having to meet a different legal standard.

The Challenge of the Future

In the 1970s and 1980s, hospitals did not need such sophistication to develop an occupational health program. Many hospitals simply developed brochures listing hospital services, assumed a brand name, appointed a marketing person, improved injured workers' emergency department treatment, and sold their "occupational health program." Often, the hospitals had no personnel specifically trained in occupational medicine and were unable to deal with basic occupational health issues. Employers often received these early programs warmly; any hospital attention directed toward work-related problems was welcomed.

This approach to occupational health is no longer sufficient. Occupational health programs are becoming increasingly competitive and specialized. Developing a successful program requires more knowledge and skills than were required just a few years ago.

This book tries to make sense out of the rapidly changing occupational health market. It covers the services, legal issues, marketing needs, and ethical concerns facing programs as we begin the 1990s. It attempts to alert hospitals to frequently encountered problems and to suggest solutions that have proved successful elsewhere.

Developing or expanding occupational health programs can be difficult work. Few fields of medicine operate in an arena of such conflicting economic and technical forces. This book provides guidelines for achieving success. Improving the health and safety of workers is vitally important. Hospital occupational programs play an important role in that process. The stakes are high for employers and employees—and also for hospitals.